Delirium:
acute confusional states in
palliative medicine

Delirium:
acute confusional states in palliative medicine

Augusto Caraceni

Rehabilitation and Palliative Care Unit, National Cancer
Institute of Milan, Italy

and

Luigi Grassi

Department of Medical Disciplines, of Communication and
Behaviour, Section of Psychiatry, University of Ferrara, Italy

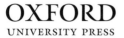
OXFORD
UNIVERSITY PRESS

OXFORD
UNIVERSITY PRESS

Great Clarendon Street, Oxford OX2 6DP

Oxford University Press is a department of the University of Oxford.
It furthers the University's objective of excellence in research, scholarship,
and education by publishing worldwide in

Oxford New York

Auckland Bangkok Buenos Aires Cape Town Chennai
Dar es Salaam Delhi Hong Kong Istanbul Karachi Kolkata
Kuala Lumpur Madrid Melbourne Mexico City Mumbai Nairobi
São Paulo Shanghai Taipei Tokyo Toronto

Oxford is a registered trade mark of Oxford University Press
in the UK and in certain other countries

Published in the United States
by Oxford University Press Inc., New York

A catalogue record for this title is available from the British Library

Library of Congress Cataloging in Publication Data
(Data available)

ISBN 0–19–263199 3 (Pbk)

10 9 8 7 6 5 4 3 2 1

Typeset by J&L Composition, Filey, North Yorkshire
Printed in Great Britain
on acid-free paper by
Biddles Ltd, Guildford and King's Lynn

This book is dedicated to
Giannina Rita and Valeria
Giuseppe and Tommaso
Cinzia and Francesca
Eleonora and Davide

Foreword

Delirium is among the most prevalent and challenging clinical problems. Its assessment and management must be individualized based on both a biomedical understanding of the disease and its comorbidities, and a more nuanced understanding of prognosis, risks, and benefits of treatment. Every intervention must be informed by a critical understanding of the changing goals of care. These complexities are critically explored in this volume.

Given the diversity of clinical presentations associated with neurological and psychiatric disorders in the medically ill, considerable efforts have been made during the past decade to derive meaningful diagnostic criteria for delirium. Consensus on diagnostic criteria is needed as a foundation for future investigations focused on the epidemiology, aetiologies, and treatments of this disorder. Even distinctions that appear simple in some populations, such as the difference between delirium and dementia, can become clouded when an underlying disease is progressing and the patient is exposed to complex therapies for the disease itself and for its consequences. If an acute confusional state that is expected to be transitory never clears, should it still be called a delirium? If one or two of the elements that together characterize delirium—for example, changes in alertness, psychomotor activity, cognition, perception, mood, or sleep–wake cycle—occur in isolation, is this delirium?

One of the most important barriers to the adequate treatment and management of delirium is the fact that it is so commonly under-recognized or misdiagnosed. It's protean manifestations make it a syndrome that is often misdiagnosed.

The development of validated measures to identify delirium, and grade its severity, has been an important advance. These developments highlight the need for additional studies that will clarify the phenomenology of delirium, establish evidence-based criteria for diagnosis, and rationalize the type of clinical assessment that is needed to define a treatment strategy. Studies that separately assess consciousness, cognition, perception, and mood potentially could define subpopulations that may benefit from more targeted interventions. Ultimately, treatable pathophysiologies linked to a particular phenomenology might be elucidated.

Even the most sophisticated research, however, will never obviate the clinical challenge in managing delirium in populations with advanced illness. Death is commonly preceded by a period of somnolence or confusion, which may be as brief as hours or as long as months. Although the decline might be attributable to specific biomedical causes, it is not considered pathological if it is perceived to be part of the normal dying process. If this is the case, interventions are limited to those necessary to ensure comfort and reassure the family. Efforts to assess and reverse the underlying causes, which are essential in other clinical settings, would be inappropriate here.

Thus, the clinical problem of delirium resonates with a broad range of profound challenges in palliative care. Clinicians are notoriously poor prognosticators; yet some understanding of the time left is needed to inform judgements about the evaluation and management of delirium. If there is a chance for meaningful survival, and the goals of care are consistent with this, the delirious patient may undergo a very aggressive evaluation and complex interventions designed to reduce contributing causes and reverse the disorder. If the patient is perceived to be imminently dying, however, the overriding concern may be the control of agitation or fear. No effort is then made to identify or treat potential causes.

Ethical considerations are prominent in this decision-making and are under intense discussion among specialists in palliative care. Should the delirious patient at the end of life empirically receive hydration, a simple intervention that would reverse one potential contributing factor? Or does the belief that death is imminent preclude this intervention? If the delirious patient is agitated, what are the ethical considerations in using sedative doses of drugs until death occurs? These are complex issues, and require case-by-case reasoning.

Delirium is not a disorder whose impact is confined to the patient alone, particularly in the palliative care setting. Recent studies (Breitbart, *et al.* 2002a; 43: 183–94) suggest that delirium in the palliative care setting is distressing for patients, family members and health care providers. While patients experience high levels of delirium-related distress, particularly when delirium is accompanied by delusions and paranoia, family members score even higher than their loved ones who are delirious, on measures of distress. Many family members become distraught at the thought that in addition to a terminal physical illness, their loved one now has a 'psychiatric' illness and has 'lost his/her mind'; an emotional or cognitive death where they have lost the patient as a 'human being'. Then they experience a 'second death' when the patient physically dies. Nurses are highly distressed as well when caring for dying delirious patients. Caring for these patients is very emotionally difficult work for all concerned. These data suggest that educational interventions for families and caregivers on the true medical nature of delirium and what can be expected in the dying process regarding delirium may be beneficial. They also make the case, as is made in this text, that delirium can be expected to occur as part of the dying process and that not only should families and caregivers be prepared for this event they should also be aware of it as a harbinger of decline and impending death. Important discussions regarding treatment preferences and advanced directives, rituals of reconciliation and forgiveness, and other practical issues should take place in advance of the inevitable delirium. The events of delirium, given their potential for causing distress in families, inevitably influence the bereavement process, and must be considered in the aftercare of family members.

In conclusion the scientific and clinical characterization of delirium is as yet rudimentary, but clinicians must do the best they can. The need for mutual and comprehensive cooperation by a variety of disciplines (i.e. medicine, palliative care practitioners, neurologists, and psychiatrists) emerges as an important message from this book in which Caraceni and Grassi offer a critical evaluation of the existing literature and recommendations for a holistic approach to this complex syndrome. The authors' personal experience, as shown by a number of clinical examples, provide a good foundation for the challenges faced at the bedside. The addition of appendices with many of the most utilized delirium tools is a great advantage of this textbook.

February 2003

Russell K. Portenoy MD
Chairman, Department of Pain
Medicine and Palliative Care
Beth Israel Medical Center
New York, NY Professor of Neurology
Albert Einstein College of Medicine
Bronx, New York

William Breitbart, MD, Chief,
Psychiatry Service, Department of
Psychiatry and Behavioral Sciences,
Attending Psychiatrist, Pain and
Palliative Care Service, Department of
Neurology, Memorial Sloan-Kettering
Cancer Center, New York, NY and
Professor of Psychiatry, Department of
Psychiatry, Weill Medical College of
Cornell University, New York.

Preface

Delirium is a complex syndrome with a multifactorial aetiology and is characterized by marked disturbances of consciousness, attention, memory, perception, thought, and the sleep–wake cycle, and by fluctuation of symptoms. Over the last few years, clinicians, especially in geriatric and intensive care settings, have concentrated on delirium. However, since delirium is also very frequent in palliative care settings, attention to this topic has progressively increased among palliative care physicians. In fact, patients who are affected by serious and incurable diseases, have multiple organ failures, receive multiple pharmacological treatments, and are often advanced in age and are at an increased risk for the development of the disorder.

A good description of what could correspond to prodromal symptoms of delirium and to a pre-delirium state in a patient with a rapidly disseminating disease, is given by Alessandro Manzoni (1840; English translation 1972) in the last part of the famous novel *I promessi sposi* [*The Betrothed*]. At the height of the pestilence, which affected Milan in the second decade of 1600, Don Rodrigo, one of the co-protagonists, who is already affected by plague, is returning home at night: 'as he walked along', Manzoni writes, 'he began to feel a discomfort, a fatigue, a weakness in the legs, a difficulty in drawing breath, and a feeling of internal burning which he would have been only happy to attribute to the wine he had drunk. . . .' Then, when Don Rodrigo is going to bed,

> the blankets seemed to weigh a ton. He threw them back, curled up and tried to doze off, for he was half dead with the need for sleep. But his eyes had only been shut for a moment when he woke up again with a jerk, as if someone had spitefully given him a shake . . . . After much tossing and turning, he finally got to sleep, and began to dream the ugliest and most tangled dreams in the world. As they went on, he seemed to find himself in a great church, right in the middle of it, among a huge crowd. He stood there, without any idea of how he had got there, especially at that time; and this infuriated him. He looked at those who were around him. All of them had yellowish emaciated faces, with dazed, unseeing eyes and hanging lips. The rags in which they were clad where falling off them, and through the gaps he could see the bubonic swellings and discoloured patches that were the symptoms of the plague. 'Out of my way, you swine!' he cried in his dream, looking at the door, which was a great way off. Though he accompanied the words with a threatening scowl, he did not raise his hand, but rather shrank into himself, to avoid further contact with those filthy bodies, which already pressed upon him all too closely from every side. But none of those crazy figures showed any sign of wanting to get out of his way, or even of having heard him. In fact they crowded in upon him more tightly than ever, and one of them in particular seemed to be jabbing him with something, perhaps an elbow, in the left side, between heart and armpit. Don Rodrigo felt a painful pricking sensation there, a feeling of heaviness. And as he twisted away to try and free himself from it,

something else, at once, seemed to prick him in the same spot. Angered by this, he felt for his sword; but it seemed to have been jostled half out of its scabbard by the crowd, so that it was its hilt that had been pressing against his side. But he put his hand there, there was no sign of the sword, and he felt a yet sharper stab. He shouted; he was all out of breath; he was trying to shout louder still; and then it seemed as if all those faces suddenly turned to look in one direction. He glanced that way too, and saw a pulpit, over the edge of which appeared something round and smooth and shining. Then a bald cranium rose clearly to view, followed by a pair of eyes, the rest of a face, and the long white beard. A friar stood there, visible from the waist upwards above the edge of the pulpit. It was Father Cristoforo. His threatening gaze passed all round the whole audience, and finally seemed to fix itself on Don Rodrigo. The friar's hand was raised in the same attitude as when he had denounced Don Rodrigo in one of the great rooms of his palace. Then Don Rodrigo raised his own hand quickly and made a violent effort trying to leap forward and grab that outstretched arm. Words which had been choking in his gullet burst forth in a terrible scream and he woke up . . . he had some difficulty in regaining consciousness.

Manzoni continues:

he felt violent stifling palpitations of the heart, a constant buzzing or whistling in his ears, a burning in his body and a heaviness in his limbs, worse than when he had gone to bed. . . . he was aware that his mental processes were growing darker and more confused, and felt the approach of a moment when he would have no thought left in his head except the thought of abandoning himself to utter despair.

That Don Rodrigo is severely ill and his physical and mental status is rapidly deteriorating is apparent, since, as the novel continues, we find Don Rodrigo dying in the lazzareto, where he has been cast by *monatti*: 'The unhappy man was stretched out motionless. His eyes were wide open, but unseeing, his face pale and covered with dark blotches. His lips were black and swollen. It might have been the face of a corpse, except for a violent contraction of the features which bore witness to a tenacious will to live. His chest heaved from time to time in a painful struggle for breath.'

In spite of its prevalence and the relevance and the distressing nature of its symptoms for the patient (and his/her family), and the high mortality, delirium goes often unrecognized and is not properly treated in palliative care settings.

In starting to write this book, we had some considerations in mind and some challenges to address. First, as neurologists and psychiatrists, we are often involved in palliative care programmes on a consultation basis, while the integration of these disciplines in palliative care might greatly contribute to the field, as far as delirium is concerned. Second, regarding the assessment of delirium, most of the available instruments were elaborated by psychiatrists and geriatricians and tested on specific populations other than patients in an advanced phase of illness, including terminally ill patients. Therefore, testing these instruments on the more heterogeneous palliative care population and training palliative care teams on the use of the assessment methods are important aims for both clinical and research reasons. Third, in considering the dying population, the actual prevalence of delirium is unknown. If brain failure is part of the process of dying and the dying process is not an acute event, it is likely that delirium could be considered as part of the dying process itself. This condition has not been fully described. Fourth, often delirium cannot be promptly reversed both in the terminal cases and in patients with potential for recovery. It is distressing for the patient and the family and palliative treatment is required. Palliative care professionals have therefore more than one responsibility in mastering the diagnosis, management, and treatment of this disorder. Fifth, the development of home-care assistance for terminally ill patients in many countries, including Italy, run by primary care physicians and/or primary care teams coordinated by general practitioners, makes evident the need for specific training in this underrecognized clinical area.

This book is designed to address these problems and to provide palliative care professionals with what our experience and the most recent literature can offer in terms of theory and clinical practice with regard to the classification, aetiology, phenomenology, and management of delirium. We hope this book will also provide a stimulus to further exploration of this area and to a more integrated approach in daily assistance to terminally ill patients and their families.

In Chapter 1, we focus attention on the definition and conceptualization of delirium over time, starting with the historical roots of Hippocratic medicine, through the first attempt of classification during the nineteenth and early twentieth centuries, to the most recent classifications of the World Health Organization (1992; *International classification of disease*—ICD-10) and the American Psychiatric Association (2000; *Diagnostic and statistical manual of mental disorders*—DSM-IV-TR).

Chapter 2 addresses the neuropathophysiology of delirium, including the anatomical, neurotransmitter, metabolic, and molecular levels of dysfunction, which are considered to be involved in the pathogenesis of the disorder.

Chapter 3 deals with the problem of incidence and prevalence of delirium in clinical settings, while, in Chapter 4, the core clinical symptoms and signs of the prodromal phases of delirium (pre-delirium) and full-blown delirium are presented and discussed in detail.

Chapter 5 discusses the relevant problem of differential diagnosis between delirium and other significant neurological and psychiatric disorders, such as dementia and psychiatric disorders with psychotic features.

The different clinical subtypes of delirium and the populations at risk of delirium are the themes of Chapters 6 and 7. Chapter 6 examines the most common forms of delirium, such as alcohol withdrawal delirium (delirium tremens) and other withdrawal deliria, delirium due to metabolic causes, and delirium due to structural brain lesions. Chapter 7 looks at the populations that are particularly exposed to the development of delirium, such as advanced cancer patients, HIV-infected subjects, the elderly, and patients who have undergone surgery. The problem of terminal delirium is also discussed here.

In Chapter 8, we examine the main diagnostic examinations, including laboratory (e.g. blood chemistry, urine analysis, drug level screening) and instrumental diagnostic tests (e.g. electroencephalogram, computed tomography, magnetic resonance imaging). We also review the most used delirium assessment tools to be applied in clinical practice (e.g. diagnostic algorithms, rating scales, and other tests).

Chapter 9 considers the management of delirium and presents the most useful strategies, examining the characteristics of psychotropic drugs, especially antipsychotics, and their correct use. The application of educational and environmental strategies by health staff professionals is also discussed.

The final chapter is dedicated to the often neglected area of the family of terminally ill patients. It provides a synthesis of the struggle of family members to adjust and respond to the multiple demands both in the terminal phase of illness of their loved one and bereavement, including the problems that can emerge during this phase, such as complicated grief.

Finally, a consideration that supports the comprehensive character of the book. While we are more than aware of the relevance that terminal care has within the frame of palliative care, we strongly support the view that palliative medicine and palliative care are not to be considered equivalent to 'end-of-life care', because, on the contrary, they cover a much wider span of the evolution of progressive incurable illnesses crossing the fields of oncology, neurology, anaesthesiology, and internal medicine at least and building an autonomous and specific area of cultural and practical development in medicine.

We are indebted to all the patients and families we have encountered in our clinical activity for what they have taught us. We would like to thank all the clinical units of the National Cancer Institute of Milan and of the S. Anne University Hospital in Fenase for their continuous trust in referring their patients to us. A special thank you goes to the Diagnostic Radiology Unit A and its director Professor Renato Musumeci (National Cancer Institute, Milan) for their friendly collaboration in reproducing many of the radiological images presented. We are also grateful to Paul Packer for his valuable contribution in editing the manuscript and to Lea Baider for her thoughtful comments and suggestions on Chapter 10.

Augusto Caraceni   February 2003
Luigi Grassi

Contents

Appendices

Abbreviations

5-HT	5-hydroxytryptamine (serotonin)
ACh	acetylcholine
AChE	acetylcholinesterase
ADS	Agitation Distress Scale
APA	American Psychiatric Association
ARAS	ascending reticular activating system
b.i.d.	twice a day
BZD	benzodiazepine
CABG	coronary artery bypass graft
CAM	Confusion Assessment Method
CAM-ICU	CAM for use in intensive care units
CDCG	clinical descriptions and diagnostic guidelines (ICD-10)
CI	confidence interval
C–L	Consultation–Liaison (psychiatry)
COPD	chronic obstructive pulmonary disease
CS	Communication Capacity Scale
CSE	Confusional State Evaluation
CTD	Cognitive Test for Delirium
DA	dopamine
DI	Delirium Index
DIC	disseminated intravascular coagulation
DSI	Delirium Symptom Interview
DSM	*Diagnostic and statistical manual (of mental disorders)* (American Psychiatric Association)
DRS	Delirium Rating Scale
DT	delirium tremens
DWT	Delirium Writing Test
ECT	electroconvulsive therapy
EEG	electroencephalography
ESRS	Extrapyramidal Symptom Rating Scale
GABA	γ-aminobutyric acid
GBL	gamma-butyrolactone
GHB	gamma-hydroxybutyric acid
ICD	*International classification of disease* (WHO)
ICD-10-DCR	*ICD-10 Classification of mental and behavioural disorders— diagnostic criteria for research* (WHO)
ICDSC	Intensive Care Delirium Screening Checklist

ICIDH-2	*International classification of functioning and disability* (WHO)
ICU	intensive care units
IL-2	interleukin 2
IM	intramuscular
IV	intravenous
LOS	length of stay (in hospital)
LSD	lysergic acid diethylamide
MAO	monoamine oxidase
MCS	minimally conscious state
MDAS	Memorial Delirium Assessment Scale
MMSE	Mini-Mental State Examination
NA	noradrenaline
NCSE	non-convulsive status epilepticus
NMS	neuroleptic malignant syndrome
OR	odds ratio
OSAS	obstructive sleep apnoea syndrome
PaP	palliative prognostic (score)
PCA	patient-controlled anaesthesia (pump)
PCP	phencyclidine
PEG	polyethylene glycol
PET	positron emission tomography
pMHPG	plasma-free 3-methoxy-4-hydroxyphenyl (ethylene)glycol
p.r.n.	*pro re nata* ('as circumstances may require'; of dosage)
q.h.s.	*quaque hora somni*, before going to sleep
q.i.d.	four times a day
REM	rapid eye movement
SAA	serum anticholinergic activity
SAS	Specific Activity Scale
SC	subcutaneous
SCLC	small-cell lung cancer
SIADH	syndrome of inappropriate antidiuretic hormone secretion
SPECT	single-photon emission computerized tomography
SSRIs	selective serotonin re-uptake inhibitors
TCAs	tricyclic antidepressants
TdP	torsades de pointes
TICS	telephone interview for cognitive status
t.i.d.	three times a day
TRP	tryptophan
VS	vegetative state
WHO	World Health Organization

Chapter 1

Delirium: historical concepts and current definitions

1.1 Historical note

The first chapter of Lipowski's (1990*b*) seminal book on delirium is a magnificent source for the history of the definition, taxonomy, and fluctuating denominations of this syndrome through the centuries.

Celsus (first century AD) was the first to use the term 'delirium' to describe a mental condition developing in different contexts, but often in association with fever, and to unify the conditions already known as 'phrenitis' and 'lethargus' by observing the frequent transition between the two. The detection of mental or psychic changes due to medical illnesses had already been established by Hippocrates who described the occurrence of delirium due to fever, meningitis, trauma, and pneumonia. Hippocratic medicine is based on observation and its merit can be well appreciated today as 2500 years ago clinical findings were already being clearly described and their association with disease and prognosis correctly interpreted. Hippocrates uses different words (παραφροσύνη, παράνοια, ἔκπληξισ, παραλήροι, φρενίτισ) to describe an altered mental status with incoherence of thought, altered sleep–wakefulness pattern, inability to recognize known people, and psychomotor agitation. Most of these words have been translated into English using the word 'delirium' (Hippocrates [English translation] 1931). He distinguishes this condition from cases characterized by sleepiness and immobility often evolving into coma, pointing out also that agitated states can often evolve into lethargic conditions and vice versa. It is likely that the most commonly used word, παραφροσύνη, corresponds to delirium secondary to fever, while φρενίτισ is a primary brain infection such as meningitis.

It is interesting to quote a few original statements from Hippocrates.

When in continued fevers occur difficulty of breathing and delirium (παραφροσύνη), it is a fatal sign. (*Aphorisms*, IV, L)

As to the motion of the arms I observe the following facts. In acute fevers, pneumonia, phrenitis and headache, if they move before the face, hunt in the empty air, pluck nap (κροκύδασ) from the bedclothes, pick up bits (καρφολογεούσασ), and snatch chaff from the walls—all these signs are bad, in fact deadly. (*Prognostic* IV)

Acute pain of the ear with continuous high fever is dangerous for the patient is likely to become delirious and die. (*Prognostic* XXII)

These and other examples and the clinical descriptions found in the *Books of epidemics* show that Hippocrates attributed the aetiology of delirium to the brain, described most of the relevant clinical findings with words still used today (such as crocidismus and carphology), and associated its onset with the presence of unresolving fevers of several aetiologies. He observed that agitated deliria often evolved into lethargic states and that the resolution of delirium was a favourable prognostic sign. It is also likely that his interpretation included cases of primary brain origin (phrenitis), and others originating secondarily from other infections such as pneumonia and fever. Galenus (Galen 1978) clearly distinguishes cases due to noncerebral causes, which give rise, by 'sympathetic' effect on the brain, to 'a certain type of delirium', from those due to primary brain affections, causing lethargy or phrenitis. Galen's understanding of medicine mainly reflected Hippocratic theories and his own fascinating clinical observations and intuitions.

The dualism between the word phrenitis—which is increasingly used to describe acute mental insanity—and lethargy was common in the medical literature until the eighteenth century (Fredreriks 2000).

Many good clinical descriptions of the phenomena that characterize delirium can be found throughout medical literature from Roman times until the eighteenth century, including those of Areteus from Cappadocia who distinguished chronic conditions (dementias) from acute deliria and recommended boiled poppy and rest as therapy (Adams 1861; Azorin *et al.* 1992; Ey *et al.* 1989; Lipowski 1990*b*). The main topics that made a unitary concept of delirium so difficult to come by were clearly delineated: primary versus secondary cerebral infection; differential diagnosis with psychoses; constant association with fever; acute onset versus chronic conditions such as dementia and mania. Over this time and more recently, core concepts were elaborated that led to the modern understanding of delirium.

In the nineteenth century, the terminology describing delirium exhibited significant ambiguity. In France, a number of authors used different terms to describe similar syndromes, such as Pinel's *idiotisme acquis* (1809), Esquriol's *démence aiguë* (1814), Georget's *stupidité* (1820). In Germany, Wille (1888) described *Verwirrtheit* as a functional disorder of the brain, usually with acute or, more rarely, chronic features, characterized by confusion, hallucinations, delusions, disturbances of the consciousness, and stupor. Later on, Meynert (1890) described a similar syndrome by introducing the term 'amentia'. In England, Norman (1890) described 'acute confusional insanity' as a syndrome with a rapid evolution characterized by hallucinations and disturbances of the consciousness.

Greiner (1817) pioneered the concept of the clouding of consciousness (*Verdunkelung des Bewusstseins*) as the main pathogenetic feature of delirium in a treatise that gave a very comprehensive picture of the psychopathology of the syndrome. Chaslin's (1895) account of 'la confusion mentale' (mental confusion is a French definition) identified the inability to think coherently, reduced perceptual discrimination, and memory failure as the unifiying features of the syndrome with the possibility that oneiric aspects were superimposed as in delirium tremens. This definition has remained quite constant in French literature after the term *délire* was restricted to the description of thought pathology (delusion), and confusion has come to occupy the conceptual space of delirium up to the present time (Berrios 1981; Gil 1989).

Bonhoeffer (1908–1912; in Neumarker 2001) described acute organic brain disorders as acute exogenous reactions (symptomatic psychoses) that included a group of different syndromes, such as epileptic excitement, crepuscular states, hallucinosis, amentia, and catatonic psychosis. Bonhoeffer's contribution was very important in suggesting that the brain could react in a similar way to very many exogenous noxae due to physical illnesses in what he called 'acute exogenous reaction types', which were all characterized by a clouding of consciousness. From his work came the concept of the dysergastic reaction (Wolf and Curran 1935). The contribution of Hughling Jackson, and of his theory of a hierarchical organization of the central nervous system (CNS), should also be acknowledged as he defined consciousness as one function of the CNS that could be disturbed by different agents leading to positive and negative signs of disturbance (Jackson 1932).

It is only in the twentieth century that Engel and Romano (1959) made one of the most important observations to date on the pathogenesis of delirium, by showing that delirious patients were affected by a reduction of consciousness that corresponded to a slowing of electroencephalographic (EEG) activity and, in their interpretation, to a general cerebral metabolic insufficiency. In their unitary interpretation the disturbance of consciousness could result in failure at different cognitive tasks, fluctuating levels of awareness, psychomotor hyper- or hypoactivity, agitation, or lethargy.

Lipowski categorized all the psychic manifestations due to a direct, specific, demonstrable aetiology residing in brain dysfunction under the taxonomy of organic brain syndromes. Delirium in his view is a 'transient, global disorder of cognition, consciousness and attention regardless of the level of consciousness (awareness) or psychomotor activity that a given patient exhibits which may often change from one extreme to another in the course of a single day' (Lipowski 1990b, p. 44) or 'a transient organic mental syndrome of acute onset, characterized by global impairment of cognitive functions, a reduced level of consciousness, attentional abnormalities, increased or decreased psychomotor activity and disordered sleep–wake cycle' (Lipowski 1990b, p. 41). His thought is in accordance with the established meaning of the word delirium in English medical literature by the end of the nineteenth century. In *Tuke's Dictionary of Psychological Medicine* (1892) delirium is defined as a condition complicating a wide range of nonmental diseases manifesting with intellectual and cognitive impairment (Lipowski 1990b). Lipowski's definition has been very influential on the most recent psychiatric nosological systems, such as the *Diagnostic and statistical manual of mental disorders* (DSM), developed by the American Psychiatric Association (APA; see next paragraph). However, this definition is broad and further research is needed to establish how well it identifies various clinical conditions from a pathophysiological point of view. Still open to discussion is the question as to whether delirium tremens has peculiar clinical and pathophysiological features, deserving a specific taxonomy. In our opinion, the definition should be judged from an empirical point of view by evaluating its ability to identify a homogeneous group of patients in terms of psychopathology whilst more research is conducted to identify the exact or more precise aetio-pathogenetic subgroups (Camus *et al.* 2000).

1.2 International terminology—differences and similarities

Medical and lay terminology should be viewed differently from diagnostic concepts. We are not able to review here how the word delirium translates in all languages but a few examples will explain where the semantic diversity is only at linguistic level and where it could reflect more profound changes in meaning (see Table 1.1). In the Italian version of the different versions of DSM-III and DSM-IV the word delirium is not translated and the Italian term is endorsed as it is. The medical term in Italian corresponds to Lipowski's definition of 'acute confusional state' (*Stato confusionale acuto*; Caltagirone and Carlesino 1990), even though the closest medical term to delirium in Italian is *delirio*. However, '*delirio*' and also the French term *délire* correspond to the English term 'delusion' and the German term *Wahn*, as a specific thought disorder that

Table 1.1 International terminology related to the vocabulary of delirium

Delirium	English word for acute mental change secondary to exogenous noxae affecting the brain
Delirio	Italian word for delusion
Délire	French word for delusion
Acute confusional state	Synonym of delirium accepted by anglophone authors but used mainly in non-anglophone textbooks (French, Italian)
Encephalopathy	Neurological term that identifies brain syndromes not due to focal lesions or to specific neurological diseases, characterized by generalized suffering of brain structure often manifesting with delirium
Oneirism	From the French literature, it describes those clinical aspects of delirium-acute confusional state that resemble dreaming such as hallucinations and complex hallucinatory and delusional behaviours
Clouding of conscioussness	A term from the German literature that was useful when coined since it pointed to one important pathophysiological aspect of delirium, but it soon became a source of confusion and is now of limited clinical usefulness
Toxic psychosis	Acute mental syndrome caused by drug or poison—term now obsolete
Exogenous, organic or symptomatic psychoses	Acute mental syndromes due to systemic illnesses, a term often used in German neurology (*hirnorganisches Psychosyndrom*)

can be found in many different psychiatric disorders, including schizophrenia, acute psychotic states, mood disorders with psychotic features, as well as in delirium. To add to the confusion, the Italian *delirio* in the lay vocabulary can be considered a translation of the Latin 'delirium'—and has a nonmedical meaning very close to that of the English 'delirium'.

In one Italian neurology textbook (Capitani 1985) 'confusional state' is described in the chapter on consciousness alterations as: 'a condition where the patient suffers a generalized alteration of the content of consciousness, time and often space disorientation, memory impairment, perceptual errors (mainly visual); it is fluctuating, with the possibility of lucid phases. Sleep–wakefulness cycle imparment is possible, agitation or reduced level of consciousnees with sensory obtundation and somnolence'. A well known French short textbook of psychiatry (Lemperiere and Feline 1977) reports all the clinical characteristics of delirium in the chapter on confusional states. For the French authors the principal clinical features are disturbances of vigilance, memory, and orientation to space and time. Additional findings include oneirisim (alteration of perception and behaviour resembling that of dreams), which French tradition prefers to keep as a separate concept (Sellal and Collard 2001). These conditions have organic causes and are acute and generally transient.

We think that authors of many different linguistic and cultural backgrounds will recognize that the DSM-IV definition of delirium can be used to describe acute confusional states well. The history of the words used to define the syndrome is intertwined with the origins of many psychopathological concepts and in its complexity is beyond the scope of this chapter. Table 1.2 summarizes some of the important conceptual steps made by different authors and shows how, across the different languages, the present clinical definition was born through contributions, in the nineteenth and twentieth centuries, from at least three cultural areas: anglophone, French, and German.

1.3　Recent classification systems

The most remarkable change in the concept of delirium occurred in conjunction with the significant revolution in psychiatry in the early 1970s and again in the early 1980s with the introduction of diagnostic criteria and the development of psychiatric nosological systems, in particular, due to the American Psychiatric Association (APA) and the World Health Organization (WHO). There are several reasons for introducing diagnostic criteria and implementing psychiatric diagnostic classification (Dilling 2000; Lindesay 1999; Tucker 1999; Williams 1999).

◆ There is a need to bring some order to the chaotic psychiatric terminology that has been in use for decades, secondary to the different theoretical models and existing schools. As we have already pointed out, delirium was beset by this problem for many years.

◆ There is a need to create a common language and better communication between clinicians when describing psychiatric disorders.

◆ Classification has the advantage of allowing psychiatrists to approach mental disorders in a more constructive way, in terms of epidemiology (e.g incidence and

Table 1.2 Important steps in the evolution of the modern concept of delirium in the nineteenth century

Concept	Significance
Acute versus chronic	Delirium was separated from the concept of psychoses before the latter were nosologically identified as such, by distinguishing the acute insanity associated with fever, i.e. delirium (*délire aiguë* in French), from chronic insanity, i.e. madness (*délire chronique*)
Fever	Acute onset and fever were often required as necessary adjuncts of delirium; the absence of fever was a differential diagnostic criterion for separating madness from delirium, although in the nineteenth century it was already clear that fever was not a condition *sine qua non* for delirium (Berrios 1981)
Consciousness and confusion	The concepts of a consciousness and of its disturbances as expressed by 'clouding of consciousness' resulted in the nineteenth century in another important differential criterion for separating delirium from other forms of insanity. Complementary to the new definition of clouded consciousness, oneiric consciousness, or narrowing of consciousness, French psychiatry coined the term *confusion mentale*, while *délire* came to be restricted specifically to 'delusion'. Similarly, German authors used the terms *Verwirrtheit*, amentia, or dysnoia. Chaslin (1895) gave unitary form to the concept and linked it to organic causes
Exogenous cause	By the beginning of the twentieth century an exogenous cause was finally considered essential for the diagnosis of delirium or acute confusion as systematized by Bonhoeffer (see Neumarker 2001)

prevalence), comprehension of underlying mechanisms, clinical differences, course, and response to treatment.

During the last 2 decades, the diagnostic criteria and the consequent classification of delirium have changed in accordance with the new data that research and clinical experience have accumulated. Thus, the most recent classification of delirium and the related criteria are the result of efforts to create a nomenclature sharing a common conceptual and clinical construct within the entity of the former confusional states. A review of the two nosological systems currently used in psychiatry, the *Diagnostic and statistical manual of mental disorders* (DSM) of the APA and the *International classification of disease* (ICD) of the WHO, follows.

1.3.1 DSM classification

DSM-III and DSM-III-R

The third edition of the DSM (DSM-III; American Psychiatric Association 1980) had a significant impact on psychiatric classification in many respects. It explicitly introduced diagnostic criteria for each mental disorder and it provided a multiaxial system to evaluate patients (axis I for main psychiatric disorders; axis II for personality disorders; axis III for medical disorders; axis IV for coding stressful events; axis V for coding individual psychosocial functioning on a 0–100 scale).

In the DSM-III delirium was entered for the first time as a specific diagnostic entity, under the rubric 'Organic mental disorders'. The chapter included, along with delirium, dementia, amnestic syndrome, organic delusional syndrome, organic hallucinosis, organic mood syndrome, organic personality syndrome, intoxication of and withdrawal from substances, and mixed or atypical organic mental syndrome. It was conceived that: (1) delirium could be determined by a specific aetiology or physiopathological process (e.g. a medical disorder classified on axis III according to the ICD) or by an unknown cause; (2) it could be superimposed on to a diagnosis of dementia (primary degenerative dementia, pre-senile onset or senile onset, and multi-infarct dementia); (3) it could be secondary to intoxication from substances (amphetamine or similarly acting sympathomimetic; phencyclidine or similarly acting arylcyclohexylamine) or to withdrawal from substances (alcohol, barbiturates or similarly acting sedative, and hypnotics); (4) it could be secondary to other or unspecified substances. The diagnostic DSM-III criteria for delirium are presented in Table 1.3.

In the revised version of the DSM-III (DSM-III-R; American Psychiatric Association 1987), delirium remained under the rubric 'organic mental syndromes and disorders', which was similar to the DSM-III classification—apart from the introduction of the new diagnosis of organic anxiety syndrome and the modification of mixed or atypical organic mental syndrome into 'organic mental syndrome not otherwise specified'. The classification of delirium also remained quite similar, as presented in Table 1.4. However, the criteria for delirium changed in comparison with the DSM-III. In particular, criterion A replaced 'clouding of consciousness' with 'reduced ability to

Table 1.3 DSM-III diagnostic criteria for delirium

A   Clouding of consciousness (reduced clarity of awareness of environment), with reduced capacity to shift, focus, and maintain attention to environmental stimuli

B   At least two of the following:

1   perceptual disturbance, e.g. misinterpretations, illusions, or hallucinations

2   speech that is at times incoherent

3   disturbance of sleep–wake cycle with insomnia or daytime drowsiness

4   increased or decreased psychomotor activity

C   Disorientation and memory impairment (if testable)

D   Clinical features develop over a short period of time (usually hours to days) and tend to fluctuate during the course of the day

E   Evidence from the history, physical examination, or laboratory tests of a specific organic factor judged to be aetiologically related to the disturbance

Reprinted with permission from the Diagnostic and Statistical Manual of Mental Disorders, III edition. Copyright 1980 American Psychiatric Association.

Table 1.4 DSM-III-R disorders in which a diagnosis of delirium is possible and relative codes

Code	Disorder
Dementias	
290.30	Primary degenerative dementia of the Alzheimer type, senile onset, with delirium
290.11	Primary degenerative dementia of the Alzheimer type, presenile onset, with delirium
290.41	Multi-infarct dementia, with delirium
Psychoactive substance-induced organic mental disorders	
Withdrawal	
291.00	Alcohol withdrawal delirium
292.00	Sedative, hypnotic, or anxiolytic withdrawal delirium
Intoxication	
292.81	Amphetamine or similarly acting sympathomimetic delirium
	Cocaine delirium
	Phencyclidine (PCP) or similarly acting arylcyclohexylamine delirium
	Other or unspecified psychoactive substance delirium
Axis III disorders (or aetiology unknown)	
293.00	Delirium secondary to physical disorder and conditions to be registered on axis III

maintain and to shift attention to external stimuli'. The criteria for the diagnosis of delirium according to DSM-III-R are presented in Table 1.5.

DSM-IV and DSM-IV-TR

The development of the fourth edition of the DSM (DSM-IV; American Psychiatric Association 1994) was complementary to the work of the WHO on the new edition of the ICD, the ICD-10. Major changes occurred throughout the DSM-IV in comparison with the DSM-III-R in regard to the conceptualization, classification, and diagnostic criteria of mental disorders, including delirium. With regard to classification, the term 'organic mental syndrome and disorder' has been deleted from DSM-IV on the basis that it incorrectly implied the existence of 'non-organic' mental disorders that do not have a biological basis. Thus, in DSM-IV, the disorders formerly called 'organic mental syndromes and disorders' were grouped into three distinct sections: (1) 'delirium, dementia, and amnestic and other cognitive disorders'; (2) 'mental disorders due to a general medical condition'; and (3) 'substance-related disorders'. In the first category the predominant element is a clinically significant deficit in cognition or memory implying a significant change from a previous level of functioning. For each disorder, the aetiology is considered as either a general medical condition (although the specific general medical condition may not be identifiable) or a substance (i.e. a drug of abuse, medication, or toxin), or a combination of these factors. Thus, delirium is classified according to presumed aetiology into the following categories: 'delirium due to a general medical condition', 'substance-

Table 1.5 DSM-III-R diagnostic criteria for delirium

A	Reduced ability to maintain attention to external stimuli (e.g. questions must be repeated because attention wanders) and to appropriately shift attention to new external stimuli (e.g. perseverates answer to a previous question)
B	Disorganized thinking, as indicated by rambling, irrelevant, or incoherent speech
C	At least two of the following:

    1   reduced level of consciousness, e.g. difficulty keeping awake during examination

    2   perceptual disturbance: misinterpretations, illusions, or hallucinations

    3   disturbance of sleep–wake cycle with insomnia or daytime sleepiness

    4   increased or decreased psychomotor activity

    5   disorientation to time, place, or person

    6   memory impairment, e.g. inability to learn new material, such as the names of several unrelated objects after 5 minutes, or to remember past events, such as history of current episodes of illness

D	Clinical features develop over a short period of time (usually hours to days) and tend to fluctuate during the course of the day
E	Either (1) or (2):

    1   evidence from the history, physical examination, or laboratory findings of a specific organic factor (or factors) judged to be aetiologically related to the disturbance

    2   in the absence of such evidence, an aetiological organic factor can be presumed if the disturbance cannot be accounted for by any non-organic mental disorder, e.g. manic episode, accounting for agitation and sleep disturbance

Reprinted with permission from the Diagnostic and Statistical Manual of Mental Disorders, III edition revised. Copyright 1987 American Psychiatric Association.

induced delirium' (with the variants 'substance intoxication delirium' and 'substance withdrawal delirium'), 'delirium due to multiple aetiologies', and 'delirium not otherwise specified' (if the clinician is unable to determine a specific aetiology for the delirium) (Table 1.6).

With regard to the diagnostic criteria (Table 1.7), the essential characteristic of delirium is considered to be the disturbance of consciousness (i.e. reduced clarity of awareness of the environment) with impairment in the ability to focus, sustain, or shift attention (criterion A), accompanied by a change in cognition (e.g. memory deficit, disorientation, language disturbance) or the development of a perceptual disturbance that cannot be better accounted for by a pre-existing or evolving dementia (criterion B). It is stated that the disturbance develops over a short period of time, usually hours to days, and tends to fluctuate during the course of the day (criterion C). There should also be evidence from the history and physical examination of the patient, or from laboratory tests, that the delirium is a direct physiological consequence of a general medical condition, substance intoxication or withdrawal, use of a medication, or toxin exposure, or a combination of these factors (criterion D).

Both the classification and the diagnostic criteria are retained in the text revision of the DSM-IV (DSM-IV-TR; American Psychiatric Association 2000), in which new

Table 1.6 DSM-IV (and DSM-IV-TR) classification of delirium (and relative codes)

Code	Description/comments
Delirium due to a general medical condition	
293.0	Indicate the general medical condition and code it on axis III
290.41	Vascular dementia, with delirium
Substance-induced delirium	
Substance intoxication delirium	
291.0	Alcohol
292.81	Amphetamine (or amphetamine-like substance), cannabis, hallucinogen, inhalant, opioid, phencyclidine (or phencyclidine-like substance), sedative, hypnotic, or anxiolytic; other (or unknown substance) (e.g. cimetidine, digitalis, benztropine)
Substance withdrawal delirium	
291.0	Alcohol
292.81	Sedative, hypnotic, or anxiolytic; other (or unknown) substance
Delirium due to multiple aetiologies: multiple codes reflecting specific delirium and specific aetiologies, e.g.	
293.0	Delirium due to viral encephalitis
291.0	Alcohol withdrawal delirium
Delirium not otherwise specified	
780.09	

information has been introduced according to the research data accumulated over the last 10 years. In particular, data concerning the prevalence of delirium, the course of the disturbance, and its consequences in terms of medical complications and mortality have been updated. The DSM-IV-TR diagnostic criteria for the different forms of delirium are presented in Tables 1.7 to 1.11. As far as the differential diagnosis, the DSM-IV-TR indicates the need to ascertain if the person has a dementia rather than a delirium, has a delirium alone, or has a delirium superimposed on a pre-existing dementia. From a clinical point of view, although memory impairment is common to both delirium and dementia, the disturbance in consciousness is characteristic of a delirium.

Other psychiatric disorders that should be distinguished from delirium, especially if vivid hallucinations, delusions, language disturbances, and agitation are present, are 'brief psychotic disorder', 'schizophrenia', 'schizophreniform disorder', 'other psychotic disorders', and 'mood disorders with psychotic features'. Usually, fragmentation and poor systematization of psychotic symptoms are more typical of delirium. When anxiety and mood changes are significant, differential diagnosis with 'anxiety and mood disorders' should also made, while, when delirium is associated with fear, anxiety, and dissociative symptoms (e.g. depersonalization), a diagnosis of 'acute stress reaction' (secondary to traumatic event) should be ruled out. In delirium, psychotic, anxiety, mood, and dissociative symptoms tend to fluctuate, occur in the context of a reduced ability to appropriately maintain and shift attention, and are usually associated with

Table 1.7 Diagnostic criteria for 293.0, 'Delirium due to . . . (indicate the general medical condition*)'

A   Disturbance of consciousness (i.e. reduced clarity of awareness of the environment) with reduced ability to focus, sustain, or shift attention

B   A change in cognition (such as memory deficit, disorientation, language disturbance) or the development of a perceptual disturbance that is not better accounted for by a pre-existing, established, or evolving dementia[†]

C   The disturbance develops over a short period of time (usually hours to days)and tends to fluctuate during the course of the day

D   There is evidence from the history, physical examination, or laboratory findings that the disturbance is caused by the direct physiological consequences of a general medical condition

* Coding note. Include the name of the general medical condition on axis I, e.g. 293.0 'Delirium due to hepatic encephalopathy'; also code the general medical condition on Axis III (see Appendix G for codes).

† Coding note. If delirium is superimposed on a pre-existing vascular dementia, indicate the delirium by coding the 290.41, 'Vascular dementia, with delirium'.

Reprinted with permission from the Diagnostic and Statistical Manual of Mental Disorders, IV edition, Text revision. Copyright 2000 American Psychiatric Association.

Table 1.8 Diagnostic criteria for substance intoxication delirium*

A   Disturbance of consciousness (i.e. reduced clarity of awareness of the environment) with reduced ability to focus, sustain, or shift attention

B   A change in cognition (such as memory deficit, disorientation, language disturbance) or the development of a perceptual disturbance that is not better accounted for by a pre-existing, established, or evolving dementia

C   The disturbance develops over a short period of time (usually hours to days) and tends to fluctuate during the course of the day

D   There is evidence from the history, physical examination, or laboratory findings of either (1) or (2):

  1   the symptoms in Criteria A and B developed during substance intoxication

  2   medication use is aetiologically related to the disturbance[†]

* Note: This diagnosis should be made instead of a diagnosis of 'substance intoxication' only when the cognitive symptoms are in excess of those usually associated with the intoxication syndrome and when the symptoms are sufficiently severe to warrant independent clinical attention.

† Note: The diagnosis should be recorded as 'substance-induced delirium' if related to medication use. The codes for (specific substance) intoxication delirium are: 291.0, alcohol; 292.81, amphetamine (or amphetamine-like substance); 292.81, cannabis; 292.81, cocaine; 292.81, hallucinogen; 292.81, inhalant; 292.81, opioid; 292.81, phencyclidine (or phencyclidine-like substance); 292.81, sedative, hypnotic, or anxiolytic; 292.81, other (or unknown) substance (e.g. cimetidine, digitalis, benztropine).

Reprinted with permission from the Diagnostic and Statistical Manual of Mental Disorders, IV edition, Text revision. Copyright 2000 American Psychiatric Association.

EEG abnormalities. Other differential symptoms are represented by memory impairment and disorientation, which are more typical of delirium, and the evidence of an underlying general medical condition, substance intoxication or withdrawal, or medication use. Delirium must be distinguished also from 'malingering' and from 'factitious disorder', given the often atypical presentation in 'malingering' and 'factitious

Table 1.9 Diagnostic criteria for substance withdrawal delirium*

A   Disturbance of consciousness (i.e. reduced clarity of awareness of the environment) with reduced ability to focus, sustain, or shift attention

B   A change in cognition (such as memory deficit, disorientation, language disturbance) or the development of a perceptual disturbance that is not better accounted for by a pre-existing, established, or evolving dementia

C   The disturbance develops over a short period of time (usually hours to days)and tends to fluctuate during the course of the day

D   There is evidence from the history, physical examination, or laboratory findings that the symptoms in Criteria A and B developed during, or shortly after, a withdrawal syndrome

* Note. This diagnosis should be made instead of a diagnosis of 'substance withdrawal' only when the cognitive symptoms are in excess of those usually associated with the withdrawal syndrome and when the symptoms are sufficiently severe to warrant independent clinical attention. Code for (specific substance) withdrawal delirium: 291.0, alcohol; 292.81, sedative, hypnotic, or anxiolytic; 292.81, other (or unknown) substance.

Reprinted with permission from the Diagnostic and Statistical Manual of Mental Disorders, IV edition, Text revision. Copyright 2000 American Psychiatric Association.

Table 1.10 Diagnostic criteria for 'delirium due to multiple aetiologies'*

A   Disturbance of consciousness (i.e, reduced clarity of awareness of the environment) with reduced ability to focus, sustain, or shift attention

B   A change in cognition (such as memory deficit, disorientation, language disturbance) or the development of a perceptual disturbance that is not better accounted for by a pre-existing, established, or evolving dementia

C   The disturbance develops over a short period of time (usually hours to days) and tends to fluctuate during the course of the day

D   There is evidence from the history, physical examination, or laboratory findings that the delirium has more than one aetiology (e.g. more than one aetiological general medical condition, a general medical condition plus substance intoxication or medication side-effect)

* Coding note. Use multiple codes reflecting specific delirium and specific aetiologies, e.g. 293.0, delirium due to viral encephalitis; 291.0, alcohol withdrawal delirium.

Reprinted with permission from the Diagnostic and Statistical Manual of Mental Disorders, IV edition, Text revision. Copyright 2000 American Psychiatric Association.

Table 1.11 Criteria for 'delirium not otherwise specified' (code 780.09)

This category should be used to diagnose a delirium that does not meet criteria for any of the specific types of delirium described in this section.

Examples include:

1   A clinical presentation of delirium that is suspected to be due to a general medical condition or substance use but for which there is insufficient evidence to establish a specific aetiology

2   Delirium due to causes not listed in this section (e.g. sensory deprivation)

Reprinted with permission from the Diagnostic and Statistical Manual of Mental Disorders, IV edition, Text revision. Copyright 2000 American Psychiatric Association.

disorder' and the absence of a general medical condition or substance that is aetio-logically related to the apparent cognitive disturbance. Individuals may present with some but not all symptoms of delirium. Subsyndromal presentations need to be care-fully assessed because they may be harbingers of a full-blown delirium or may signal an as yet undiagnosed underlying general medical condition. Such presentations should be coded as 'cognitive disorder not otherwise specified'.

1.3.2   ICD-10

A few years before the publication of the DSM-IV, the World Health Organization (1992) published the tenth revision of the *International classification of diseases* (ICD-10), with substantial changes with respect to the former ICD-9, published in 1979. The number of categories available for the classification were obviously higher. ICD-9 numeric codes (001–999) were replaced by an alphanumeric coding scheme (codes with a single letter followed by two numbers at the three-character level (A00–Z99).

With regard to the 'Classification of mental and behavioural disorders' (Chapter V–F) the ICD-9 categories were replaced by 100 categories in the ICD-10. There are many similiarities between the ICD-10 (Chapter V) and the DSM-IV, not surprisingly in view of the mutual contributions from the two task forces that worked on the systems. However, unlike the DSM-IV:

◆ the multiaxial system is conceptualized in a different way, with one axis for psychi-atric and medical diagnosis, one axis for disability (similar to the DSM axis V),[1] and one axis covering psychosocial and environmental stressors (similarly to the DSM axis IV);

◆ the terms neurosis and psychosis are maintained in a number of syndromes;

◆ the terms organic mental syndrome and organic mental disorder are retained;

◆ the diagnostic criteria are more flexible (Dilling 2000).

However, as a general rule, the codes and terms provided by the ICD-10 are compat-ible with the DSM-IV and DSM-IV-TR (Appendix H of the DSM-IV-TR), as a result of co-joint consultations between the WHO and APA and the mutual coordination in the development of the two systems.

A clinical modification of the ICD-10 (ICD-10-CM) is, however, expected to be implemented in the USA in 2004, making it easier for clinicians to use both systems as well as having conversion tables available for clinical and administrative purposes.

Clinical description and diagnostic guidelines for delirium

In the ICD-10 classification, delirium is in part subsumed under the rubric, 'organic, including symptomatic, mental disorders' (categories F00–09), and in part under

---

[1] The WHO (World Health Organization 2001) has recently published the draft full version of the *International classification of functioning and disability* (ICIDH-2), which groups functional states associated with health conditions (i.e. a disease, disorder, injury or trauma, or other health-related state) with the aim of providing a unified and standard language and framework for the description of human functioning and disability as an important component of health, including mental health.

Table 1.12 ICD-10 classification of delirium

F00-F09: Organic, including symptomatic, mental disorders	
F05	**Delirium, not induced by alcohol and other psychoactive substances**
	F05.0 Delirium, not superimposed on dementia, so described
	F05.1 Delirium, superimposed on dementia
	F05.8 Other delirium
	F05.9 Delirium, unspecified
F10-F19: Mental and behavioural disorders due to psychoactive substance use*	
F1x.03	Acute intoxication, with delirium
F1x.4	Withdrawal state with delirium
F1x.40	Without convulsions
F1x.41	With convulsions

* 'x' in the entries stands for the psychoactive substance as follows. Mental and behavioural disorders due to: use of alcohol (F10); opioids (F11); cannabinoids (F12); sedatives or hypnotics (F13); cocaine (F14); other stimulants, including caffeine (F15); hallucinogens (F16); tobacco (F17); volatile solvents (F18); other psychoactive substances (F19).

Reproduced with permission from World Health Organization, The ICD-10 Classification of Mental and Behavioral Disorders: Clinical Descriptions and Diagnostic Guidelines, WHO Publications, Geneva, 1992.

the rubric, 'mental and behavioural disorders due to psychoactive and other non-prescribed substance use' (categories F10–19; Table 1.12).

The rubric, 'organic, including symptomatic, mental disorders' (categories F00-09), consists of 'dementia in Alzheimer's disease' (F00), 'vascular dementia' (F01), 'dementia in other diseases classified elsewhere' (F02), 'unspecified dementia' (F03), 'organic amnesic syndrome, not induced by alcohol and other psychoactive substances' (F04), and 'delirium, not induced by alcohol and other psychoactive substances' (F05). According to the ICD-10, 'the term "organic" used in this section does not mean that the other psychiatric disturbances are "non-organic", in the sense of not having a cerebral substrate', but 'organic means simply that the syndrome so classified can be attributed to an independently diagnosable cerebral or systemic disease or disorder' (World Health Organization 1992).

As far as the rubric 'mental and behavioural disorders due to psychoactive substance use' is concerned, it is stated that delirium can also be a complication of all the *acute intoxication* states of the substances listed in Table 1.12 (specification of the code F1x.03) or *withdrawal* from the substance (F1x.40 without convulsions; F1x.41 with convulsions) where x in these codes refers to the particular substance (see footnote to Table 1.12). The latter category includes also alcohol withdrawal syndrome or *delirium tremens*, described as a toxic confusional state that is short in its length, can be life-threatening, and is characterized by the classical triad of reduced level of consciousness, intense hallucinations or illusions, and marked tremor.

The ICD-10 general clinical descriptions and diagnostic guidelines (CDCG) for delirium are quite similar to those proposed by the DSM-IV and DSM-IV-TR, as indicated in Table 1.13. The ICD-10-CDCG defines delirium as

Table 1.13 ICD-10 clinical guidelines for the diagnosis of delirium

To meet the diagnosis symptoms (mild or severe) must be present in each of the following areas:

1   Impairment of consciousness or attention on a continuum from clouding to coma; reduced ability to direct, focus, sustain, and shift attention

2   Global disturbance of cognition (perceptual distortions, illusions, hallucinations, most often visual; impairment of abstract thinking and comprehension with or without transient delusions, but typically with some degree of incoherence; impairment of immediate recall and recent memory but with relatively intact remote memory; disorientation for time as well as, in more cases, for place and person)

3   Psychomotor disturbances (hypo- or hyperactivity or unpredictable shifts from one to the other; increased reaction time; increased or decreased flow speech; enhanced startle reactions)

4   Disturbances of the sleep-wake cycle (insomnia or, in severe cases, total sleep loss or reversal of the sleep-wake cycle; daytime drowsiness; nocturnal worsening of symptoms; disturbing dreams or nightmares that may continue as hallucinations after awakening)

5   Emotional disturbances, e.g. depression, anxiety or fear, irritability, euphoria, apathy, or wondering perplexity

Reproduced with permission from World Health Organization, The ICD-10 Classification of Mental and Behavioral Disorders: Clinical Descriptions and Diagnostic Guidelines, WHO Publications, Geneva, 1992.

an etiologically non specific syndrome characterized by concurrent disturbances of consciousness, and attention, perception, thinking, memory, psychomotor behaviour, and the sleep–wake cycle. It is stated that the syndrome can develop at any age, even if it is more common after the age of 60. The delirious state is transient and of fluctuating intensity; most cases recover within four weeks or less. Delirium lasting, with fluctuations, for up to six months is not uncommon, however, especially when arising in the course of chronic liver disease, carcinoma, or subacute bacterial endocarditis. The distinction that is sometimes made between acute and subacute is of little clinical relevance; the condition should be seen as a unitary syndrome of variable duration and severity ranging from mild to very severe. A delirious state may be superimposed on, or progress into, dementia. The onset is usually rapid and the course fluctuating during the day. The total length of the syndrome is less than six months.

If delirium is superimposed on dementia, this should be registered (F05.1). Delirium with multiple aetiologies and subacute confusional states includes 'other delirium' (F05.8), while a diagnosis of 'unspecified delirium' (F05.9) is given when it is not possible to specify clinical or aetiological aspects of delirium. In the differential diagnosis approach delirium should be distinguished from other organic syndromes, specifically 'dementia' (F00–F03), 'acute transient psychosis' (F23), 'acute states of schizophrenia' (F20), and 'confusional states possibly present in affective syndromes' (F30–39).

Diagnostic criteria for research

In 1993, the *ICD-10 Classification of mental and behavioural disorders—diagnostic criteria for research* (ICD-10-DCR) was published (World Health Organization 1993).

This not only had the obvious aim of helping clinicians in research settings, but also had the aim of increasing the congruence and reducing the differences between the DSM and ICD systems. The criteria of the ICD-10-DCR are more restrictive, although they are completely compatible with the ICD-10-CDDG. Regarding delirium, the ICD-10-DCR indicates six criteria (A–F):

A Impairment of consciousness, i.e. reduced awareness of the environment, with reduced ability to focus, sustain, and shift attention

B Global disturbance of cognitive functions consisting in both of the following aspects:
1 impairment of immediate recall and recent memory but with relatively intact remote memory;
2 disorientation for time, place, or person

C At least one of the following psychomotor disturbances:
1 rapid and unpredictable shifts from hypoactivity to hyperactivity;
2 increased reaction time;
3 increased or decreased flow in speech;
4 enhanced startle reactions

D Disturbances of the sleep or the sleep–wake cycle, as indicated by the presence of at least one of the following:
1 insomnia that, in severe cases, can cause total sleep loss, with or without daytime drowsiness, or reversal of the sleep–wake cycle;
2 nocturnal worsening of symptoms;
3 disturbing dreams or nightmares, which may continue as hallucinations or illusions after awakening

E Rapid onset and fluctuations of symptoms during the day.

F Evidence (from the history, physical and neurological examination, or instrumental and laboratory findings) of an underlying cerebral or systemic disease or disorder (not due to psychoactive substances) that can be responsible for the clinical symptoms described in the criteria A–D.

The ICD-10-DRC notes also that emotional disturbances (e.g. depression, anxiety or fear, irritability, euphoria, apathy, or wondering perplexity), perceptual distortions (illusions, hallucinations, most often visual), and transient delusions are typical but are not specific criteria for the diagnosis.

1.4 Conclusions

According to Liptzin (1999) some caveats should be taken into account in the discussion of delirium classification and the criteria currently used.

1 Delirium is now recognized and systematized as a nosological entity, even if the classification of the disorder and its diagnostic criteria have changed over the last decade. Table 1.14 summarizes the significant differences among the several DSM versions and ICD-10 in the criteria for the diagnosis of delirium, according to Smith *et al.* (1994).

Table 1.14 Differences in the criteria for the diagnosis of delirium throughout the DSM and ICD-10 classifications

DSM-III	DSM-III-R	DSM-IV/DSM-IV-TR	ICD-10
Attention, awareness, consciousness criteria			
Clouding of consciousness; reduced clarity of awareness of environment, with reduced capacity to shift, focus, and maintain attention to environmental stimuli	Reduced ability to maintain attention to external stimuli (e.g. questions must be repeated because attention wanders) and to appropriately shift attention to new external stimuli (e.g. perseverates answer to a previous question)	Disturbance of consciousness (i.e. reduced clarity of awareness of the environment) with reduced ability to focus, sustain, or shift attention	Impairment of consciousness or attention on a continuum from clouding to coma; reduced ability to direct, focus, sustain, and shift attention
Cognitive disturbance criteria			
Disorientation and memory impairment (if testable)	Disorganized thinking, as indicated by rambling, irrelevant, or incoherent speech	A change in cognition (such as memory deficit, disorientation, language disturbance) or the development of a perceptual disturbance that is not better accounted for by a pre-existing, established, or evolving dementia	Global disturbance of cognition (perceptual distortions, illusions, hallucinations, most often visual; impairment of abstract thinking and comprehension with or without transient delusions, but typically with some degree of incoherence; impairment of immediate recall and recent memory but with relatively intact remote memory; disorientation for time as well as, in more cases, for place and person)
Chronological criteria			
Clinical features develop over a short period of time (usually hours to days) and tend to fluctuate during the course of the day	Clinical features develop over a short period of time (usually hours to days) and tend to fluctuate during the course of the day	The disturbance develops over a short period of time (usually hours to days) and tends to fluctuate during the course of the day	

Table 1.14 (cont.)

DSM-III	DSM-III-R	DSM-IV/DSM-IV-TR	ICD-10
Associated symptom criteria			
At least two of the following: (a) perceptual disturbance (e.g. misinterpretations, illusions, or hallucinations; (b) speech that is at times incoherent; (c) disturbance of sleep–wake cycle with insomnia or daytime drowsiness; (d) increased or decreased psychomotor activity	At least two of the following: (a) reduced level of consciousness, e.g. difficulty keeping awake during examination; (b) perceptual disturbance (i.e. misinterpretations, illusions, or hallucinations; (c) disturbance of sleep–wake cycle with insomnia or daytime sleepiness; (d) increased or decreased psychomotor activity; (e) disorientation to time, place, or person; (f) memory impairment, e.g. inability to learn new material, such as the names of several unrelated objects after 5 minutes, or to remember past events, such as history of current episodes of illness	None	Psychomotor disturbances (hypo- or hyperactivity or unpredictable shifts from one to the other; increased reaction time; increased or decreased flow speech; enhanced startle reactions); disturbances of the sleep–wake cycle (insomnia or, in severe cases, total sleep loss or reversal of the sleep–wake cycle;daytime drowsiness; nocturnal worsening of symptoms; disturbing dreams or nightmares that may continue as hallucinations after awakening); emotional disturbances, e.g. depression, anxiety or fear, irritability, euphoria, apathy, or wondering perplexity

Table 1.14 (cont.)

DSM-III	DSM-III-R	DSM-IV/DSM-IV-TR	ICD-10
Criteria for judging if there is an organic factor			
Evidence from the history, physical examination, or laboratory tests of a specific organic factor judged to be aetiologically related to the disturbance	Either (1) or (2): (1) evidence from the history, physical examination, or laboratory findings of a specific organic factor (or factors) judged to be aetiologically related to the disturbance; (2) in the absence of such evidence, an aetiological organic factor can be presumed if the disturbance cannot be accounted for by any non-organic mental disorder, e.g. manic episode accounting for agitation and sleep disturbance	There is evidence from the history, physical examination, or laboratory findings that the disturbance is caused by the direct physiological consequences of a general medical condition	Not expressly required but presumable: the presence of an underlying medical condition

2 In spite of the tendency to define explicit criteria for delirium based on the specificity of the symptoms, it has to be remembered that certain clinical situations
can be a source of confusion in the diagnosis. For example, hospitalization and
diagnostic procedures, as well as physical symptoms, such as pain or breathing
difficulties, can produce pseudodelirium symptoms such as sleep disorders and
psychomotor disturbances in hospitalized elderly and physically ill patients (Liptzin
1999).

3 Subsyndromal delirium should be considered an entity to be recognized in clinical
practice when dealing with confused patients (Levkoff et al. 1996). Subsyndromal
delirium is described as a disorder that has some symptoms of delirium (e.g. clouding of consciousness, disorientation), but does not meet the full diagnosis. It also
falls on a continuum between delirium and 'normality', and has risk factors identical to those for delirium.

4 The balance between different nosological systems is necessary to avoid the risk of
false-positives or false-negatives in making the diagnosis of delirium. With respect
to this, Liptzin et al. (1991), in a study of 325 hospitalized elderly patients, demonstrated that a diagnosis of delirium was possible in 38.4% ($n = 125$) by using the
DSM-III, in 32.6% ($n = 106$) by using the DSM-III-R, and in 9.2% ($n = 30$) by
using the ICD-10 criteria. In a recent study of elderly patients in an emergency
room, the prevalence of delirium was 24% using the DSM-III-R, 20% using the
DSM-IV, and 21% by using the physician's clinical impression (Monette et al. 2001).
These results indicate, obviously, that too inclusive or too restrictive criteria can
cause marked differences in prevalence rates of a disorder. Similar problems
emerge, for example, in diagnosing depressive disorder in the terminally ill. By
using different systems (DSM-III and the Research Diagnostic Criteria) and different threshold levels in the criteria, Chochinov et al. (1994) found a total prevalence
of depressive disorder ranging from a minimum of 13% to a maximum of 26%,
with a prevalence of major depression between 9.2% and 16.9%.

A final caveat stems from the fact that knowledge about the diagnosis and treatment
of delirium is still limited to certain medical fields, such as psychiatry, neurology, geri-
atrics, and palliative medicine. As stated by Francis (1999), there is a strong need to
expand the level of awareness of the problem of delirium of all health professionals
who care for patients who can develop this disorder (e.g. intensive care professionals,
anaesthetists, surgeons, internal medicine physicians, oncologists, and general practitioners working in the home setting). With regard to this, the involvement of medical
disciplines, other than psychiatry, specifically primary care, has been the aim of recent
publications of the APA (DSM-IV-TM, primary care version; American Psychiatric
Association 1995) and the WHO (ICD-10-DMCG, primary care version; World
Health Organization 1996). The two systems represent an opportunity for primary
care physicians to familiarize themselves with the most important psychiatric
disorders, in terms of both diagnosis and management.

Chapter 2

Pathophysiology

2.1 General considerations

The pathophysiology of delirium is not fully understood but several mechanisms, namely, neurophysiological pathways, anatomical and neurotransmitter substrates, are important in interpreting clinical findings and can be discussed in some detail.

From the DSM-IV and previous definitions, delirium is an affection of cognition, arousal, and attention. The usefulness of the definition is to correctly classify patients with similar clinical features and to allow communication among professionals minimizing taxonomic ambiguity. In this respect the accepted DSM IV definition has the advantages of encompassing a broad spectrum and being lucid and clear, but it also implies great complexity. The areas of neurological function identified are indeed very wide and can hardly be attributed to the activity of discrete cerebral structures. Also controversial is the interpretation that the syndrome is caused by the ability of different aetiological factors to impact on a final common pathway producing stereotyped clinical consequences.

2.2 Delirium as a disorder of consciousness

A discussion of the definition of consciousness is beyond the scope of this book, but it is certainly relevant to the DSM-IV definition of delirium (Giacino 1997; Zeman 2001). Consciousness can be defined as the brain function that allows awareness of oneself and of the environment and is characterized by two main aspects: the level of consciousness and the content of consciousness (Plum and Posner 1980*b*). The level of consciousness reflects arousal and vigilance: being awake, asleep, or comatose. The content of consciousness, or part of it, is experienced by the subject as awareness of him or herself and of the environment when awake and normally alert. Delirium can be interpreted as an abnormality of the level of consciousness (Plum and Posner 1980*b*).

One fundamental aspect of the pathophysiology of delirium is the recognition of the functional dissociation of cognition and awareness from arousal on clinical and neuroanatomical grounds. In simplistic terms, arousal is a general activation of the cortical and subcortical functions that is a prerequisite for cognition and awareness, and it is also related to the regulation of the sleep–wakefulness cycle. Arousal and the sleep–wake cycle can be intact in patients with profound cognitive failure, e.g. in the demented and even more dramatically in patients without any sign of active cognition including awareness, such as those in a vegetative state (Plum and Posner 1980*b*).

Another compelling clinical observation is that, in most of the cases presenting with delirium, if the cause cannot be removed, the condition evolves into stupor and then into a coma, which has led to the interpretation that the cerebral structures involved in the modulation of alertness and arousal must be affected in delirium (Young 1998). In this case, delirium, as a condition characterized by selective altered arousal, is considered to be the trigger of all or most of the other disordered brain functions.

This concept depends on being able to distinguish between brain structures or functions of structures responsible for a basic form of brain activation (crude consciousness, wakefulness, arousal—the level of consciousness) and other structures responsible for higher cognitive processes (emotion, memory—the content of consciousness). Arousal is the prerequisite for the content of consciousness to be experienced and expressed.

Any type of lesion diffusely affecting the brain will impact on the level of consciousness. It has been shown that integrative brain functions are lost proportionally to the amount of brain matter lost but also to the rapidity of onset of the pathological insult (Plum and Posner 1980b). This observation agrees with current evidence of the relevance of brainstem and medial thalamic structures together with cortical brain areas (especially associational areas) for the development of delirium.

2.3 Delirium as a disorder of attention

Attention is the second main concept to define when dealing with delirium. Attention is the ability to focus, sustain, and switch mental activity in response to environmental or internal stimuli. Arousal and attention are linked. Arousal is the most generic neurophysiological term used to define brain activation. Arousal is necessary for vigilance and alertness, which have been defined as the tonic and phasic components of attention, respectively (Seltzer and Mesulam 1990). Vigilance, the tonic component, is characterized by circadian physiological fluctuations, including the sleep–wake cycle, that can overlap with the level of consciousness. Alertness, the phasic component, can be enhanced or diminished by physiological activation for the performance of cognitive or praxic activities or by pathological conditions in the hyper- or hypoalert states that are typical of delirium (see also Chapter 4).

A failure of selective attention, the ability to select in the environment significant stimuli and to focus attention on them for a protracted time, is found in all cases of delirium and has also been suggested as the essential feature of the syndrome (Mesulam 1985). This is easier to demonstrate in the early stages and in mild cases allowing detailed neuropsychological examination. Selective lesions of cortical association areas in the right (non-dominant) cerebral hemisphere (posterior parietal, inner temporooccipital, and prefrontal) can produce attention failure and acute confusional states (Mesulam et al. 1976). Other symptoms that characterize delirium, such as language and memory alterations, writing and constructional apraxia, disruption of the wakefulness–sleep cycle, or hallucinations, can be early findings in the course of the syndrome and also in isolated findings of partial syndromes. These symptoms suggest focal origins. This emphasis on the phasic component of attention is not completely accepted. In fact, the more general definition now accepted in DSM-IV includes attention and level of consciousness, which, in the terminology used in this section, correspond more closely to alertness (phasic component of attention) and vigilance (tonic component of attention), respectively (Sellal and Collard 2001).

The observations that both diffuse metabolic states and focal lesions of cortical association areas important for the attentional process can produce delirium are not contradictory. Diffuse metabolic causes can affect first the most sensitive cerebral structures and give rise to symptoms that will subsequently combine in the full delirium syndrome or evolve into more severe states of impaired consciousness.

Arousal and attention are the products of the integrative function of different cerebral structures, which will be affected by acute events both diffuse and focal. In particular, the primary impairment of attention could be due to the dysfunction of the association cortical areas of the right hemisphere, but a lesion of the reticular activating system will also impact on both arousal and attention. The combination of diffuse cause with focal sensitivity and with the ability of cerebral structures to substitute for the function of the affected regions will result in the final clinical picture. Clarifying the complexity of the previous two examples can be helpful. For example, in the case quoted earlier (Mesulam *et al.* 1976), a focal vascular lesion of a cortical area crucial for the higher integration of attention abilities can manifest with delirium. In contrast, thiamine deficiency will affect diffusely all the brain neurons and produce early dysfunction of sensitive structures in the medial thalamus, hypothalamic mammillary bodies, and oculomotor nuclei, with subsequent memory deficit and ocular palsy. The full clinical effects will result in the Wernicke–Korsakoff syndrome, a form of dementia, but in earlier phases delirium may be the only clinical manifestation (Barbato and Rodriguez 1994; O'Keeffe *et al.* 1994).

2.4   Cerebral structures implied in the pathogenesis of delirium

2.4.1   Arousal

The CNS structures responsible for arousal, attention, and for regulating the sleep–wake cycles are partially known and their functions overlap. Several brainstem neural groups are important for these functions and some neurostransmitters are linked to the functions of these cells.

The ascending reticular activating system (ARAS) was described more than 50 years ago by Moruzzi and Magoun (1949; see Fig. 2.1). These authors demonstrated that the dorsal mesencephalic reticular formation with its rostral projection system is necessary to sustain arousal, that its lesion is associated with coma, and that its stimulation produces behavioural and electroencephlographic arousal. The same authors demonstrated that the dorsal hypothalamus and the subthalamic region could also modulate (increase) the arousal level (Magoun 1952). Other relevant brainstem structures with different functions are the locus ceruleus and the raphe nuclei. The ARAS projects to the intralaminar and the reticular nuclei of the thalamus, which in turn regulate the thalamic-specific nuclei outflow to the cortical mantle and also project to the cortex itself (Brodal 1981). These areas overlap with neurons that are relevant to the

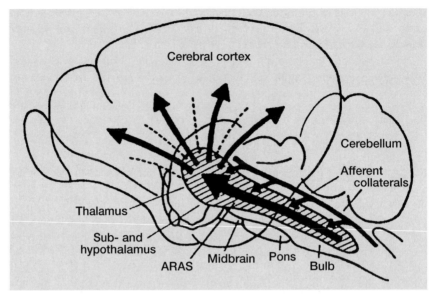

Fig. 2.1 One of the first representations of the ascending reticular activating system (ARAS). The schematic drawing shows how the brainstem and thalamic reticular formation should, by means of their cortical projections, influence the maintenance and regulation of the level of consciousness. The connections, called 'afferent collaterals', would serve to explain how peripheral inputs can modulate the activity of the ARAS and be carried to the conscious level in the cortex after being filtered by the ARAS itself and the thalamus. (From Starzl *et al.* (1951).)

regulation of the sleep–wakefulness cycle. Cases of persistent vegetative state confirm that the preservation of brainstem and hypothalamic structures can be sufficient to sustain arousal and sleep–wake cycles while cognition is lost (Kinney *et al.* 1994). The importance of brainstem structure for the regulation of normal wakefulness is supported also by cases of delirium proven on autopsy to be associated with degeneration of the reticular formation, raphe nuclei, and locus ceruleus (Fukutani *et al.* 1993). The anatomical model of Moruzzi and Magoun (Fig. 2.1) integrated with a modern understanding of neurochemistry and neurophysiology is still valid today.

2.4.2 Attention

Attention is closely related to arousal. Lesions in the same brainstem areas as those affecting arousal will also affect attention. As it is mostly implicated in the selection of relevant stimuli, attention has to rely on the ability of the brainstem and thalamic structures to distinguish between relevant and irrelevant external stimuli, in letting them influence the higher cortical area. At the cerebral cortical level, the right parietal lobe, the cingulate gyrus, and the dorsolateral prefrontal cortex are all important areas for directing and sustaining attention. Ischaemic lesions of some of these areas and reduced metabolism in the same structures have been associated with cases of delirium (Mesulam *et al.* 1976; Trzepacz 1994*a*). Two studies have shown that visuospatial attention and visual memory tests could discriminate delirious patients from demented patients (Hart *et al.* 1997; Mach *et al.* 1996). These types of visual cognitive abilities are associated with right hemisphere functions.

2.5 Neurophysiological and functional studies in humans

Electroencephalography (EEG) makes it possible to assess the activity of a great number of neurons in order to understand the function of the mass of cortical neurons and their interconnections. As already shown, this activity is modulated by subcortical structures. Engel and Romano (1959) in their pioneering work described the EEG findings typical of delirium. They demonstrated that, independently of the aetiology of delirium, the EEG showed a diffuse slowing of its frequency that paralleled the severity of the disease. In mild cases the EEG could be slowed in comparison with the patient baseline, albeit being within normal ranges, and at recovery the EEG rhythm could be restored.

An increase of fast EEG rhythms in the beta frequency[2] range (13–35 counts/s) can be found as a typical sign of delirium tremens and other drug withdrawal deliria. This inhomogeneity is the basis for the major criticism of the unifying theory of delirium as a syndrome of cerebral insufficiency.

Similar findings were reproduced experimentally by injecting anticholinergic drugs in normal volunteers (Itil and Fink 1968). Depending on the dose, the subjects experienced delirium with reduced arousal, hallucinations, and agitated behaviour or stupor and their EEG showed typical changes (alpha rhythm disruption, delta and theta rhythms, and superimposed fast activity). When the same subjects experiencing anticholinergic toxicity were challenged with other drugs, some cholinergics could reverse both the clinical and EEG findings and amphetamines improved alertness, while LSD aggravated the agitated and hallucinated clinical picture when the EEG showed increased fast activity. Chlorpromazine abolished psychomotor agitation and hallucinations and produced stupor with slow EEG frequencies (Itil and Fink 1968). This experiment was considered an example of anticholinergic delirium and is a useful model to suggest the presence of EEG excitatory phenomena associated with hyperactive delirium, while a dominant slow EEG rhythm was the hallmark of reduced alertness and psychomotor activity.

A few studies (Trzepacz 1994*a*) suggest that evoked potentials are affected in delirious patients at a subcortical level (Trzepacz *et al.* 1989*b*). More recently, single-photon emission computerized tomography (SPECT) studies (Trzepacz *et al.* 1994) showed reduced global cerebral metabolism in some cases and, in others, selective areas of reduced energy consumption in the orbitofrontal and prefrontal cortical areas, while enhanced cerebral metabolism characterized delirium tremens. It is important, however, to remember that the techniques employed to date are still not sensitive enough to document with precision the brainstem and thalamic physiological activity.

---

[2] EEG recording is conventionally classified according to the frequency of the electrical signal as follows: alpha (α), 8–13 Hz; beta (β), 13–35 Hz; delta (δ), < 4 Hz; theta (θ), 4–8 Hz.

2.6 Neurotransmitters

The neurochemical characterization of the arousal and sleep–wake cycle regulation points to the importance of several neurotransmitters, namely, acetylcholine, catecholamines, serotonin, and histamine (Flacker and Lipsitz 1999a; Trzepacz 1994a, 1999).

2.6.1 Acetylcholine (ACh)

Cholinergic transmission from the basal forebrain and from the brainstem-activating system to cortical areas is one relevant biochemical substrate of some aspects of arousal and sleep, attention, and memory (Perry *et al.* 1999; Robbins and Everitt 1995; see Fig. 2.2). The importance of the cholinergic system as the potential final common pathway of many deliriogenic conditions is suggested by its impairment in dementia and in ageing of the brain, both of which are conditions that lead to a higher risk of delirium. Anticholinergic drugs are, indeed, among the most frequent causes of

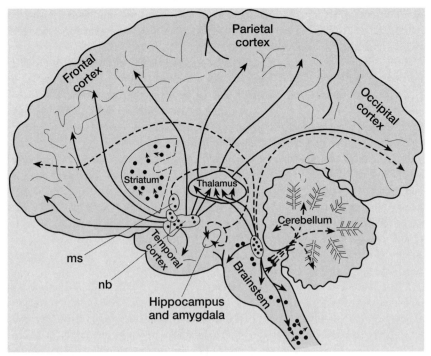

Fig. 2.2 Major cholinergic systems in the human brain with diffuse cortical projections from the basal forebrain, hypothalamic areas (nb, ms, and adjacents), from the thalamus, and from the brainstem to the thalamus. The role of acetylcholine in cognition, dementia, and delirium is discussed in the text. This picture represents the evolution from anatomy (Fig. 2.1) to neuropharmacology in interpreting the regulation of consciousness. (Reproduced with permission from Perry E., Walker, M., Grace, J., and Perry R., (1999) Acetylcholine in mind: a neurotrasmitter correlate of consciousness, Trends Neurosci, 22, 273–80. Copyright 1999, with permission from Elsevier Science.)

delirium. The use of drugs with anticholinergic effects is associated with delirium especially in the elderly (Han *et al.* 2001) and in the postoperative period (Tune *et al.* 1993).

2.6.2   Serum anticholinergic activity

Several studies have tried to demonstrate a link between the level of serum anticholinergic activity (SAA; Tune *et al.* 1992) and the risk of developing delirium; they have given ambiguous results. Serum anticholinergic activity should be hypothetically absent in humans and has been considered to reflect the effect of drugs or other substances (Flacker and Lipsitz 1999*a*; Tune *et al.* 1992). Some studies have shown that SAA is associated with an increased risk of delirium (see Flacker and Lipsitz 1999*b* for a review). Acute changes in SAA status were seen during febrile illnesses but could not be related to the development of delirium (Flacker and Lipsitz 1999*b*). Another study recently found that SAA and the use of neuroleptics and benzodiazepines were independently associated with the occurrence of delirium in a group of 61 elderly patients (Mussi *et al.* 1999). Anticholinergic activity due to endogenous substances, independent of any drug effect, has been demonstrated in elderly patients with acute illness (Flacker and Wei 2001). Differences in study results may depend on different assay methods for determining SAA, but it is more likely that they reflect the complex interaction of external factors with the individual patient response and it is probable that SAA reflects an aspecific stress response of elderly subjects to illness (Flacker and Lipsitz 1999*b*).

2.6.3   Dopamine

The role of dopaminergic and noradrenergic pathways is closely linked to the cholinergic system in regulating sleep–wakefulness states (Zeman 2001). An imbalance between the activities of these systems is likely to contribute to delirium symptoms with a relative overactivity of the dopaminergic system and hypoactivity of cholinergic transmission. Agents that block dopamine (DA) activity and, in particular, DA2 receptors are used to control delirium symptoms, whereas certain substances (such as cocaine) or conditions (such as electroconvulsive therapy, ECT) that enhance DA levels can cause delirium Interestingly, ECT often causes hyperactive deliria and has also been used to resolve untreatable delirium (Fink 1993; Levin *et al.* 2002; Liston and Sones 1990; Rao and Lyketsos 2000). On the other hand, the central activating system pharmacology involves at least ACh, DA, noradrenaline (NA; also called norepinephrine), serotonin (5-hydroxytryptamine, 5-HT), and histamine in a complex and integrated network (see also Fig. 2.3 and comments). For instance, ACh and NA seem to serve different aspects of attention functions (Robbins and Everitt 1995).

2.6.4   Serotonin (5-HT)

The raphe nuclei in the brainstem also have a cortical projection and contain serotonin. Serotonergic neurons in the raphe nuclei and in the hypothalamus are considered important for sleep regulation, in particular, for those phases of sleep characterized by dreams (rapid eye movement (REM) sleep), and perhaps in the genesis of

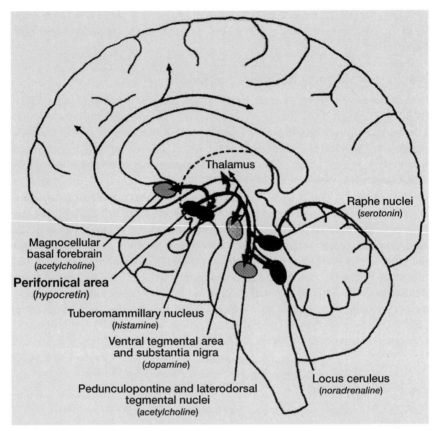

Fig. 2.3 This schematic drawing highlights the relationship between several areas considered important for the regulation of vigilance and sleep–arousal cycles and their associated neurotransmitters (acetylcholine, dopamine, serotonin, histamine), together with the most recent projections (black arrows) demonstrated from and to most of these areas containing hypocretin. (Reproduced with permission from Silber, M.H. and Rye D.B. Solving the mystery of nacolepsy. The hypocretin story, *Neurology*, 56 (2001) 1616–18. Copyright 2001 American Academy of Neurology.)

hallucinations as supported by the observation that lysergic acid diethylamide (LSD)-like drugs exert their hallucinogenic activity by probably acting as 5HT-2 agonists (Ross 1991). The serotonergic syndrome is a recognized complication of drugs that selectively enhance 5-HT transmission and is characterized by delirium (Gillman 1999).

A number of studies have tried to link 5-HT or 5-HT metabolites to delirium in postoperative, septic, and hepatic deliria and in elderly populations. Both high and low levels of 5-HT have been associated with delirium. The balance of 5-HT CNS availability can be compromised by the reduced uptake by the brain of tryptophan, which is the precursor of 5-HT, due to an altered metabolism of amino acids. In particular, the increase of phenylalanine and large-chain neutral amino acids in certain pathological conditions, such as liver failure, postoperative stress, and poor general condition, could be the initial cause of 5-HT reduction and simultaneously of increased noradrenergic and dopaminergic function and, finally, could predispose to delirium (van der Mast and Fekkes 2000; van der Mast *et al.* 1991). On this basis, branched amino acid infusions have been tried with some success in septic and hepatic failure deliria (Flacker and Lipsitz 1999*a*). The stress response and immune activation may also influence the levels of plasma amino acids. This mechanism may be involved in the development of postoperative delirium in the elderly more vulnerable patients (van der Mast and Fekkes 2000).

2.6.5   Gammaaminobutyric acid (GABA)

GABAergic thalamic interneurons have an inhibitory effect on the thalamocortical projection, and GABA is, in general, the major inhibitory transmitter within the central nervous system. The anxiolytic and hypnotic effects of benzodiazepines and barbiturates are mediated by GABAergic effects. In patients with hepatic encephalopathy, circulating benzodiazepine-like substances are found that could act on the GABA inhibitory system at the cortical level to produce EEG and behavioural signs of reduced arousal and delirium. While a role of the GABAergic system in producing hepatic encephalopathy is confirmed (Meyer *et al.* 1998), the role of benzodiazepine-like substances is uncertain (Macdonald *et al.* 1997). In fact, the benzodiazepine antagonist flumazenil is effective in improving clinical and EEG findings in only a minority of patients with hepatic encephalopathy (Annese *et al.* 1998; Barbaro *et al.* 1998; Gyr *et al.* 1996; Laccetti *et al.* 2000).

2.6.6   Histamine, other neurotransmitters, and recent findings

Histamine-containing neurons are also present in the hypothalamus, and H2 histamine receptors in the cortex and hippocampus mediate sedative effects. In particular, the activity of histaminergic neurons in the anterior hypothalamus promotes vigilance, while activity in the posterior hypothalamic areas promotes sleep.

Recently, a new peptide was identified in the hypothalamus and named hypocretin 1 (Silber and Rye 2001). This peptide or, more accurately, its receptors, is present in all areas that are important for regulating arousal and the sleep–wake cycle, including cholinergic neurons of the basal forebrain and of the brainstem, histaminergic neurons in the hypothalamus, dopaminergic neurons of the ventral tegmental area, serotonergic neurons of the raphe nuclei, and noradrenergic neurons of the locus ceruleus (Fig. 2.3). Hypocretin 1 is now thought to play an important role in activating the ascending reticular activating system, and its deficiency seems to be a cause of daytime somnolence and abnormalities of REM sleep found in narcolepsy (Silber and Rye 2001). The role of this peptide in many other disorders of arousal, including some forms of delirium, should be investigated. The activity of a relatively new drug, modafinil, which has been used to improve vigilance in hypersomnic and sedated states due to different neurological diseases (narcolepsy, Parkinson's disease, depression; Holder *et al.* 2002; Nieves and Lang 2002; Rammonah *et al.* 2002), has been linked to the function of histaminergic neurons within the anterior hypothalamus (Scammell *et al.* 2000).

2.7 Metabolic and molecular levels of dysfunction

The cholinergic hypothesis on the pathogenesis of delirium tends to demonstrate that both predisposing factors (age, dementia) and exogenous insults (thiamine deficiency, exogenous toxic substances, hypoxia, ion disturbances) act on a final common pathway at cellular and molecular level, which has one unifying step, namely, the failure of cholinergic transmission (Gibson *et al.* 1991). Altered cerebral metabolism due to different causes such as hypoxia, ageing, and nutritional deficiency would impact on the cholinergic system causing the symptoms of delirium (Blass and Gibson 1999). Changes in other neurotransmitters such as dopamine and glutamate may also occur and the second-messenger systems are implicated in fundamental damaging mechanisms at cellular level.

2.7.1 The role of thiamine deficiency

Wernicke–Korsakoff encephalopathy is characterized by memory loss, ocular movement disturbances, and dementia. Often, peripheral neuropathy is an associated symptom, which is related to nutritional thiamine (vitamin B1) deficiency in patients with alcohol abuse. Recently, partial syndromes have been thought to be more frequent than the classic full-blown encephalopathy. Elderly institutionalized patients with poor general health are considered at risk of malnutrition. Therefore, thiamine deficiency should be frequently suspected in cases presenting with a change in cognition and reduced food intake or absorbtion. A different question is whether thiamine deficiciency is frequent or is a relevant risk factor for the development of delirium in the elderly or severely ill patients. In this case also an unequivocal answer is lacking because the method (thiamine pyrophosphate effect) used to assess thiamine levels is relatively arbitrary. However, in the hospitalized elderly a definite thiamine deficiency can be found in between 17% (O'Keeffe *et al.* 1994) and 5% of patients (Papersack *et al.* 1999). In a group of 50 subjects admitted to a palliative care unit, 28% had significant thiamine deficiency defined with the same level of assay sensitivity (Barbato and Rodriguez 1994). Cognitive performance correlated with thiamine levels in the palliative care setting and was associated with delirium in one study of the elderly (O'Keeffe *et al.* 1994) but not in a more recent in-depth study (Papersack *et al.* 1999).

2.8 Stress and the immune response

2.8.1 Endogenous steroids

A relationship between delirium and cortisol is suggested by the potential development of delirium, sometimes also called steroid psychosis, during the therapeutic administration of glucocorticoids and by observation of psychoses and delirium occurring in the course of Cushing's syndrome. An impaired regulation of the hypothalamo-pituitary-adrenal axis resulting in increased cortisol levels or activity, has been observed in delirious patients (Robertsson *et al.* 2001) and, according to one study (O'Keeffe and Devlin 1994), was considered to be a risk factor for the development of delirium in the elderly. The theory that delirum can be caused by endogeous cortisol and favoured by a low threshold to stress is hypothetical (Flacker and Lipsitz 1999*a*).

2.8.2   Cytokines

The therapeutic administration of interleukins (IL-2) can cause delirium (Denikoff *et al.* 1987) and can cause subclinical cognitive changes (Caraceni *et al.* 1992). IL-1 and prostaglandin D2 play a role in sleep regulation. The role of cytokines as potential direct or indirect toxic factors in the development of postsurgical or infectious delirium is unknown (Flacker and Lipsitz 1999*a*). Studies on the relationships, if any, between neuroendocrine and immune system dysfunction in the course of delirium are lacking (Broadhurst and Wilson 2001; Stefano *et al.* 1994).

2.9   Conclusions

The pathogenesis of delirium is still controversial. However the DSM-IV definition requires altered states of arousal and attention to be present. Physiological and anatomical knowledge suggests a main role for brainstem-thalamocortical connections for the regulation of arousal and the sleep–wakefulness cycle. A useful model can identify in this system the main target for most, if not all, of the noxae that can cause delirium. The discussion on the roles of different neurotransmitters in the pathogenesis of delirium has been thus far mainly academic and supported by almost no animal models (Flacker and Lipsitz 1999*a*; Gibson *et al.* 1991; Ross 1991; Trzepacz 1994*a*, 1999). The availability of cholinesterase inhibitors for treating the symptoms of Alzheimer's disease is an opportunity to test the cholinergic hypothesis in deliria of different aetiologies (Slatkin *et al.* 2001). The same is true for nutritional factors such as thiamine, or endogenous response to stress, though the available evidence remains again slightly beyond the territory of hypotheses. However, in definite risk categories, such as the elderly or the severely ill, it would seem sensible to assess the usefulness of reducing anticholinergic effects, supplementing thiamine, and introducing stress-modifying interventions as a means of reducing the risk of developing delirium.

Chapter 3

Epidemiology

3.1 Incidence/prevalence

The difficulties encountered in defining diagnostic criteria, the fluctuating clinical course, and uneven methods of assessment explain the delay in the development of valid epidemiological research on delirium. While it has been clearly demonstrated that, as expected, retrospective chart studies are totally unreliable (Johnson *et al.* 1992), it is important to realize that the population under analysis is a crucial epidemiological factor. In fact, the risk of developing delirium varies enormously across different patients and contexts of care. This chapter will review studies that used prospective methods and specific criteria for diagnosis and will distinguish as far as possible the populations at risk.

3.1.1 The elderly

The epidemiology of delirium in the elderly population has received more attention recently, due to the high frequency of the syndrome, its impact on hospital care and costs (Inouye *et al.* 1999*b*), and its evident link with senile dementias. In a study of 2000 consecutive admissions of patients aged 55 or older, 9% were demented, of whom 41% were delirious at admission (Erkinjutti *et al.* 1986). A number of studies have described the prevalence of delirium at the time of hospital admission, and the incidence of cases developing during the hospital stay in elderly patients admitted to general medical and surgical wards over significant periods of time. Table 3.1 summarizes this data (Brauer *et al.* 2000; Francis *et al.* 1990; Inouye *et al.* 1999*a*, 1993; Inouye and Charpentier 1996; Levkoff *et al.* 1992; Pompei *et al.* 1994). It has to be pointed out that all of the above-mentioned studies excluded terminal patients. Although not identical, the design of these studies was homogeneous in respect to the diagnostic criteria employed. In fact all studies used DSM-III or DSM-III-R criteria for diagnosis (the Confusion Assessment Method (CAM) is based on DSM-III-R criteria). Therefore the variability in prevalence, greater still in the number of cases observed to occur after admission, is very interesting.

In more heterogeneous populations of the elderly with chronic debilities, the prevalence can increase. For instance, in a recent cross-sectional survey of patients aged 75 or more admitted to emergency hospital, nursing-homes, long-term geriatric facilities, or receiving home-care the prevalence of delirium reached 43.9% (Sandberg *et al.* 1999).

The number and the complexity of risk factors, individual vulnerability, and environmental factors identified by these authors and by other studies can explain this

Table 3.1 Prevalence and incidence of delirium in elderly patients admitted to medical and surgical wards

Reference	Prevalence (%)	Incidence (%)	Population age (years)	Method* Screening	Diagnostic
Francis et al. 1990	16.0	6.0	≥ 70	Daily MMSE	DSM-III
Lefkoff et al. 1992	10.5	31.3	≥ 65	Daily DSI	DSM-III
Pompei et al. 1994	4.8	10.0	≥ 65	Daily MMSE, digit span, vigilance A test, CAC, CAM	DSM-III-R
Inouye et al. 1993		25	≥ 70	Daily CAM	CAM
Inouye and Charpentier 1996		18	≥ 70	Every other day CAM	CAM
Inouye et al. 1999a		12.4	≥ 70	Daily MMSE, digit span CAM	CAM
Brauer et al. 2000		9.5	85 †	CAM	CAM

* CAC, Clinical Assessment of Confusion; CAM, the Confusion Assessment Method (see Appendix 2); DSI, Delirium Symptom Interview; MMSE, Mini-Mental State Examination (see Appendix 1).

† Median age. Patients were admitted for hip fractures.

variability. In the series of studies performed at Yale University, the number of incident cases decreased over time, and is lower still in the most recent reports. However, it must be remembered that this study selected a population at intermediate or high risk for developing delirium according to previously identified risk factors. Time-related changes of environmental factors may have contributed to this variability (Inouye *et al.* 1999*a*; McCusker *et al.* 2001*a*). Risk factors identified by several authors are summarized in Table 3.2.

One model recently identified the role of predisposing vulnerability factors, combined with the role of precipitating factors. In independent groups of elderly patients ($\geq$ 70 years old), vision impairment, pre-existing cognitive impairment, severity of illness, and high blood urea nitrogen/creatinine ratio were defined as vulnerability factors (Inouye *et al.* 1993) and were used to assign patients to different risk groups (Inouye and Charpentier 1996). The effect of precipitating factors was then assessed on these risk groups (Inouye and Charpentier 1996). Precipitating factors were represented by the patients' need for physical restraints, their malnutrition, the use of more than three medications, the use of a bladder catheter, and any iatrogenic event (Inouye and Charpentier 1996). The model demonstrates the interaction of vulnerability factors (the background) with precipitating factors (potentially aetiological) in contributing to the final individual risk of developing delirium (Inouye and Charpentier 1996), therefore confirming an early intuition of Lipowski (1990*a*).

The role of environmental factors, for a long time thought to be relevant in the onset of delirium episodes in the elderly, has recently been confirmed in an article that identified number of room changes, absence of a clock or watch, and absence of reading glasses as potentially modifiable risk factors (McCusker *et al.* 2001*a*).

It is worth saying that statistical associations leading to the definition of risk factors or precipitating factors are not substitutes for the recognition of aetiological factors or true biological causes, but they can suggest the role of potential causes or conditions that are associated with such causes. The same authors demonstrated that, by acting on some of the environmental/physiological factors identified, it was indeed possible to reduce the incidence of delirium (Inouye *et al.* 1999*a*).

3.1.2   Postoperative delirium

The frequency of postoperative delirium is highly variable depending on preoperative vulnerability factors, type of surgery, and intra- and postoperative factors. For elective non-cardiac surgery, the incidence of delirium in the first 5 postoperative days is 9% (Marcantonio *et al.* 1994*a*). A clinical prediction score has been developed and validated showing that preoperative factors and type of surgery will affect enormously the incidence of cases (Table 3.3; see Marcantonio *et al.* 1994*a*; Williams-Russo *et al.* 1992). This model was also validated in a consecutive series of 138 patients operated on for head-and-neck cancer (Weed *et al.* 1995).

Very high incidences have been observed in emergency surgery for the higher-risk elderly (42.5% after hip fracture, 42.3% after bypass surgery for lower limb ischaemia; Sasajima *et al.* 2000), after open-heart surgery (14 to 59%; van der Mast *et al.* 1999), and lung transplant (73%; Bitondo Dyer *et al.* 1995).

Table 3.2 Risk factors for the development of delirium in the elderly hospitalized patients determined by multivariate analyses

Variable	Francis et al. 1990	Levkoff et al. 1992	Schor et al. 1992	Inouye et al. 1993	Pompei et al. 1994	McCusker et al. 2002
Age (years)		* (> 80)	* (> 80)			
Previous cognitive failure	*	*	*	*	*	
Fracture/illness severity	*	*	*	*	*	
Psychoative drugs, neuroleptics, opioids	*	*	*			
Fever, infection	*					
Renal function	*			*		
Abnormal sodium	*					
Institutionalization, vision impairment, environmental factors		*				*
Male sex			*			
Depression					*	
Alcoholism					*	

* Indicates that the study found variable to be a risk factor.

Table 3.3 Score for the prediction of postoperative delirium (modified from Marcantonio *et al.* (1994*a*))

Risk factor	Points
Age ≥ 70 years	1
Alcohol abuse	1
Cognitive impairment (TICS score < 30) *	1
SAS class IV †	1
Markedly abnormal serum sodium, potassium, or glucose‡	1
Aortic aneurysm surgery	2
Non-cardiac thoracic surgery	1

Risk of developing postoperative delirium according to preoperative score

Score	Level of risk	Percentage developing postoperative delirium
0	Low risk	2
1	Medium risk	8
2	Medium risk	13
≥ 3	High risk	50

* TICS, Telephone interview for cognitive status, a modification of the Mini-mental Status Examination.
† SAS, Specific Activity Scale; it measures physical function (class IV represents severe physical impairment).
‡ Sodium, < 130 or > 150 mmol/l; potassium, < 3.0 or > 6.0 mmol/l; glucose, < 3.3 or > 16.7 mmol/l.
Reproduced with permission from Marcantonio, *et al.* (1994). A clinical prediction rule for delirium after elective noncardiac surgery. *J Am Med Ass* **271**(2): 134–9. Copyright 1994 American Medical Association.

Intra- and perioperative factors contributing to the risk of postoperative delirium are: the use of psychoactive drugs, especially benzodiazepine, meperidine, and drugs with anticholinergic activity (Berggren *et al.* 1987; Marcantonio *et al.* 1994*b*); low postoperative oxygen saturation (Berggren *et al.* 1987); and blood loss with haematocrit reduction during and immediately after surgery (Marcantonio *et al.* 1998).

The presence of more severe postoperative pain has also been associated with the occurrence of delirium while opioid type and dose were not (Lynch *et al.* 1998). This finding combines with other observations documenting: a higher incidence of delirium in patients with poorly controlled pain (Schor *et al.* 1992); no difference in delirium incidence in patients randomized to IV opioids versus epidural analgesia (Williams-Russo *et al.* 1992); and higher pain score with more postoperative confusion in patients treated with intramuscular (IM) morphine injection as compared to those using patient-controlled analgesia (Egbert *et al.* 1990). Pain, or factors that are associated with more severe pain, increases the risk for delirium more than opioid medication in the postoperative period.

3.1.3 Delirium tremens

The frequency of delirium tremens (DT) reflects the specificity of this withdrawal syndrome but also its continuity with other general factors implied by the mechanisms underlying acute confusional reactions. Among 200 alcoholics hospitalized for alcohol withdrawal or detoxification, 24% developed DT (Ferguson *et al.* 1996). At multivariate analysis, the number of days since the last drink was a risk factor for DT (odds ratio (OR), 1.3; 95% confidence interval (CI), 1.09–1.61) but a significantly higher risk was associated with comorbidity of an acute medical illness (OR, 5.1; CI, 2.07–12.55). Patients with no risk factors had a 9% probability of developing DT. Those with one or two risk factors had a 25% and 54%, respectively, chance of developing DT during hospitalization. In a recent study on patients admitted for alcohol withdrawal (334 cases), 6.9% developed alcohol withdrawal delirium after admission. The patients at risk of developing delirium were those diagnosed as having concurrent infections, tachycardia (above 120 beats/min), a history of seizures and delirium, or serum alcohol levels of more than 1g/l (Palmstierna 2001).

3.1.4   Cancer

The most quoted statistics on the epidemiology of delirium in cancer settings come from the work done by Derogatis and his collegues (1983) on the prevalence of psychiatric disorders among cancer patients.This study was a prospective cohort assessment of all new admissions of patients with a Karnofsky performance status of 50 or more, engaged in active treatment in in- or outpatient facilities at three major US cancer centres. In this sample, based on DSM-III definitions, 32% of patients had a diagnosis of adjustment disorder and 4% of organic brain syndrome, the latter representing 8% of all psychiatric diagnoses. From the article it is impossible to say how many of these patients would have fulfilled the criteria for delirium. At present, no data are available about the prevalence or incidence of delirium in the cancer population undergoing treatment. Indirect data shows that change in mental status is a common reason for neurological and psychiatric (Levine et al. 1978) consultations in oncology (17% of neurological consultations) and toxic/metabolic encephalopathy the most frequent final diagnosis (Caraceni et al. 1999; Clouston et al. 1992; Tuma and DeAngelis 2000), which often corresponds to the clinical features of delirium.

Patients with advanced cancer admitted to palliative care units or hospices are nowadays assessed more carefully in the area of cognitive function, and recent data confirm earlier anecdotal observations about the high prevalence of delirium in this population (Massie et al. 1983). Cognitive failure developed in 83% of patients before death in one palliative care unit (Bruera et al. 1992b). Using specific clinical criteria for delirium, prevalence was found to be 28% at hospice admission (DSM-III-R; Minagawa et al. 1996; Morita et al. 1999) and 27.7% at referral to palliative care units in an Italian multicentre study (CAM criteria (Appendix 2); Caraceni et al. 2000). In this study the diagnosis of delirium at referral was associated with brain metastases, lower performance status, male gender, and poorer clinical prediction of survival. Recently, two prospective studies found the prevalence of delirium to be 42% at admission to a tertiary palliative care unit (Lawlor et al. 2000b) and 20% in a hospice (Gagnon et al. 2000), with incidence thereafter rising to 45% (Lawlor et al. 2000b) and 33% (Gagnon et al. 2000), respectively, among patients monitored until death.

3.2 Prognosis

Two main issues relate to the prognosis of a delirium episode—its reversibility and the potentially increased mortality risk.

3.2.1 Reversibility and outcome

It is obvious that acute confusional states related to readily identifiable causes or conditions, such as drug intoxication or acute febrile illnesses, are to be counteracted by reversing or withdrawing the cause. It is less obvious in more complex situations in the elderly and the severely ill where the cause can be more difficult to identify and the explanation of the course of delirum is not so easily found. In these cases the precipitating cause is likely to be combined with a number of comorbidities or predisposing factors. In one study only 4% of elderly patients with delirium had complete recovery from the syndrome at discharge and about 30% still fulfilled the DSM-III criteria for delirium (Levkoff *et al.* 1992).

Patients diagnosed with delirium had a greater probability of a longer stay in the hospital or of being placed in an institution after discharge (Francis and Kapoor 1992; Levkoff *et al.* 1992) and of more severe cognitive and functional decline at follow-up independently of other risk factors or morbid conditions (Francis and Kapoor 1992; McCusker *et al.* 2001*b*). Furthermore, higher scores on the delirium rating scales, reflecting more severe cases, are associated with poorer clinical outcome (Wada and Yamaguchi 1993; Marcantonio *et al.* 2000, 2002).

In advanced cancer patients delirium was reversible in a minority of cases and often preceded death by about 2 weeks (Bruera *et al.* 1992*b*). Recently, 49% of delirium episodes were evaluated as reversible in an acute palliative care unit setting with a very high prevalence of delirious patients on admission. The most frequent aetiological factor associated with reversible cases was opioid toxicity, whereas factors more often associated with irreversibility were lung disease and infection causing hypoxia (Lawlor *et al.* 2000*b*).

3.2.2 Mortality

As we reported in Chapter 1, the earliest medical observations indicated that delirium was a sign of impending death. When and how this prediction is borne out is a more difficult question. Hildgard of Bingen (1098–1179; Ildegarda di Bingen 1997) observed that cases of delirium secondary to different diseases can evolve to death, but, at the same time, she stated that, if delirium resolves, the person is also likely to recover from the disease.

Several observations have indicated that mortality is more likely in patients with delirium (Curyto *et al.* 2001; van Hemert *et al.* 1994). Recent studies (Francis and Kapoor 1992; Levkoff *et al.* 1992; Pompei *et al.* 1994) have suggested that early mortality was increased in delirious patients irrespective of the medical condition, whereas long-term mortality (90 days, 6 months, 1 year) was increased in patients who developed delirium, secondarily to the severity of their medical illness. Mortality was not increased in the year following the delirium episode. More sophisticated analyses, however, could demonstrate that, in the elderly, delirium was an independent

Table 3.4 The Palliative Prognostic Score (PaP score)

Variable	Score
Dyspnoea	
No	0
Yes	1
Anorexia	
No	0
Yes	1
Karnofsky Performance Status	
≥ 50	0
30–40	0
10–20	2.5
Clinical prediction of survival (weeks)	
> 12	0
11–12	2.0
9–10	2.5
7–8	2.5
5–6	4.5
3–4	6.0
1–2	8.5
Total white blood cells	
4800–8500 cell/mm^3	0
8501–11 000 cell/mm^3	0.5
> 11 000 cell/mm^3	1.5
Lymphocyte rate (%)	
20.0–40.0	0
12.0–19.9	1.0
0–11.9	2.5

Risk group	30-Day survival probability (%)	PaP score
A, Best prognosis	> 70	0.0–5.5
B, Intermediate prognosis	30–70	5.6–11.0
C, Worst prognosis	< 3	11.1–17.5

Reproduced with permission from Caraceni *et al*. *Cancer* (2000) Copyright 2000 American Cancer Association.

predictor of mortality for patients without dementia and that this association was stronger depending on the severity of delirium (McCusker *et al.* 2002). However, preoperative delirium was not correlated with long-term survival in liver transplant candidates (Trzepacz and DiMartini 1992).

When looking at more selected acutely ill populations, such as patients with advanced cancer under palliative care, the occurrence of delirium is independently associated with a worse prognosis (Metitieri *et al.* 2000). The diagnosis of delirium in this population has been used successfully to design a prognostic model (Bruera *et al.* 1992*b*; Caraceni *et al.* 2000; Morita *et al.* 1999). In a recent case series of patients with cancer, delirium was associated with more advanced disease and had a poor prognostic impact on overall outcome. The 30-day mortality was 25%, and 44% of patients died within 6 months. Younger patients and those with hypoxaemia or kidney or liver dysfunction were more likely to die (Tuma and DeAngelis 2000).

The mortality rate in septic patients who had been admitted to intensive care units (ICU) and developed encephalopathy and delirium was found to be higher (33–39%) than that among septic patients who did not develop encephalopathy (16–27%; Eidelman *et al.* 1996).

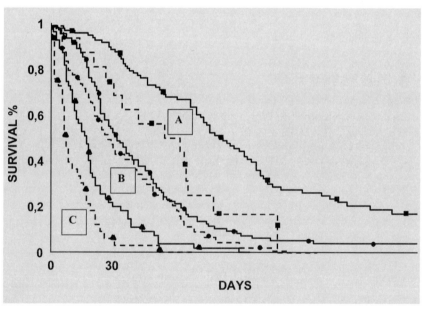

Fig. 3.1 Survival curves of three different prognostic groups of patients, admitted to a palliative care program, according to the PaP score (Table 3.4). A (squares) best prognosis, B (circles), intermediate prognosis, C (triangles), worst prognosis. The survival of delirious patient at referral is represented by the dotted lines and that-one of non-delirious patients by continuous lines. The impact of delirium on survival is evident in all groups and particularly in the best prognostic group. Reproduced with permission from Caraceni *et al. Cancer* (2000); **89**: 1145–9. Copyright 2000 American Cancer Society.

Giving an accurate prognosis is very important in palliative care. Recent research has focused on a number of clinical variables in helping to formulate accurate inter- mediate- and short-term-prognoses. A recent systematic analysis of the literature includes cognitive failure among the factors that are definitely associated with survival in terminal cancer patients (Viganò *et al.* 2001). On the other hand, the onset of delirium is, *per se*, an occasion during which an accurate prognostic assessment is of immediate value, for planning care and family counselling.

Two prognostic scores have been published so far to be used in patients with advanced cancer. The palliative prognostic index of Morita *et al.* (1999)is based on the presence of dysphagia, dyspnoea, oedema, and delirium. This score showed a 80% sensitivity and 85% specificity in predicting 3-week survival.

The palliative prognostic score (PaP score) of Maltoni *et al.* (1999; see Table 3.4) is particularly interesting for evaluating the effects of delirium on survival because it has been designed without the contribution of cognitive function assessment. This score is based on the presence of some symptoms (anorexia and dyspnoea), performance status, lymphocyte and granulocyte count, and on the clinical prediction of survival expressed by a palliative care physician (Pirovano *et al.* 1999). When the diagnosis of delirium was combined with the PaP score it proved to an independent factor in pre- dicting patients survival (Caraceni *et al.* 2000; Fig. 3.1). The PaP score can therefore be used in delirious patients to try to improve prognostication. In addition, as shown by Lawler *et al.* (2000*b*), a better understanding of irreversible delirium will certainly help in defining true terminal cases.

3.3 Conclusions

The functional and survival outcomes of different populations affected by delirium are intertwined with the undelying neuropathological and general condition. Often, delirium will be a sign of the underlying impaired brain reserves due to either primary or secondary causes and therefore will be a harbinger of different outcomes such as chronic cognitive decline in the elderly (dementia) or death in the acutely ill.

Chapter 4

Clinical phenomenology

Delirium, as we have already observed, is a syndrome and not a disease, and it is therefore defined by a cluster of symptoms and signs. Chapter 8 on diagnostic criteria will further elaborate the way to use clinical findings in a consistent classification system useful for distinguishing the clinical conditions of a single patient (see also Chapter 1.3). The clinical presentation of the subjective and objective findings is the aim of this chapter. The study of the phenomenology of delirium, in comparison with other areas of clinical interest, has received little attention in recent times. Invaluable information on phenomenology is available in old accounts (Farber 1959; Wolf and Curran 1935), but accurate clinical observations with modern methodology should help in clarifying the pathophysiology and clinical outcome (Meagher *et al.* 1998; Meagher and Trzepacz 1998).

4.1 Disordered level of consciousness

According to Plum and Posner (1980*b*), consciousness is the 'state of awareness of the self and environment'. Others have defined it as the capacity for subjective experience, while awareness is defined as the ability to react to or manifest that experience.

Arousal, alertness, or wakefulness can be used somewhat interchangeably and define one aspect of consciousness, also called the level as opposed to the content of consciousness. In the absence of wakefulness it is impossible to explore the content, if any, of consciousness and especially the patient's awareness of such content (Giacino 1997). It is difficult to separate the concept of level of consciousness from that of arousal. The relevance of the reticular formation, hypothalamus, and other structures in modulating arousal and therefore the level of consciousness has already been discussed in Chapter 2.

As a clinical concept, arousal has been operationally defined as the intensity of sensory stimulation that is needed to arouse a subject from sleep, or to keep him or her awake, and the duration of this state following stimulation. 'Easily arousable' or 'arousable only with intense stimulation' are common clinical expressions reflecting the need to quantify the arousal level. Arousal has been subdivided into tonic arousal, which explains the spontaneous fluctuations in the level of wakefulness occurring during the daylight hours, independent of sensory stimulation (equivalent to vigilance according to some authors; see Sellal and Collard 2001), and phasic arousal (equivalent to alertness; Sellal and Collard 2001), which can be understood as the orienting reaction that enhances arousal in response to new or sudden stimuli (Giacino

1997). Phasic arousal induces an attentional reaction. The ability to sustain attention has been linked to the concept of alertness, and the brain structures involved in phasic arousal largely overlap with those implied in attentional processes. The lesion of the structures responsible for tonic arousal will produce a reduced level of consciousness, while a lesion of the phasic arousal system will cause distractability or reduced ability to direct and mantain attention.

The appreciation of the theoretical boundaries between these concepts also underlines the substantial degree of clinical overlap reflected in the DSM-IV first criterion, which combines a disordered level of consciousness with attention failure. It is therefore necessary to assess the level of consciousness if delirium is to be differentiated from dementia, mania, or inattention.

The level of consciousness or arousal that can be found in delirious patients is, on the other hand, difficult to define. By definition, symptoms in delirium are fluctuating. An oscillating level of arousal identifies patients who are at times in stupor or even in coma and may be delirious when arousal improves. The arousal can be enhanced or diminished either way, pathologically, to the extent that it interferes with attention and cognition. Therefore, the patient with delirium can be hypoalert or hyperalert, which is typical of delirium tremens and other excited states. On the other hand a sufficient level of arousal or vigilance is needed to allow the assessment of attention and cognitive functions. Drawing the line of this clinical boundary may be difficult, because severely delirious patients may be unable to perform most cognitive tasks. However, delirium is certainly found in patients with a disorder of arousal on the continuum between hyperalertness, normal wakefulness, stupor, and coma or that can be classified on this continuum (Ross 1991). Folstein, in proposing the Mini-Mental State Examination (MMSE) for assessing acute or chronic changes in cognition, inserted after the questionnaire a visual analogue scale to quantify the level of arousal exactly on this continuum (Folstein *et al.* 1975).

The correct diagnosis of an abnormal level of arousal requires some familiarity with the differential diagnosis of the main syndromes of impaired consciousness (Giacino 1997; Plum and Posner 1980*b*; Young 1998), which are briefly summarized in Table 4.1. Table 4.1 also underlines how content (cognition) and level of consciousness are linked but also differentially affected in different clinical conditions.

The assessment of arousal in cases of delirium will disclose that patients can be hyperaroused and agitated, display a reduced level of arousal, and be somnolent or have mixed features at different assessment times. Lipowsky (1990*b*) in formulating a unitary concept of the syndrome proposed the adoption of the definitions of hypoactive, hyperactive, or mixed delirium. A recent study used factor analysis to confirm the existence of two types of clinical presentations characterized by the clustering of different symptoms—the hyperactive form associated with agitation, aggressiveness, hallucinations, and delusions and the hypoactive variant associated with decreased reactivity, motor and speech retardation, and facial inexpressiveness (Camus *et al.* 2000).

In one study, 58 delirious patients were assessed in terms of their arousal level as somnolent or activated: 39 were found to be hypoactive and 19 were activated (Ross *et al.* 1991). The activated group was more likely to display agitated behaviour and to

Table 4.1 Syndromes of impaired consciousness and states of unresponsiveness

Syndrome	Arousal/level of consciousness	Cognition: content of consciousness
Delirium/acute confusional state	Impaired, diminished or increased interfering with attention and cognition, often fluctuating. The patient is awake or easily arousable	Impaired
Stupor	Impaired. The patient is arousable only with vigorous stimuli. If the stimulus is withdrawn the patient lapses back into the unresponsive state. The patient lies with closed eyes, unresponsive	Not assessable
Minimally conscious state (MCS)	Preserved or slightly impaired	Impaired. Inconsistent but reproducible behavioural evidence of awareness of self and environment. Inconsistent but reproducible ability to perform easy tasks: follow command, gestural, verbal, yes/no responses
Akinetic mutism	Preserved or slightly impaired	Impaired with mainly elective failure of volitional drive. The patient is totally apathetic, shows occasional, infrequent speech or movement to command. Has been described as subcategory of MCS
Vegetative state (VS)	Preserved eye can be opened and sleep–wakefulness cycle documented on EEG	Absent. No evidence of awareness of self or environment
Coma	Absent, no sleep–wakefulness cycle on EEG recording. The patient lies unresponsive with eyes closed	Absent. No evidence of awareness of self or environment
Locked-in syndrome	Preserved	Preserved. The patient is unresponsive due to supranuclear palsy of the spinal and cranial nerves, but can usually respond by blinking nerves, but can usually respond by blinking
Dementia	Preserved	Impaired. At extreme extent of progression the condition can mimick VS
Psychogenic unresponsiveness	Preserved	Difficult to assess; preserved

have delusions, hallucinations, and illusions. In another study of 125 elderly patients with delirium, 15% were rated as only hyperactive, 19% only hypoactive, 52% had a mixed clinical picture, and 14% had neither hyper- nor hypoactivity (Liptzin and Levkoff 1992). Although this study *a priori* codified specific symptoms or behaviours as belonging to the hyper- or hypoactive series and did not specify a way of assessing the arousal state specifically, its results are useful in showing the high prevalence of mixed clinical presentations.

A more recent study used an activity scale to rate psychomotor behaviour and found that, of the 94 elderly delirous patients analysed, 21% had a hyperactive form, 29% were hypoactive, and 43% presented mixed features (O'Keeffe 1999). Patients with hypoactive deliria were more frequently affected by more severe illness and had a longer hospital stay than hyperactive cases, but the mortality rate did not differ. In the same study, patients with withdrawal syndromes and with drug toxicity had more hyperactive deliria while those with metabolic disturbances more often had hypoactive deliria (O'Keeffe 1999). In another study, deliria due to anticholinergic toxicity were more often hypoactive (Meagher *et al.* 1998, 2000). It is a repeated clinical observation that hyperactive deliria have a more favourable outcome as far as time of recovery and prognosis are concerned (Kobayashi *et al.* 1992; Olofson *et al.* 1996).

4.2 Attention

As mentioned above, the clinical assessments of attention and arousal often overlap to a significant extent. Indeed, changes in arousal level will affect performances used to assess or measure attentional abilities. Some authors consider attention deficit the core of the neurological dysfunction characterizing delirium (Geschwind 1982; Mesulam 1985). If we leave the interpretation controversy, and accept the phenomenological definition adopted by the DSM-IV, we should distinguish attention failure due to several CNS lesions affecting the cerebral cortex and especially the frontal lobes from attention failure associated with disordered arousal, as characteristic of delirium. Attention is the process that enables one to select relevant stimuli from the environment, to focus and to sustain behavioural responses to such stimuli, and to switch mental activity towards a new stimulus, reorienting the individual behaviour according to the relevance of the stimulus. Although attention, consciousness, and cognition can be variously explained, consciousness is, in general, considered the prerequisite for experiencing and expressing a cognitive content, cognition would derive from the ability to elaborate and respond to the content of consciousness, while attention is conceptualized as the processing ability related to this content and the consequent behavioural responses. The most simple clinical assessment of attention is limited to the recognition of clear-cut symptoms such as the following.

♦ Distractability is reported when the subject is unable to sustain a task for a more or less prolonged time, a very common sign of delirium, considered among its essential characteristics by the DSM-IV.

♦ Neglect is the selective failure of attention for a given sensory modality, usually due to focal brain lesion, though true neglect is seldom found in delirium.

- Perseveration is the failure to redirect behaviour toward new stimuli while perseverating in the present task. Perseverating behaviours can often be seen in severely delirious patients.

The quantitative assessment of attention capacity can rely on different test and neuropsychological measures (Deutsche Lezak 1995; Whyte 1992; Zacny 1995). It is beyond the scope of this book to review this wide area of neuropsychology. It is worth recalling that many of the tasks that are commonly included in many bedside neuropsychological tests are better explained as tests of attention. This is the case for short-term memory for numbers, objects, and easy calculations as required in the popular serial sevens. Other tests could be interesting for clinical research purposes because of their sensitivity to attention deficits, e.g. the study of reaction times that has been widely used for assessing neuropharmacological effects on attention and cognitive performance (Zacny 1995). Other types of assessments would make it possible to test the function of more defined brain areas such as the frontal lobes.

4.3 Alteration of the sleep–wakefulness cycle

The inversion of the sleep–wakefulness cycle in confused patients, with drowsiness during waking hours and insomnia during the night, is a very old clinical observation (Lipowski 1990b) and often an early sign of a developing delirium. Studies on the structure of sleep during both the course of delirium and the circadian wakefulness state are limited to one old observation of a change in the organization of the EEG during the day and night-time sleep (Lipowski 1990b). The concept of delirium as a disorder of arousal implies that sleep–wakefulness mechanisms are likely to be involved, since the structures responsible for these functions overlap in the brainstem, thalamus, and hypothalamus. This theory accords well with the clinical observation that sleep is practically always abnormal in delirious patients and that symptoms tend to worsen during the night.

The terms 'sundowning' and 'sundowner' have been used to designate the nighttime deterioration of cognitive functions and even the onset of full-blown delirium, especially in the elderly and in patients with overt or masked dementia (Vitiello *et al.* 1992; Duckett and Scotto 1992).

Palliative care patients, using breakthrough analgesia and adjusting their doses as needed, who developed delirium, were using more analgesic doses in the evening and at night, while non-delirious patients tended to use analgesia more often in the morning. The authors speculate that this may be related to an effect of delirium on the normal circadian rhythm (Gagnon *et al.* 2001).

4.4 Cognition

The definition and assessment of cognitive functions involve large fields of neurology and neuropsychology that lie outside the scope of this book. (More detail has been given concerning attention because of its potential specific implications in the clinical phenomenology of delirium.) One useful interpretation is that all aspects of cognition, higher cerebral functions in Jacksonian terms, will be affected if the arousal mechanisms in the lower, more primitive part of the brain are impaired. Depending on the severity of the delirious state, cognitive tasks will be affected in proportion to the demand on attention implied by the task. Calculation ability will be affected before immediate memories and, in serial sevens, the more difficult subtractions (usually crossing decades) will prompt more confused responses than the easiest ones. One of our patients was oriented to time, space, and person, and able to subtract 7 from 100 and from 79, but when asked to subtract 7 from 93, he was not only unable to do it, but made easily avoidable mistakes such as giving a number higher then 93. Memory for recent events will be affected, while past history can be recalled precisely. This hierarchy of mental function derangement can be used with benefit in examining patients. The same observations could be used to argue that the tests with gradually increasing demands on attention are more easily failed.

4.4.1   Orientation

Orientation to person, space, and time is the most common and first-line clinical assessment of cognition traditionally performed by physicians and nurses at the bedside, and is often considered a hallmark of confusion. In fact, 66% of patients presented defects in orientation in an old study (Farber 1959). Orientation does not explore a specific cognitive function, but represents a synthetic evaluation of attention, arousal, and memory. Though delirious patients very rarely forget who they are, they often become disoriented with regard to space and almost always to time. This hierarchical structure of the construct of orientation can be verified easily in clinical practice and is confirmed from the experience with electroconvulsive therapy showing a reverse order (person, space, time) in the recovery from the confusional state that follows the procedure. Patients may forget where they are and often locate themselves in a known, familiar place, and, if delusion occurs, they may also act out their usual occupation, according to the 'rule' of mistaking the unfamiliar for the familiar (Lipowski 1990*b*). One of our patients who sustained a long-lasting post-liver-transplant delirium and was a farmer from the valley around the Po river, was convinced he was near his barn and urged that it was time to milk his cow. Commonly, the hospital is mistaken for another hospital more familiar to the patient or for a hotel. One patient, who had just recovered from a severe delirious episode due to a sudden increase in the plasma level of an immunosuppressive agent (tacrine), went on for at least 24 hours professing that the 'waitress' (a nurse) had brought him a pill that morning.

Hospitalized elderly patients who lose their familiar environmental context may experience disorienting episodes especially at night, either unmasking previously compensated cognitive deficits or precipitating true delirious episodes in the situation often described as 'sundowning'.

The concept of orientation has no known normative data as such, but it is included in the Mini-mental State Examination, which has been accurately studied and which, with some limitations, is still a very useful tool in assessing the mental status of potentially delirious patients (see Chapter 8).

4.4.2 Language

Language is impoverished in delirium. Delirious subjects can appear silent and inhibited or they may persevere in discussing odd or irrelevant subjects, with difficulties in finding words or concepts that can lead to the inadvertent use of *passe-par-tout* words or expressions to fill in gaps ('you know what I mean'). Paraphrasias are frequent, i.e. the use of a different, but well-recalled word in place of the one not coming to explicit memory. Language difficulties are probably due more to disordered arousal and attention levels than to a specific cause or, alternatively, they can disclose an altered thought process. In severe cases of global impairment, frank confabulation can dominate, leaving little opportunity to assess language, memory, and thought content. Often language and speech, including reading, are less affected than writing, especially in mild or early cases.

Few specific observations are available on language disturbances found in the course of delirium. In one study misnamings were very frequent, as frequently as observed in demented patients, but they differed in being more often of the types of word intrusion and unrelated misnamings (Wallesch and Hundsaltz 1994). Word intrusion is in part explained by perseveration. The patient repeats a previously pronounced word (therefore perseverating) in place of the expected word that he is unable to find or pronounce. Unrelated misnaming is the use of a word that wildly differs in meaning from the intended word and therefore has no relationship with the word that is appropriate for the context.

4.4.3 Writing

Several observations have pointed out the relative importance of writing disturbances in the course of widespread brain failure and, in particular, of delirium. The fragility of writing is due to the complexity of its functional demand which integrates motor, praxic, visuospatial, linguistic, and kinaesthetic abilities. The control of this complex behaviour requires therefore the integrity of higher cortical function, high attention levels, and intact arousal. Not many studies specifically describe the frequency and type of writing disturbance that can be found in patients with delirium. Although we lack sound epidemiological data, clinical experience supports the opinion that writing is practically always and precociously abnormal (Aakerlund and Rosenberg 1994; Chedru and Geschwind 1972b; Macleod and Whitehead 1997). The following list and the associated examples can be used to classify writing abnormalities found in delirious patients.

- ◆ Motor impairments range from thin tremor affecting lines (Fig. 4.1) to unreadable grossly deformed graphic elements.
- ◆ Visuospatial control abnormalities. Letters are poorly aligned, aligned upward, downward, or diagonally, or written too close to the margins of the sheet of paper making it impossible to conclude the word (Fig. 4.2). Also characteristic is the contamination of a letter or a word with another one.
- ◆ Reluctance to write. Chedru and Geschwind (1972b) in their classic paper found that 19 of 34 patients hesitated and tried to refuse writing, excusing themselves in someway ('you know I am not much of a writer'). We observed this tendency of

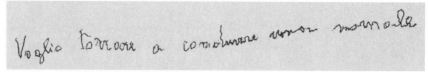

Fig. 4.1 Sample of spontaneous writing. The patient wrote 'Voglio [I want] tornare [to go back] a condurre [to have] una normale [a normal].' Tremor and lack of spatial control is evident and one word is missing [life] as the complete phrase should read 'I want to go back to have a normal life.'

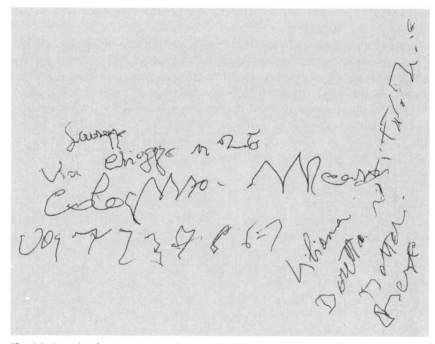

Fig. 4.2 Sample of spontaneous writing showing gross disturbance of reasoning and spatial control. The patient started to write, most probably, his address (Via Chioggia n 25 Cologno Monzese), followed by phone number, and then went on with a list of names difficult to read. However, he lost spatial control of his writing within the limits of the sheet of paper, going upwards across the lines he had already written when reaching the end of the sheet of paper.

reluctance to participate in a complex task as a general phenomenon in examining confused patients. It is probably a sign of preserved insight and emotional involvement of the patient, due to his or her perception of inadequacy and fear of acknowledging to themselves the failure of their mental integrity.

♦ Syntactic changes. When asked to spontaneously write a sentence, agrammatic or simplified phrases are preferred with the extreme being the use of single or a few words in place of a complete sentence.

- Spelling mistakes involve mainly omissions, substitutions, and reduplications or perseverations often affecting the end of the word. In a recent hospice series, reduplication of letters was the single most frequent sign of dysgraphia (Macleod and Whitehead 1997; Fig. 4.3).

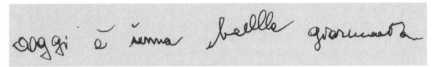

Fig. 4.3 Writing to dictation. The patient was asked to write the sentence, 'Oggi [Today] é [is] una bella giornata [a nice day].' Several perseverations can be seen.

In one study of the occurrence of postoperative delirium, writing abnormalities were a very sensitive sign of the development of an acute confusional state and a very specific index since they were not found in any patient who did not develop delirium (Aakerlund and Rosenberg 1994). A very recent study on 56 delirious patients observed that the detection of writing abnormalities was not very sensitive to the presence of delirium. By using a global rating of writing, 32.7% of delirious patients made errors, but almost no patients with a psychiatric diagnosis but without delirium had pathological writing, leading to very a high specificity for writing evaluation (98.3%; Baranowski and Patten 2000).

It is worth noting that the Mini-Mental State Examination includes the production of a written complete sentence, after command but not dictated, and the duplication of a drawing. These simple tests can be very useful for assessing the presence of writing abnormalities and constructional apraxia.

Testing writing therefore has significant value in association with other clinical findings and can be important in the differential diagnosis of delirium from other psychiatric diseases. According to one interpretation the fragility of writing could be secondary to a primary defect of attention in the pathogenesis of delirium, which could explain the errors, perseveration, and lack of spatial control in the performance (Chedru and Geschwind 1972*a*, *b*).

4.5 Perceptual disturbances

Disorders of perception are frequent but not invariably present in acutely confused patients. Earlier clinical description of the syndrome reported a high prevalence of hallucinations ranging from 50 to 75% of patients (Farber 1959; Wolf and Curran 1935). These case series included many patients with delirium tremens (Wolf and Curran 1935) or alcohol abuse, head trauma, acute fevers, and drug toxicities (Farber 1959) and are more representative of the hyperactive agitated type of delirium than of the hypoactive variant. This type of delirium is found more commonly in younger patients who do not present the complex symptoms such as multiorgan failure and metabolic derangement found in elderly patients with long-term chronic disease. A historical change in patient referral, use of clinical diagnostic criteria, and more accurate study methods explain the difference from the old stereotype of the agitated, hallucinated patient. Also a recent study based on psychiatric referrals cannot be used to give definite prevalence data due to the likelihood of referral bias (Webster and Holroyd 2000). However, in this study, of 227 patients with a DSM-IV diagnosis of delirium, 32.6% had hallucinations: 27% of the visual type; 12.4% auditory; and 2.7% tactile. No olfactory or gustatory hallucinations were found. In prevalence studies perceptual disturbances were found in only 23% of acutely confused elderly in one recent hospital series (Levkoff et al. 1992), and hallucinations in 24% in another one (Francis et al. 1990).

Perceptual changes associated with delirium include the following possibilities.

* *Perceptual distortions* usually involve visual modality and can cause changes in the number, shape, or magnitude of the perceived objects of the external world or parts of them or of the patient's own body parts.

* *Illusions* are misinterpretations of inner or external perceptions. They can be simple such as folds on the bedcover mistaken for objects or animals or more complex and fading into interpretation and delusional thoughts, as in the case of a nurse misidentified with a maid, or doctors with ghosts.

* *Hallucinations.* These will be discussed in the following subsection.

4.5.1 Hallucinations

A hallucination is a perception in the absence of an object. The definition of hallucinations covers a wide range of clinical phenomena, ranging from simple sensations, such as the vision of lights and geometrical shapes (photopsia, teichopsia, vision of fortifications) or the perception of single-tone sounds (tinnitus), which are also referred to as unformed hallucinations, to seeing people, animals, complex scenes, or hearing music or voices, which are also referred to as formed hallucinations. Hallucinations are, at times, but not always, associated with complex emotional experiences. In its broader definition phantom limb phenomena and synaesthesias can also be considered hallucinations.

Hallucination can be part of a primary psychotic disorder or be found as the effect of substance toxicity or of an identifiable structural brain pathology. Besides the quality and type of the hallucination, we can also distinguish hallucinations occurring with a clear sensorium and hallucinations with consciousness compromise, as those occurring in delirium.

Every type of lesion on a specific sensory and perceptual system, from the peripheral receptor, for instance, in the retina, to the cortical areas responsible for conscious perception and cognition, can evoke abnormal perceptions. The same is true for other sensory modalities, e.g. one patient had musical hallucinations in the context of brain metastases as an effect of partial seizures (Fenelon et al. 1993). When delirium is associated with hallucinations a more general effect on different brain functions is likely to occur, as already discussed. Some cases are, however, intriguing due to the overlap of different clinical conditions.

Cyclosporine toxicity, for example, is an interesting condition that is mainly seen in organ transplant recipients treated with cyclosporine for immune-suppression (Craven 1991; Gijtenbeek et al. 1999). Visual hallucinations are typical when neurotoxic levels of the drug are reached (Katirji 1987) and have been associated with a transitory lesion of the occipital white matter (posterior leukoencephalopathy), loss of vision (Strouse *et al.* 1998), delirium, and coma. A similar clinical course has been observed in cases of centrally acting drug toxicities (Rosenbraugh *et al.* 2001). Visual hallucinations (unformed or formed) can indeed be the only sign of opioid toxicity or be prodromal to the onset of opioid-induced delirium (Caraceni *et al.* 1994; Jellema 1987).

The phenomenology of hallucinations in the course of delirium has only been described in the early case series. In general, visual hallucinations predominate in the delirious states (Wolf and Curran 1935), they tend to occur at night, and, in some cases, they can appear during the day as soon as the patient closes his or her eyes. The content of the hallucination tends to be simple, at times just colours, lines, or shapes (metamorphopsia or teichopsia). In comparison with the more structured experiences of the psychoses, hallucinations in the course of deliria tend to be short-lived and poorly defined. Patients sometimes report seeing lots of people and confused scenes as if watching a fast-playing film, which, at times, intrude on their vision only when they close their eyes. Hallucinations, on the other hand, can be part of a delusional experience and can be coloured by negative emotions such as fear and anxiety. Hallucinations of seeing small animals, which carry an aversive emotional content, are considered typical of DT.

Auditory and tactile hallucinations are possible. Auditory hallucinations were reported by about 40% of patients in older series (Farber 1959; Wolf and Curran 1935), but are probably more frequent in DT and alcohol toxicity.

The clinical rationale of this discussion is confirmed by a recent paper on 100 patients admitted to hospice, showing that 43 had hallucinations and of these only 23% had delirium (Fountain 2001). The simpler hallucinations, such as visions of lights, shapes, people standing at the bedside, occurred more often alone and were not frightening. The vision of people occurred in about 40% of the hallucinations recalled, and in half of them were of the hypnagogic (arising when going asleep) or hypnopompic (arising when awakening) type. Complex scenes occurred in 22% of the cases. The visions of complex scenes and animals could be frightening and were more often recalled after a delirious episode. The occurrence of hallucinations in this study was associated with the use of opioids. The relevance of other factors could not be ascertained due to the small population under study.

Among the explanations given for the occurrence of hallucinations in course of delirium we identified a few useful theories.

- The reduction of the level of arousal is possibly important, together with sleep–wakefulness cycle abnormalities, in producing a cortical defect in judging or evaluating the reality of inner flow of consciousness, imagery, memories, and dream-like activity (the oneiric consciousness or dreamy state of the French authors).
- Dream-like cerebral activity can occur due to the pathological condition and be facilitated by closing one's eyes or a change in external stimuli (turning lights off). In the past, delirium has been described as a waking dream. Indeed, nightmares,

and hallucinations were connected with the content of patients' experience, which reproduced the content of previous vivid dreams (Wolf and Curran 1935).

In line with the interpretation that reality may be distorted due to reduced arousal are those cases of disperception and delusion that follow the rule of the 'known for the unknown' in which foreign places or people are interpreted as more familiar ones, e.g. the hospital as a house, the nurse as a waiter, etc.

4.6 Thought

4.6.1 Thought processing

Thought processing, i.e. the organization, flow, and production of thought, is affected by delirium in several ways. The patient seems blocked on some internal perplexity, unable to focus on, access, and marshal his/her own thoughts. This condition, together with the lack of accuracy in retrieving memories and information, has been often alluded to as 'clouding' or 'narrowing' of consciousness. Thinking can be rambling, irrelevant, and redundant and incoherent. At times though, processing can be abnormally slow or fast. Abstract concept formation is more difficult than focusing on concrete experiences. The patient with mild delirium is partially aware of the difficulty in thinking and can report it to the examiner.

4.6.2 Thought content

Thought content can be completely deranged and delusional. The patient is totally unable to criticize his/her delusional experience and acts accordingly. Delusions were reported frequently in up to 54% of cases (Farber 1959), and, in a more recent prevalence study on an elderly population admitted to a general hospital, delusion manifested in 36% of cases (Schor *et al.* 1992). The available descriptions of delusions come from a case series of patients with agitated delirium referred for psychiatric management (Wolf and Curran 1935). The delusions are invariably transient and poorly systematized. Interestingly, delusions suffered in the course of delirium can have a relationship with the patient's premorbid personality, involving important life events or conflicts, including previous psychopathology. In these cases, persecutory and paranoid ideas of imprisonment, homicide, poisoning, and jealousy are often present, probably facilitated by the unfamiliar hospital environment. One of our patients was convinced that during the night she had been abducted with the whole bed, and taken home where she found her husband with another woman. The patient was right only insofar as the bed had had to be moved to clean the room, and some conflict about her family life was also real. Another patient was very suspicious that people wanted to poison him with with some tablets, after physicians examined him and talked about the efficacy of oxycodone for his pain. In other cases, the delusion has a quiet occupational everyday quality (as in our patient who was busy milking his cow in the barn). Patients undergoing several separate delirium episodes due to different causes experienced similar delusional reactions. Amnesia can follow the delirious delusional episode, but not always as patients' reports of their delusions are available (Lipowski 1990*b*; Wolf and Curran 1935; Breitbart *et al.* 2002).

4.6.3 Suicidal ideation

Sucidal ideation or attempt has been reported in 7% of cases during delirium (Farber 1959). Premorbid psychiatric conditions are extremely important. In their own case series, Wolf and Curran (1935) described the case of a patient with a probable underlying psychopathology who was delirious due to barbiturate toxicity. Throughout his delirium he made several suicidal attempts. The acute episode was solved and the patient was discharged and went back to work. A few years later he committed suicide.

In the palliative care population with advanced cancer, the risk of suicide is probably higher than in the general population (Ripamonti *et al.* 1999). Among the few studies available, that of Farberow *et al.* (1963) suggests that delirium is a protecting factor against suicidal acts in the population with cancer. Breitbart (1987, 1990) suggests instead that delirium can facilitate impulsive behaviours and loosen control and is important in explaining cases of suicide in hospitalized patients with advanced cancer. The theory is interesting but no one has yet assessed the relevance and consequences of suicidal ideation in a delirious patient affected by a terminal disease. One recent study reported that suicidal ideation in cancer patients was associated with depression in 57% of cases and with delirium in 29% (Akechi *et al.* 1999).

In cases of thought pathology, the symptoms and the clinical course of delirium are also compounded by abnormality of arousal, attention, and fluctuations over a short time. From a unitary viewpoint, this can explain different levels of awareness and perhaps justify impulsive actions harming oneself or other people.

4.7 Psychomotor behaviour

The observation of overt behaviour can give important information. Restlessness and agitation are often combined with abnormally fast and pressured thought-processing, delusions, and hallucinations. Hypoactive patients are confused in a more defective way with fewer positive symptoms and signs. By combining the assessment of the level of arousal with the quality of observed behaviours it is possible to classify patients as suffering hypo- or hyperactive or mixed variants of delirium (Liptzin and Levkoff 1992; Ross *et al.* 1991). These definitions are, however, at present not unequivocal. Behavioural evaluation always includes the assessment of arousal level, which is linked, but not equivalent, to the concept of hyper/hypoactivity. Hypoactive patients are often lethargic. More importantly, patients often evolve from hyperactive states into lethargic hypoactive deliria, and, in some cases, this stage precedes stupor and coma.

Extreme hypoactivity can be confused with lethargy, while it could be better explained as depression, catatonia, or frontal lobe dysfunction, due to the fact that arousal compromise may be difficult to evaluate (see Fig. 6.6 and the related case report). The inconsistent association of causes with clinical manifestations can be explained by the evolving nature of the process in many cases.

Typical behaviours associated with delirium include signs originally described by Hippocrates and Soranus.

◆ *jactitatio*: purposeless movement of the hands in the air, other similar behaviour may involve searching under the bed, or in the closet;

- *crocidimus (floccilletion)*: picking at bedclothes;
- *carphology*: picking at the walls.

In general, behaviour and emotional expression are modifications of the patient's usual habits. The impression of change is often the first sign reported by relatives and people who know the patient well, occurring before florid signs can be observed. Psychomotor slowing, apathetic attitude, repetitive gestures, and lack of interest in the environment are common and may be misinterpreted as signs of depression (Farrell and Ganzini 1995). In the early phase these symptoms are far more common than the overly agitated picture. Agitation with purposeless behaviours, which can, at the extreme of the spectrum, be aggressive and dangerous for the patient and care-givers, can follow. It can also characterize a minority of cases from the onset. Preliminary observations by means of motor activity recordings make it possible to classify demented patients with delirium into different groups according to their motor activity into, e.g. a nocturnal delirium type, wandering type, hypobulic type, and lying-down type (Honma *et al.* 1998).

4.8   Affectivity

As already mentioned, perplexity is probably the most frequent mood colour apparent to the examiner. Patients often look very apathetic as if lacking drive or motivation. This would be considered a failure of frontal lobe functions. Fear, anxiety, and anger can dominate the clinical picture of the hypeactive conditions at times associated with DT or the toxicity of some drugs. Mood lability with sudden unexplained hilarity or sadness can be found. Emotions are often consonant with the impact of the underlying illness and can be influenced by the painful awareness of mental impairment. In some cases, depressive symptoms mislead the diagnosis from delirium to depression (Nicholas and Lindsey 1995). Earlier clinical descriptions reported depression in 53% of cases and constricted or flat affect in 30% (Farber 1959). In a study of an elderly population, depressive symptoms were frequent with 60% of patients showing low mood, 68% feelings of worthlessness, and 52% thoughts of death (Farrell and Ganzini 1995). The implications of these clinical observations for a population at risk of grave emotional involvement, such as the terminally ill, are unknown.

4.9   Early clinical findings

Delirium episodes often occur suddenly but can be heralded by subtle symptoms and signs that are often recalled by family members or care-givers after the episodes are full blown. Such recollections can often be elicited by careful interviewing. Table 4.2 lists potential warning signs. The value of such a list is probably higher if combined with the careful monitoring of the risk factors (baseline vulnerability) and potential causal factors characterizing the high-risk populations demonstrated by recent studies (see Chapter 3). No study has specifically addressed the relevance of these observations that are so consistently found in everyday clinical practice.

One article on patients admitted to a coronary care unit showed that delirium was preceded by anxiety, slight agitation, EEG slowing, and changes in eye movements

Table 4.2 Prodromal presentations of delirium

Symptoms and signs
Insomnia
Vivid dreams or nightmares with difficulty in distinguishing dream from reality when awake
Restlessness
Irritability
Distractability
Hypersensitivity to lights and sounds
Anxiety
Subjective sense of difficulty in marshalling own thought
Difficulty in concentrating
Behaviours
Unaccustomed behaviours
Change in behaviour
Hyper- or hypoactivity
Inappropriate behaviours

(Matsushima *et al.* 1997), but it is unclear whether these signs can be related to the classic clinical observations mentioned above and listed in Table 4.2.

4.10   Subjective perception

Systematic assessments of subjective awareness or consciousness during a delirious episode are very rare. Anecdotal reports can be found of patients' recall of the delirious experience, many of which were given by physicians recovering from a febrile illness or a postoperative delirium. Most of these patients reported unpleasant experiences, horrible dreams, waking experiences merging with dreams, and a lack of control of the waking state into which hallucinatory or dream-like experiences intruded (Lipowski 1990*b*). A more recent report confirms the usefulness of a better documentation of patients' perceptions and of their subjective awareness and recall in the fluctuating phases of the disease (Crammer 2002).

In our experience the characteristic fluctuations of severity and of level of consciousness have a significant impact on a patient's affective experience. More lucid phases may allow understanding of the potential occurrence of further mental changes, generating anxiety, anguish, and fear. Emotional reactions can include apathy, depression, perplexity when the clinical situation is perceived as worsened, and cognitive compromise as part of the inevitable grim course; this can influence the elaboration of suicidal thoughts. The quality of the patient's experience of his or her own delirium is not easy to predict and probably depends, as already mentioned, on the patient's personality structure and previous experiences (Wolf and Curran 1935).

Frequently, personal feelings are associated with themes related to the severity of the actual disease (death, torture, kidnapping). It should be significant for medical culture that most, or at least many, of the illusional or delusional interpretations of the medical environment, reported to us by acutely confused patients, had very bad and hostile qualities. One patient perceived physicians around the bed as ghosts, and therapies were seen as attempts to poison her. Another patient believed that she was in a 'laager' with a friend of hers, who was also a patient in the same ward. She recalled that they were both bald (as they indeed were due to chemotherapy) and that people (doctors and nurses) were coming to laugh at them and torture them. This patient had never had any war or imprisonment experiences.

Other experiences are possible in different situations, e.g. in post-liver transplant deliria the relationship with the donor and donor's family is often present: one patient hallucinated that the donor came to him to request the restitution of the organ. The subjective experience was very negative. Another patient had instead the vision of a kaleidoscopically coloured forest inhabited by a fantastic flora and fauna. On recall, he found it a very positive and interesting experience that he connected with his curiosity in the 1960s as to the effects of the hallucinogenic drugs that were popular among his peers and that he never tried. These two opposite reactions may reflect different ways of living the transplant experience.

In reporting his own delirium Crammer was able to recall four episodes of delirious experiences, during a 4-day period of consciousness compromise due to renal failure, one of which was clearly associated with the delusion of being attacked and having to fight for self-defence, the other three were of a relatively neutral type based on the perception of being travelling to Australia or to India by plane. In all cases some environmental elements or stimuli (such as nurses taking care of him) were misintrerpreted in a delusional way (Crammer 2002).

It is therefore likely that present circumstances, together with personality structure and more profound relationships between life events and personal feelings, play a role in producing the final quality and emotional impact of delirium. These considerations should also be valid for delirium at the end of life, but empirical data about the medical, psychological, existential, or spiritual issues characterizing delirium in this particular condition are very limited (Massie *et al.* 1983; Kubler-Ross 1969).

It is also interesting to evaluate to what extent patients are aware of being confused. Again few published experiences are useful in answering this question. In a very recent study on delirium in patients with cancer, we asked the patients if they felt confused and to rate their perceived level of confusion on a four-point scale from 'not at all' to 'very much'. While a group of patients reported to feel not confused at all while fulfilling the diagnostic criteria for delirium, the subjective report of confusion correlated, at a low level of statistical significance, with the Delirium Rating Scale (DRS; Appendix 4) and the Memorial Delirium Assessment Scale (MDAS; Appendix 6) scores for delirium. However, the patients with more severe symptoms were not able to answer the questionnaire (Bosisio *et al.* 2002).

Delirium recall has been investigated in one interesting article by Breitbart *et al.* (2002a). Over 101 delirium episodes occurring in cancer patients 53% of patients could recall their experience. Ability to recall was inversely associated with delirium severity, and consciousness compromise, but, above all, with the severity of memory impairment during the episode. Patient who recalled being confused reported often (80%) severe distress from the experience. The severity of hallucinations and mainly of delusions were the most significant predictor of distress. Spouses and care-givers were also severely distressed by witnessing the delirium of their dear-ones. Interestingly the degree of spouses distress was related to the patient's general condition compromise (Karnofsky performance score) while nurses were more distressed by caring for patients with more severe deliria.

Finally, anecdotal evidence and clinical experience favour the notion that delirium is *per se*, at least in some cases, a source of suffering, justifying the need of palliative treatment.

4.11 Involuntary movements and other neurological signs

In a book on delirium, it should be said, at least once, that the diagnosis of delirium always requires a complete neurological examination. Typically, the diagnosis of delirium does not require the presence of any specific neurological sign. However, some neurological signs, in particular involuntary movements, are common in patients with delirium. Tremor, myoclonus, and asterixis are considered typical of some clinical conditions. We will see that the specificity of these and other neurological signs is low but that their presence has significant clinical value as it can contribute to the differential diagnosis.

4.11.1 Tremor

Tremor is a classic finding in DT. Tremor is, by definition, an involuntary movement involving one joint characterized by a periodic swinging of a body segment according to the joint range of motion due to alternate contraction of antagonist muscles. Tremor is characterized by its frequency, amplitude, occurrence, and the conditions provoking it. The tremor of DT is a thin, high-frequency tremor that is thought to be due to overactivity of the adrenergic system inducing a pathological exacerbation of the physiological tremor.

A thin tremor can also be found in the course of uraemia and other metabolic abnormalities (metabolic tremor) but it is not specific to any clinical condition. In states of emotional or organic excitement, increased tremulousness can be seen as part of an adrenergic activation as the enhancement of physiological tremor (Elble 2000).

4.11.2 Myoclonus

Myoclonus is an involuntary, sudden, brief, shock-like movement caused by muscle contraction (positive myoclonus) or inhibition (negative myoclonus) sufficient to displace a limb or a body segment (Fahn *et al.* 1986). It is different from a fasciculation, which is the contraction of only some fascicles in a muscle not able to move the limb, and from tremor because the contraction is not rhythmic and will affect antagonist muscles at the same time. This confers on myoclonus its 'jerky' feature. Myoclonus is characteristic of some neurological diseases. It can be segmental (only one muscle or muscle group is involved), multifocal (different muscles are involved randomly), or generalized (all body muscles are involved). Myoclonus can also be classified according to its pathophysiology as cortical, subcortical, spinal, and peripheral. In this classification it is recognized that myoclonus can originate at many different levels in the peripheral and central nervous system. Myoclonic jerks are typical of several toxic metabolic encephalopathies and often present together with delirium. Renal failure, hyponatraemia, and drug toxicity can cause myoclonus. Usually, in these types of encephalopathies, myoclonus is multifocal or generalized and has cortical subcortical aetiologies. At times it can precede or be complicated by seizures. Generalized myoclonus has the appearance of the muscle fits that are experienced randomly by any one in the phases preceding sleep. A typical example is holding a book when lying down in bed and suddenly finding oneself jumping from sleep with the book again in the hands. A similar reaction can be obtained by waking somebody up briskly (startle reaction). The same contraction in a fully awake state is usually pathological.

Opioid-induced myoclonus is increasingly reported in the palliative care literature, perhaps due to the more liberal use of higher doses of opioid drugs (Daeninck and Bruera 1999). Its pathophysiology has to do with the excitatory effects of opioids at the CNS level where they are also able to produce hyperalgesia and seizures but it needs to be studied in greater depth (see also Chapter 6).

4.11.3 Asterixis

Asterixis, also known as flapping tremor or hepatic tremor, is a negative myoclonus. With the patient keeping his arms and hands extended at the level of its eyes, the first movement to be seen is a coarse tremor in the horizontal plane giving a kind of rotation to the hands. After a little while (the position should be kept for at least a minute), the hands drop due to the resolution of the anti-gravitary muscle tone and abruptly rise back as the muscles automatically correct the position in response to the tone resolution. This failure of maintaining the muscle tone is due to central inhibition and is considered a negative myoclonus. Asterixis is seen in hepatic failure but also in other metabolic disorders and drug toxicities (ifosfamide, opioids, acyclovir). It can be shown in the legs by having them in hip, leg-flexed position, foot against foot with the knees in an external suspended posture. For the very ill and exhausted patient, it is more comfortable to try to observe asterixis by just having him or her extend their index finger. The flapping movement of the finger is equivalent to the more demanding traditional manoeuvre.

4.11.4 Aspecific motor signs

These signs are thought to be related to cortical damage and are often referred to as frontal liberation signs as they are often associated with frontal syndromes. They are also referred to as primitive reflexes that would be released in pathological conditions affecting the cerebral cortex and consciousness, by the control of higher structures in

Jacksonian terms. They are frequent in different types of dementias and are physiological in newborn babies. Their finding in a patient known for not manifesting such reactions before is valuable in diagnosing the recent onset of encephalopathy. A list of these signs follows.

- *Palmomental reflex.* By gently but firmly scratching with a blunt instrument against the palm of the hand, a contraction of the mentalis and orbicularis otis muscles is evoked homolaterally to the stimulation side.
- *Sucking reflex.* By presenting a tactile stimulus to the lips and mouth, lip protrusion, as if in the process of sucking, is evoked.
- *Grasping.* Tactile stimulation of the palm causes the patient to grasp the examiner's hand. The response cannot be inhibited voluntarily by the patient.
- *Snouting.* Tactile stimulation of the perioral area evokes a mimic reflex comparable to animal snouting.
- *Paratonia* or *gegenhalten.* This is a paradoxical reflex increase of the muscle tone by semivoluntary contraction in opposition to passive stretching of the muscles, usually tested on the arm flexory muscles. It is not easy to distinguish from true voluntary opposition.
- *Glabella.* When gently tapping the glabella area in the forehead a physiological blinking of the eyelids results that usually disappears after a number of trials. The inability to naturally block this reflex in time is pathological.

4.12 Clinical course

Delirium was traditionally considered to be an acute event, with a fluctuating course that should lead to a relatively quick recovery, or a transitory condition on the worsening course towards coma and death. This is still true for deliria developing in young relatively healthy individuals due to acute conditions or stressing events, which have a favourable course and last usually for a few days. The duration is longer in the elderly with stroke, metabolic disorders, and structural brain disease (19.5 ± 15.4 days in one study, (Koponen and Riekkinen 1993)). Another study (Manos and Wu 1997) suggests that longer duration is associated with dementia, and that duration is shorter in postoperative delirium (mean 7.6 days) than in medically ill cases (13.2 days). The study by Levkoff *et al.* (1992), mentioned in Section 3.2.1, showed that full recovery was rare before discharge, only 4% of cases, and more than 50% of the patients who were diagnosed according to DSM-III criteria during their hospital stay still fulfilled criteria for delirium after 6 months. In such cases the differential diagnosis with dementia can be difficult (Lipowski 1990*b*). It is possible that cognitive symptoms that persist after the delirium episode resolves are due to an underlying structural brain disorder (Hill *et al.* 1992). Indeed, in a recent case series, an episode of delirium in the elderly was followed by a diagnosis of dementia either immediately or within the subsequent 2 years in 55% of 51 patients (Rahakonen *et al.* 2000). As already mentioned, in patients admitted to a specialized palliative care unit, 49% of the delirious episodes were reversible (Lawlor *et al.* 2000*b*).

Chapter 5

Differential diagnosis

The most important differential diagnoses of delirium are dementia; psychoses (Table 5.1); focal neurological disorders affecting higher brain functions such as attention, memory, and language; psychogenic reactions; and epilepsy.

5.1 Dementia

The clinical picture of dementia can be very similar to that of delirium due to the widespread failure of higher cerebral functions, and to the overlap of some pathogenic mechanisms involving the failure of cortical activity and, in particular, of cholinergic transmission (Perry *et al.* 1999).

Conversely, patients with dementia, as already discussed, are at increased risk of developing delirium. In a recent thematic symposium on delirium in the elderly, some authors (Blass and Gibson 1999; MacDonald 1999) questioned the need to distinguish

Table 5.1 The principal differential diagnoses of delirium

Clinical feature	Delirium	Dementia	Acute psychosis
Onset	Acute	Slow	Acute
Circadian course	Fluctuating	Stable	Stable
Level of consciousness	Affected	Spared except in severe cases	Spared
Attention	Impaired	Initially spared	Can be impaired
Cognition	Impaired	Impaired	Can be impaired
Hallucinations	Usually visual	Often absent	Often auditory
Delusions	Poorly systematized and fleeting	Often absent	Sustained and systematized
Psychomotor activity	Increased, reduced, mixed with alternating course	Often normal	Can vary with bizarre behaviour depending on the psychosis
Involuntary movements	Asterixis, myoclonus, or tremor can be present in some subtypes	Absent in most forms	Absent
EEG	Abnormal *	Abnormal *	Normal

* See text for more details.

between the clinical concepts of delirium and dementia, at least in the special population of the elderly demented patients.

The classic distinction between dementia and delirium is based on the acute onset and the disturbance of the level of consciousness (in ICD–10, 'clouding of consciousness') characterizing delirium, as opposed to the chronic process sparing the level of consciousness, at least initially and for a period that potentially can be very long, which is typical of dementia.

The underemphasis of the transitory failure of the arousal system and therefore of consciousness in delirium can lead to a de-emphasis of this clinical distinction (Lindesay 1999) and can lead to the conclusion that the global dysfunction of cognitive process can affect the elderly brain via different processes leading to a similar final condition. This view can be supported by clinical observations in the elderly with severe dementia, but also in other states of failure of the brain functions such as the preterminal phases of chronic debilitating illnesses, and in patients with severe but fluctuating compromise of state of consciousness. Yet we think that the distinction between dementia and delirium is very useful and nosologically sound for at least two reasons.

- Delirium can affect many different clinical conditions, acute illnesses as well as chronic, besides dementia as considered in this book, and some acute conditions can also be well recognized when superimposed on chronic comorbidities.

- Delirium can be reversible. The effect of psychotropic drug toxicity, which is so common among the elderly, can acutely impair their function and be promptly reversed even in demented or terminally ill patients, confirming the therapeutic usefulness of the concept of delirium in these cases (Lawlor *et al.* 2000*b*).

The case of the patient with dementia, however, is a special one and poses specific clinical difficulties. As described earlier, many elderly demented patients have prolonged courses after delirious episodes with incomplete reversibility of symptoms and functional compromise. The diagnosis of delirium may apply, but in some cases the change in mental status is the manifestation of cognitive failure heralding the onset of dementia, or the worsening of an already established dementia. These challenging cases notwithstanding, we see very good reasons in agreement with the available and up-to-date diagnostic systems to maintain a clear-cut distinction between delirium and dementia.

5.2 Psychoses

An acute behavioural change with altered cognition and attention can be the result of a psychosis. Often the patient has an history of psychiatric disease but he or she could present for the first time with a dramatic bizarre course (*pousseé delirant*). Toxicity from amphetamines or amphetamine-type street drugs often can mimic this type of reaction.

A particular challenge is posed by the patient with a psychiatric diagnosis who develops delirium. This event is not totally rare. In one study of psychiatric admissions over 3 years, delirium was found in 1.4% cases, most often due to drug toxicity (Huang *et al.* 1998). A good knowledge of the patient's pre-delirious behaviour and the observation of the sudden change of this behaviour, especially if associated with a change in the level of consciousness, can guide the diagnosis, which, however, can still be difficult. Buchman *et al.* (1999) reported a very informative example of a schizophrenic patient who developed acute psychotic symptoms after pneumonia and was found to be deficient in vitamin B12 and folic acid. After the appropriate vitamin therapy, the acute symptoms disappeared. Another case report highlighted the need to suspect toxic effects, in this situation from the recurrence of psychiatric disease (Brown and Rosen 1992).

Another important differential diagnosis in the area of psychiatric expertise is the possibility of a fully psychogenic condition mimicking delirium or altered states of consciousness The range of psychogenic reactions goes from pseudostatus epilepticus (Makker and Yanny 2000) to psychogenic unresponsiveness (Plum and Posner 1980*a*). Psychogenic excitement with bizarre behaviour and movements can be mistaken for delirium with hyperactive characteristics. Alternatively, catatonia or unresponsiveness can be confused with stupour or coma. The most important aspect of these conditions is that they are quite rare and that organic causes need first to be accurately ruled out, as delirium is far more common (Makker and Yanny 2000). In all of these cases, the history of psychiatric disease is very important. In the past, very interesting cases were described by using the amytal interview. This type of procedure is unlikely to be appropriate nowadays and certainly not in the palliative care setting (Plum and Posner 1980*a*).

Depression has to be considered also among the important differential psychiatric diagnoses of delirium. As already documented, many delirious patients, perhaps up to 50%, report depressive symptoms and, more importantly, in the elderly medically ill, up to 42% of the patients referred for depression were finally diagnosed with delirium (Farrell and Ganzini 1995).

Case report

A 75-year-old patient with a known history of manic psychosis was admitted for pain management because of advanced intrapelvic recurrence of rectal cancer with infiltration of the pelvic bone and sciatic nerve compression on the right. He had been on lithium (300 mg/day) for 12 years. On oxycodone 5 mg every 6 hours, pain was not controlled and, because of his psychiatric disease, antidepressants were not tried, Carbamazepine had not been tolerated before. Therefore, mexiletine was added for the neuropathic component of the pain. At 1200 mg of mexiletine per day he started to be ataxic, pain was not much better, and mexiletine was discontinued. Oxycodone was substituted with morphine slow-release tablets at the dose of 40 mg b.i.d (twice daily). During the night the patient started to have hallucinations and to present with delusions and grandiose behaviours (he wanted to invite all the staff to a dinner with the son of the ex-king of Italy and his ministers). This type of behaviour was not totally new for him and characteristic of his manic phases and the night-shift nurse considered it to be part of his chronic psychiatric illness. In the morning he was disoriented in respect to time but not to space and person, although he had some difficulties in naming objects and no focal neurological signs. A computerized tomography (CT) scan of the head was immediately taken and showed a cortical atrophy. Morphine was stopped and changed to oxycodone with complete recovery of cognitive function.

Subsequently, due to insufficient pain control, a young fellow in the pain service prescribed methadone at the dose of 10 mg t.i.d. (thrice daily), a very high dose if compared with his previous opioid exposure (20 mg per day of oxycodone and 40 mg per day of morphine). After 12 hours he was acutely confused, he started to be agitated again, and the grandiose delusion previously observed (the patient's wish to invite the staff to a party with the ex-king of Italy and his ministers) reappeared. Shortly afterwards, stuporous, respiratory frequency decreased to 9 per minute. Naloxone was administered (0.05 mg intravenously (IV)) with recovery of consciousness and of respiratory rate. The confusional state persisted for a few hours. Laboratory examinations showed no metabolic or haematological abnormalities and lithium levels were within therapeutic ranges (0.84 mEq/l, therapeutic range 0.4–1.5 mEq/l). Therapy was modified again to oxycodone 5 mg every 6 hours plus p.r.n. (*pro re nata*; ('as circumstances may require'), and palliative radiation therapy was started on the tumour mass with analgesic benefit.

There are several points to consider in the light of this case report.

1 The differential diagnosis of the initial presentation of delirium, which was interpreted initially as a manifestation of psychosis. Indeed, the night-shift nurse did not even call the physician on duty.

2 The potential metabolic interference of lithium causing toxic effects with morphine and with methadone but not with oxycodone (Brown and Rosen 1992).

3 The presence of brain atrophy, which is also common in psychiatric patients, and may be another risk factor for toxic reactions to opioid drugs.

5.3   Focal neurological syndromes

Both vascular and tumour-related focal damage of the CNS can be associated with delirium (see Chapter 6) or can be confused with it, especially when focal neurological deficits affect language, memory, attention, and thought, making the assessment of the patient's level and content of consciousness very difficult. In fact, patients with fluent aphasia and a preserved level of consciousness are not delirious, while patients with severe amnesic syndromes and attention failure may be confabulating and apparently very confused. Also, a selective impairment of attention that is not associated with a change in the level of consciousness should not be diagnosed as delirium. A frontal lobe lesion can cause attention failure, perseveration, and inappropriate behaviour (Deutsch and Eisemberg 1987; Deutsche Lezak 1995). All these symptoms are often found in delirum. Nevertheless, a clearcut diagnosis can be difficult, but we would recommend being as clear as possible about the relative role of focal neurological impairment on one side and consciousness impairment on the other side, recognizing that clinical overlap exists. Some acute cerebral events can present with delirium (see below) and it is important to identify and correct general metabolic or nutritional factors that might contribute to or complicate the neurological condition. Typical of this situation is the Wernicke–Korsakoff syndrome, which is due to a deficit of thiamine that manifests as failure of recent memory and eye movement abnormalities and is often associated with confabulation.

Selective, severe impairment of short-term memory can impair function and be superficially confused with delirium as in the following very short case example.

Case report

A patient with non-Hodgkin's lymphoma with a lesion of the corpus callosum (Fig. 5.1) presented with amnesia and was not able to recall the whereabouts of his room in the hospital, the date, or why he was there. He was often found wandering in the hospital, apparently confused. Consciousness was preserved and he was able to perform most cognitive tests adequately if his memory was not challenged. Nevertheless, he was immediately labelled 'confused' by the medical and nursing staff of the oncology ward.

5.4   Epilepsy

Most cases of epileptic seizures cannot be confused with delirium when clinical presentation includes clear-cut convulsive generalized or partial seizures. Medical history will be helpful in patients who have suffered from a seizure disorder independently of the present illness.

On the other hand, any type of seizure is usually followed by a post-ictal confusional state that can last for hours and can be associated with headache. Seizures that are secondary to metastases or other general medical conditions are more often partial

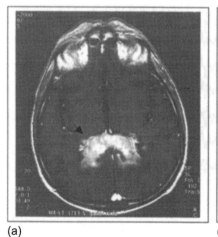 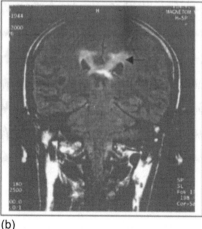

(a)   (b)

Fig. 5.1 This patient was affected by non-Hodgkin's lymphoma and metastases to the splenium of the corpus callosum. (a) Axial view of MRI with contrast (gadolinium) showing the lymphomatous lesion at the level of the splenium (arrow). (b) Coronal view showing the diffused periventricular white matter infiltration (arrow). This type of lesion is interfering with the main circuits of short-term memory.

than generalized. If consciousness is compromised we talk of partial complex seizures as opposed to partial simple seizures, which imply a normal level of consciousness.

Partial complex seizures and petit mal seizures can be more difficult to distinguish from delirium because they present with an altered state of consciousness and may be associated with limited and poorly defined motoric abnormalities such as visuofacial automatism. The specific clinical features are that consciousness is compromised while vigilance is apparently retained and the duration is short, lasting only a few seconds.

Non-convulsive status epilepticus (NCSE) is a situation of continuous or discontinuous but very frequent seizure activity, as documented by EEG recordings, that does not allow consciousness recovery and lasts for hours or days. It is not totally rare in patients who are in markedly poor physical condition and in those who have had brain injury due to metabolic disorders (Towne *et al.* 2000). There are two main types of NCSE that are relevant to delirium: the petit mal type NCSE and the partial complex NCSE. Both manifest with an altered state of consciousness, bizarre behaviours, and/or psychotic symptoms. The substantial difference is that petit mal status implies a generalized EEG abnormality typical of petit mal seizures, while partial complex status is due to prolonged epileptic activity in discrete brain areas, often the temporal lobe, that produces behavioural and psychomotor symptoms without convulsions. At the other extreme of consciousness compromise, there are cases of coma that are explained by NCSE (Towne *et al.* 2000). Seizure activity can be continuous or discontinuous. In this last case partial seizures are recorded in cycles but no complete consciousness recovery is seen between single seizures. The clinical findings will completely overlap with the continuous type.

The possibility of partial complex seizures or NCSE should not be disregarded when considering altered states of consciousness in palliative care and in patients with complex structural, toxic, and metabolic abnormalities affecting the CNS. The diagnosis can only be made by EEG recordings. One well described case of NCSE is ifosfamide toxicity (Fig. 5.2). Ifosfamide toxicity manifests with confusion and myoclonus

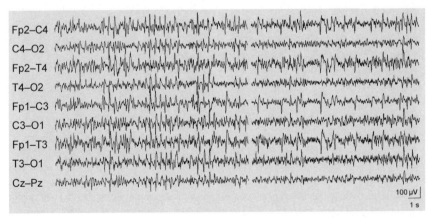

Fig. 5.2 EEG recording during acute ifosfamide toxicity (see text). Periodic diffuse peak groupings can be seen on most derivations. This recording is compatible with status epilepticus. (Courtesy of Dr Franceschetti.)

and is caused by subsequent partial seizure activity that can be abolished by the use of diazepam. Recently, methylene blue has proved to be an effective antidote for ifosfamide central toxicity (Kupfer *et al.* 1996).

Case report

The case whose EEG is reported in Fig. 5.2 is that of a 65-year-old woman affected by a pelvic carcinosarcoma who underwent a course of chemotherapy with adriamycin 25 mg/m^2 (total dose, 41 mg) and ifosfamide 3 g/m^2 (total dose, 5 g). Within 12 hours after administration, she developed perseveration, inappropriate behaviours, and reduction of vigilance. She did not have abnormal movements, convulsion, or focal signs. The EEG recordings taken during the confusional state showed continuous periodic spike-type activity(mainly triphasic) compatible with the diagnosis of status epilepticus.

5.5 Incomplete syndromes

Recent epidemiological studies have highlighted the frequency of partial syndromes. In a study on elderly ($\geq$ 65 years old) hospitalized patients, some cognitive symptoms of disorientation, disturbance of consciousness, psychomotor abnormalities, speech disorders, sleep problems, and perceptual disturbances were found as often as the full syndrome without fulfilling the criteria for delirium (Levkoff *et al.* 1992). In a validation study of delirium scales in 105 cancer patients referred for neurological or psychiatric opinion for suspected delirium, 66 patients received the diagnosis of delirium, whereas, of the remaining 39, 13 had acute mental symptoms without fulfilling all the criteria for delirium (Grassi *et al.* 2001*b*).

The finding of symptoms of acute confusion without fulfilling the criteria for delirium is not, therefore, uncommon. Hallucinations are often reported as one effect of opioid toxicity that may be part of a developing delirium or not. One patient of ours with moderate renal failure developed visual hallucinations after increasing the morphine dose, and recovered after renal function improved (Caraceni *et al.* 1994). The findings of Fountain (2001) were reported in Chapter 4 and show a prevalence of 30% for hallucinations in the hospice patient population.

The DSM-III allowed the use of the terminology, 'organic hallucinosis', for a patient with these characteristics. The condition would have been classified under the organic brain disorders. In the DSM-IV, the classification of such symptoms is more complicated requiring that they are identified within either the mental disorders related to a general medical condition or a substance-related disorder and therefore lack generality.

Partial syndromes represent, at times, cases at risk of developing the full syndrome, 'quasi-delirious', or the more selective ability of some causal factor to induce a symptom (Trzepacz 1994*a*).

An illustrative case report

A 72-year-old lady affected by breast cancer and non-Hodgkin's lymphoma with spinal cord compression at D1–D2 level was admitted for radiation therapy, chemotherapy, and symptom control. Pain in the legs and dorsal spine was treated with tramadol, initially 50 mg in oral drops t.i.d., which was substituted at admission by transdermal fentanyl 25 µg/h patch. Therapy included dexamethasone 16 mg/day. After about 24 hours on this regimen she developed her first hallucinations described as bees entering her room through the window and Talibans on top of her television set. Durogesic and dexamethasone were stopped and tramadol given as IV infusion at the dose of 300 mg/day with morphine 5 mg rescue dose for p.r.n. medication. Hallucinations disappeared for 2 days. Chemotherapy for her lymphoma was given including prednisolone 100 mg/day for 3 days. At this time a new episode occurred and she saw her friends in the room who were changed into salt statues, and people coming in the room who fell asleep in strange positions. When examined and questioned about what was going on, she reported that, due to some radio waves still persisting within the room, the people coming in were very pale with black lips. The only way to solve this problem was that she put on a special suit that you could buy in the hospital and that she had bought the evening before for about 15 Euros. At the same time, she pointed at the television set on top of which one nurse was asleep. Her vigilance was intact, visuospatial orientation perfect, memory and cognition not affected, and she could write and copy designs properly. No neurological signs were found and a head CT scan and laboratory examinations were normal.

Her drug regimen was kept unchanged as regards the intake of opioids, while steroids were tapered. In the following days, hallucinations and delusions were absent, she was disoriented to time, and had night-time insomnia and agitation. For her symptoms she also received haloperidol 2 mg at night with benefit. When asked again about the complex hallucinations experienced, she was quite irritated and replied shortly that, although what had happened was real, it was not happening any longer. She developed febrile neutropenia and pneumonia and died about a week after the first hallucinatory episode.

The role of opioids in this case is uncertain. The episodes are characterized mainly by hallucinations and the patient's report about them is still delusional when examining her after the full-blown episode had ended. Other areas of cognition were not affected and consciousness was not compromised. It would be possible to emphasize the role of corticosteroids, perhaps in combination with fentanyl, in the first episode and to classify the case as steroid psychosis, using an old definition. Using DSM IV language one should talk of a 'substance-induced psychosis'. The subjective reaction of the patient to the episodes underlines the need for a better understanding of this area of subjective feelings and the need to be prepared to help patients in coping with this type of experience.

5.6 Role of the EEG in differential diagnosis

EEG recordings can be used to differentiate delirium from seizures and from psychoses. The main EEG features found in delirium are the increase of the percentage of slow frequencies, possibly finding delta (< 4 Hz) and theta ($4–8$ Hz) rhythms together with the disruption of the physiological alpha rhythm ($8–13$ Hz). These characteristic features can be used to differentiate the delirious from the non-delirious and from demented elderly patients (Jacobson *et al.* 1993*a*, *b*; Koponen *et al.* 1989). The slowing of the EEG in the range of the alpha frequency that is still considered normal would be a significant sign of encephalopathy, but its usefulness is limited because the normal appearance of the alpha before the onset of delirium is usually unknown unless an EEG under 'control conditions' is taken. This situation is clarified in the following case example.

Case report

A 22-year-old patient affected by medulloblastoma of the posterior fossa that was surgically resected had a course of chemotherapy that included high-dose IV thiotepa. She developed consciousness impairment associated with complex forelimb movements and eye rowing. Lorazepam 5 mg IV was given in several doses and phenytoin 18 mg/kg infusion was started. Consciousness improved and pathological movement stopped but psychomotor slowing persisted for a few hours. After 6 hours she started to be confused again, and, later on, became stuporous. For better monitoring of her vital function, the patient was transferred to the intensive care unit where, in spite of antiepileptic medications, she had more episodes of involuntary movements and disturbances of consciousness. Brain magnetic resonance imaging

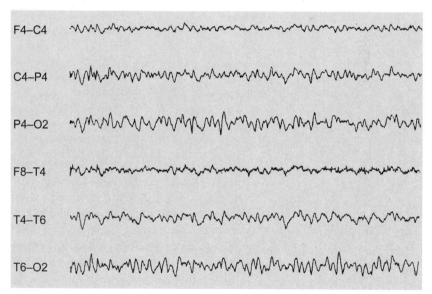

Fig. 5.3 This patient had toxicity due to chemotherapy with delirium and probably non-convulsive status epilepticus. The EEG shown corresponds to the phase of recovery of mental status, several days after the acute episode. It shows a persistent slowing (8 Hz) of the physiological alpha rhythm (13 Hz), primarily over the occipital areas where this type of frequency is physiologically mostly represented. The traces represent electrical activity recorded from only the right hemisphere. A significant slowing of the EEG frequency (8 Hz) can be seen principally in the recordings from the occipital areas (P4–O2 and T6–O2).

(MRI) showed no change, in comparison with her previous imaging. In 2 days her level of consciousness improved and the patient was awake and oriented. However, she was somnolent and slow in performing mental tasks. The EEG, taken on two different occasions when the patient's consciousness was only slightly impaired, showed that the alpha rhythm on the occipital derivations was a relatively slow 8–9 Hz (Fig. 5.3). On one occasion, during spontaneous sleep, the EEG showed the onset of slow waves in the delta rhythm range and of peaks. Thiothepa-induced encephalopathy was the final diagnosis. Consciousness compromise was attributed to potential NCES (although seizure activity was never recorded) on the basis of the sparse ictal activity (peaks) seen in the EEG, with intercurrent phases of recovery associated with delirium and encephalopathy as documented by slow waves and slowing of the physiological alpha rhythm.

Chapter 6

Frequent aetiologies

In this chapter a more detailed description is given of some clinically defined delirious syndromes. Not every cause or condition is examined, but only those that are more frequent or particularly relevant in the palliative care settings. The clinical conditions that follow are grouped according to aetiology.

6.1 Alcohol withdrawal delirium (delirium tremens) and other withdrawal deliria

Withdrawal from substances is a frequent cause of delirium. As indicated in Chapter 2, the most recent classifications of delirium indicate that delirium can occur as a consequence of withdrawal from alcohol or substances with sedative, hypnotic, or anxiolytic properties. It is important to recognize that, although full-blown withdrawal syndromes (such as DT) are relatively rare, symptoms of withdrawal are more common and can be associated with delirium.

6.1.1 Delirium tremens

Alcoholism is an important public health problem throughout the world. Individuals who excessively and continuously consume alcohol, have been drinking for years, and maintain a high alcohol intake, shifting from alcohol abuse to alcohol dependence (Ashworth and Gerada 1997; Langenbucher *et al.* 2000), commonly experience withdrawal symptoms 1 or 2 days after substantial reduction or complete withdrawal from alcohol (Chang and Steinberg 2001; Hall and Zador 1997).

Symptoms include general malaise, signs of autonomic hyperactivity (i.e. tremors, especially of hands, legs, and trunk, tachycardia and hypertension, sweating, nausea, insomnia) and psychological symptoms (i.e. anxiety and agitation, irritability and mood lability, transient perceptual disturbances, such as illusions and visual and tactile hallucinations) in a condition in which reality testing is, however, intact. These symptoms may last about 1 week and are rapidly relieved by alcohol intake. However, in some forms, alcohol withdrawal can be complicated by the onset of seizures, with a peak at 24 hours after the last consumption of alcohol. In these cases, the onset of a full-blown delirium state, diagnosed as alcohol withdrawal delirium, or delirium tremens (DT), is not uncommon (30%). Thus the onset of DT is usually gradual (2–3 days after cessation of alcohol intake, with a peak at 4–5 days), with early and prodromic symptoms represented by uncomplicated alcohol withdrawal syndrome, although sudden forms of DT are also possible (Erwin *et al.* 1998).

Risk factors for developing DT in patients with alcohol withdrawal syndrome have been suggested to be concurrent infections, tachycardia (heart rate above 120 beats/min at admission), signs of alcohol withdrawal accompanied by an alcohol concentration of more than 1 gram per litre of body fluid, a history of epileptic seizures, and a history of delirious episodes (Palmstierna 2001). It has also been suggested that patients with alcohol dependence who present with prefrontal atrophy and frontal cortical and temporal (sub)cortical atrophy at CT scan may be at higher risk of developing DT (Maes *et al.* 2000).

The clinical features of DT are represented by alcohol withdrawal symptoms, complicated by the typical symptoms of delirium—reduced level of consciousness, disorientation in time and place, impairment in recent memory, insomnia. In DT significant perceptual disturbances and thought disorders are present. The patient appears agitated and frightened by visual, but also tactile and auditory, vivid hallucinations (mostly insects or small animals) and misinterpretations of environmental stimuli. Marked autonomic arousal is also a typical feature of DT, with tremors, tachycardia, hypertension, sweating, mild fever, complicated sometimes by seizures. DT usually lasts 3 days, followed by a deep sleep from which the patient frequently awakes with no memory of the delirium. However, it has also been reported that DT may fluctuate for several weeks. Metabolic disorders, infections, poor general physical condition, and concomitant physical illness are all risk factors for the more severe complications associated with DT (Wojnar *et al.* 1999).

Mortality ranges from very low percentages to a maximum of 5%, according to the clinical severity of delirium, predisposing factors, and response to treatment (McCowan and Marik 2000).

Thus, obtaining an alcohol consumption history, identifying possible risk factors, recognizing alcohol withdrawal symptoms, and early treatment with benzodiazepines are significant steps in the prevention of DT among hospitalized patients, especially those in the advanced stages of physical illness (Mayo-Smith 1997; Schumacher *et al.* 2000).

6.1.2 Other forms of withdrawal delirium

As indicated in both the DSM-IV-TR and the ICD-10, other forms of delirium can develop because of withdrawal from substances, including sedative, hypnotic, or anxiolytic drugs.

The persistent use (or abuse) of anxiolytics and hypnotics has been reported to favour the onset of delirium upon abrupt discontinuation of these drugs (Heritch *et al.* 1987). However, Bruera *et al.* (1996) showed that, among cancer patients in an advanced phase of illness, a rapid decrease in the dosage of hypnotic drugs was not followed by withdrawal syndrome or rebound phenomena, as expected. This experience is not, however, sufficient, in our opinion, to justify neglecting caution in withdrawing benzodiazepine therapy in patients who have been using it for significant periods of time. We saw several cases presenting with signs of withdrawal, including delirium, after abrupt discontinuation of benzodiazepine that had been habitually taken for months or years.

Nicotine can also be considered a possible cause of withdrawal delirium. Mayer *et al.* (2001) reported five cases of nicotine withdrawal delirium among patients with a history of heavy tobacco usage who were treated in a neurological intensive care unit for brain injury. Transdermal nicotine replacement was shown to be effective in helping patients recover from delirium within a few hours (Gallagher 1998).

Recently, cases of withdrawal from the new drugs of abuse (because of their similarities to sedative-hypnotic or alcohol intoxication), gamma-hydroxybutyric acid (GHB) and gamma-butyrolactone (GBL), have been reported. These substances not only cause disturbances of consciousness due to overdose, but also cause delirium-like symptoms upon rapid discontinuation by high-frequency users. A withdrawal syndrome that presented with anxiety, agitation, tremor, and delirium was shown in a study carried out by Miotto *et al.* (2001) in GHB abusers. Sivilotti *et al.* (2001) reported cases of delirium with tachycardia, hypertension, paranoid delusions, hallucinations, and rapid fluctuations in sensorium, secondary to abrupt GBL discontinuation. While high doses of lorazepam proved to be ineffective, pentobarbital resulted in excellent control of behavioural, autonomic, and psychiatric symptoms.

Delirium has been reported in association with withdrawal from various drugs and case reports of this stype are always increasing, such as withdrawal from valerian root (Garges *et al.* 1998), alprazolam (Zalsman *et al.* 1998), amantadine (Factor *et al.* 1998), clozapine (Stanilla *et al.* 1997), and gabapentin (Norton 2001) to give a by no means comprehensive list.

6.2 Delirium due to metabolic causes

Together with drug-induced toxic deliria, metabolic abnormalities are likely to account for the most common group of aetiologies encountered in medically ill patients. This condition is one of the most common diagnoses in consultation or liaison psychiatry and neurology at general and tertiary care hospitals (Tuma and DeAngelis 2000). The term metabolic encephalopathy is often used as a synonym for metabolic delirium and can be considered to be, in the neurologist's vocabulary, its neuropathogenic equivalent (Lipowski 1990*b*; Plum and Posner 1980*b*). In palliative care, metabolic encephalopathy is often found in the very terminal phases of disease, as shown in a postdoctoral thesis dissertation on the result of a home-care programme for advanced cancer patients, where metabolic encephalopathy was considered the principal final cause of coma and death in 56% of cases (Groff 1993).

Metabolic encephalopathy is the result of several general metabolic abnormalities producing diffuse brain damage through mechanisms that finally cause dysfunction of the brain's cellular metabolism. Brain metabolism is particularly sensitive to oxygen and glucose demands. In general, all the causes of metabolic encephalopathy result in a reduction of oxygen and glucose consumption by the brain leading to initially reversible cellular damage and, finally, to cell death. An accurate mechanistic classification of metabolic encephalopathies is reproduced, in its general terms, from Plum and Posner (1980*b*) in Table 6.1. Table 6.2 summarizes a few principles that hold valid through the review of most metabolic encephalopathies.

Table 6.1 Classification of metabolic encephalopathies. (Modified from Plum and Posner (1980*b*, pp. 178–80))

A	**Deprivation of oxygen or substrate or metabolic cofactors**
	Hypoxia (reduction of brain oxygen supply of pulmonary or haematological origin)
	Ischaemia (of cardiac, circulatory, or rheological origin)
	Hypoglycaemia
	Cofactor deficiency (thiamine, niacine, pyridoxine, cyanocobalamin, folic acid)
B	**Diseases of other organs**
	Liver
	Kidney
	Lung
	Pancreas
	Endocrine hypo- or hyperfunction (pituitary, thyroid, parathyroid, adrenal)
C	**Exogenous toxic substances (poisons and drugs)**
D	**Ionic or acid–base imbalances**
	Water and sodium imbalances hypo- or hypernatraemia
	Acidosis
	Alkalosis
	Hyper- or hypomagnesaemia
	Hyper- or hypocalcaemia
	Hypophosphataemia
E	**Temperature dysregulation (hypothermia, heat stroke, fever)**
F	**Infections and inflammation of CNS**
G	**Primary neuronal or glial disorders**
H	**Miscellaneous disorders**
	Seizures, post-ictal state
	Posttraumatic encephalopathy
	Sedative drug withdrawal
	Postoperative delirium

Modified with permission from Plum, F. and Posner, J.B., *The diagnosis of stupor and coma*, Vol. 19, F.A. Davis, Philadelphia, 1980. Copyright Oxford University Press.

6.2.1   Hepatic encephalopathy

Hepatic encephalopathy occurs in patients with either advanced liver disease and evidence of hepatic failure or when, for different reasons, including liver disease, the bloodstream from the enteroportal cycle due to portosystemic shunt bypasses liver circulation. The clinical picture of hepatic encephalopathy can range from mild cognitive failure, drowsiness, and memory lapse to full-blown delirium. Delirium due to

Table 6.2 General principles of metabolic encephalopathies

- The more rapid the development of the toxic state, the less perturbed do the chemical findings need to be to produce symptoms

- No morphological brain abnormalities are found and, when found, they are due to secondary effects

- Non-specific motor signs are common: paratonia or gegenhalten, snouting, sucking, palmomental reflex, grasping

- Characteristic motor signs, e.g. asterixis, multifocal myoclonus, seizures, can be found independently of the underlying aetiology

- In coma resulting from metabolic encephalopathy, pupillary reactivity is preserved

- Focal signs, eye deviation, and asymmetrical extensor plantar responses can rarely be found and do not rule out metabolic encephalopathy as opposed to brain structural disease

- Hyperventilation is not always present but is rather specific, compensating for metabolic acidosis, or primary, driven by toxic state (respiratory alkalosis)

---

hepatic failure is more often of the hypoactive type (Ross *et al.* 1991) with lethargy evolving into a comatose state if not treated. However, this is only partially true, as hallucinations and hyperactive delirium are reported in up to 10–20% of the cases (Plum and Posner 1980*b*). Asterixis can be seen in many metabolic encephalopathies. It was first described in liver failure—hence the denomination 'hepatic tremor' (Adams and Foley 1953). Preclinical changes in the EEG and evoked potentials have been shown preceding more pronounced clinical findings, and the combined use of EEG,and cognitive testing has been shown to improve the accuracy of the clinical assessment (Trzepacz *et al.* 1989*a*, *b*). The pathogenesis of hepatic encephalopathy is not completely understood. Most explanations refer to the neurotoxic activity of substances coming from the portal circulation system that would normally be inactivated by the liver. Only in extreme cases (Muller *et al.* 1994) and in newborn babies, can bilirubin cross the blood-brain barrier and be toxic for the brain.

Recent studies pinpointed the role of endogenous benzodiazepine-like substances in causing sedation, cognitive dysfunction, delirium, and, eventually, coma in patients with hepatic failure. The use of the benzodiazepine antagonist flumazenil was therefore proposed to improve cognitive functions and treat comatose patients in the advanced phases of hepatic failure. The most recent evidence shows that, although an increase in the GABA-ergic tone is likely in the pathogenesis of hepatic encephalopathy (Meyer *et al.* 1998), flumazenil administration gave conflicting results in humans and had no effect on animals (Meyer *et al.* 1998), therefore bringing into question the pathogenic role of benzodiazepine-like ligands (Macdonald *et al.* 1997). Randomized trials on the use of flumazenil in patients with hepatic encephalopathy of differing severity show that only a minor percentage of patients—about 30%—show clinical or EEG improvement (Annese *et al.* 1998; Barbaro *et al.* 1998; Groeneweg *et al.* 1996; Laccetti *et al.* 2000), and no improvement was seen on cognitive and neurophysiological assessment of patients with subclinical cognitive impairment (Amodio *et al.* 1997). Also recently, no correlation was found between benzodiazepine-like substances levels and the degree of encephalopathy (Venturini *et al.* 2001). Traditional chronic management relies on lactulose, neomycin, and protein restriction with an uncertain role for the administration of branched-chain amino acids.

In progressive hepatic failure, encephalopathy will present as an inevitable progressive final evolution. When the portosystemic shunt of the venous intestinal blood is the main pathogenic mechanism, an acute excess of nitrogen due to increased alimentary intake, bleeding of oesophageal varices, and protein catabolism can acutely precipitate encephalopathy. The speed of the change may be more important than the actual ammonia level, which only partially parallels the severity of the encephalopathy (Venturini *et al.* 2001). There is a considerable degree of overlap between the levels of ammonia recorded in patients with liver disease and hepatic encephalopathy and those without signs of encephalopathy (Plum and Posner 1980*b*). Although absolute ammonia levels do not correlate well with the degree of encephalopathy (Venturini *et al.* 2001), ammonia still remains the best biochemical correlate of hepatic encephalopathy. The evidence reported, however, must lead to the conclusion that it is not ammonia *per se* that causes brain toxicity. Interestingly, MRI spectroscopy may help us to find more accurate metabolic counterparts of clinical findings but this research is at the moment only in progress (Jenkins and Kraft 1999).

Liver failure is not uncommon in advanced cancer due to metastatic disease and ammonia should be tested when cognitive symptoms are found and also when other liver function tests are not excessively abnormal or different than usual. The contribution of liver failure to the mortality of palliative care patients is unknown. In one series of patients with advanced cancer followed-up to death by a home-care-based palliative care service, hepatic failure was considered the main cause of death in 18% of cases (Groff 1993).

6.2.2   Uraemic encephalopathy

Renal failure is known to cause delirium but the cause of brain dysfunction in the course of uraemia is unknown (Tyler 1968). Urea is not responsible for brain toxicity and the relationship between blood levels of uraemia and encephalopathy is not linear. In general, plasma urea levels should be above 200 mg/dl to produce signs of encephalopathy, but delirium has been seen in cases whose levels were as low as 48 mg/dl, as in the case reported by Plum and Posner (1980*b*). In this situation the rapidity of the metabolic change is also very important, more than the absolute abnormality level. EEG changes correlate with uraemia (Hughes 1980; Lipowski 1990*b*). Parathormone and brain calcium abnormalities are one potential pathogenic mechanism that probably accounts for some clinical phenomena. Several guanidine-compounds, of which creatinine is one, may also play a role in uraemic encephalopathy. These substances accumulate in uraemia and have excitatory effects at the CNS level by activation of *N*-methyl-D-aspartate receptors (De Deyn *et al.* 2001).

Multifocal myoclonus is typically associated with uraemic encephalopathy and seizures are also frequent. Renal failure can be associated with electrolyte imbalance, metabolic acidosis, hypertensive encephalopathy, and, in the medically ill patient not affected by a primary renal illness, with other complications of the underlying primary pathological process. It can therefore be difficult to identify the aetiology of the delirium. Non-convulsive status epilepticus should also be suspected in acutely confused or stuporous patients in the terminal phases of renal failure (Chow *et al.* 2001). In patients with advanced terminal illness, dehydration, oliguria, or anuria are common terminal events. Some patients will have specific causes of renal failure such as bilateral hydronephrosis, infections, and drug toxicity. Low renal perfusion pressure is likely to intervene in most cases due to hypotension and low systolic stroke volume. The role of renal failure in characterizing the final phases of many progressive diseases is unknown, although Bruera and co-workers (1995) suggested that moderate hydration can be useful to preserve the renal clearance of drugs and metabolites in order to prevent agitated deliria.

6.2.3 Pulmonary encephalopathy and acid-base imbalances

Pulmonary encephalopathy is also defined as hypercapnic encephalopathy, and it is characteristic of advanced pulmonary disease such as chronic obstructive pulmonary disease (COPD). In this respect, it is worth considering that COPD and tobacco smoke are very frequent comorbidities in the palliative care patient, and extremely frequent in patients affected by lung cancer.

In pulmonary encephalopathy, the relative roles of hypercarbia, hypoxia, and respiratory acidosis may be difficult to ascertain. In general, CO_2 is narcotic due to its effect on the brain pH. Posner *et al.* (1965) suggested that neurological symptoms are probably related to the degree of brain cellular acidosis. Acute hypercarbia is less tolerated than a slow increase in pCO_2, as develops in cases of COPD. In patients with acute hypercarbia, 70 mm Hg of pCO_2 is sufficient to produce cerebral symptoms while the same level of hypercarbia can be well tolerated in COPD patients (Dulfano and Ishikawa 1965). The best correlate of encephalopathy in the disturbance of acid-base balance is cerebrospinal fluid (CSF) pH, which is controlled by homeostatic mechanisms that are very efficient, especially in metabolic acidosis, metabolic alkalosis, and respiratory alkalosis, and less so in respiratory acidosis (Posner and Plum 1967; Posner *et al.* 1965).

Intercurrent minor events can be crucial for the fragile balance of compensatory systems in the compromised patient. One typical example of this situation is the use of sedative drugs. Respiratory failure can develop in the progression of incurable illnesses in different patterns, depending on the patient's history and present disease. Acute dyspnoea can be suddenly caused by pleural effusion or superior vena cava syndrome or, more slowly, by progressive pulmonary parenchyma metastatic substitution or carcinomatous lymphangitis. Pulmonary infections are very common both in cancer and AIDS patients. Lawlor and co-workers (2000*b*) found that hypoxia associated with lung cancer or infection was a factor associated with irreversible deliria in advanced cancer patients. Dyspnoea is a severe and particularly distressful symptom associated with hypoxia, and has a compensatory role by stimulating ventilation in the attempt to keep pO_2 and pCO_2 within physiological limits. In the advanced patient with irreversible dyspnoea who is in high distress, palliative therapy with opioids and/or neuroleptics is often considered. One has to be aware that the delicate balance between respiratory frequency, pCO_2, and acidosis can be affected by the use of opioids or neuroleptics and by any modification of the internal milieu that decreases the respiratory centre's response to pCO_2 (Mercadante 1997). The relief of dyspnoea may parallel a slow increase of pCO_2 and acidosis, although this is not clinically evident, and hypoxia will not occur in most cases (Bruera et al. 1990). Hypercapnic encephalopathy can ensue and a vicious irreversible cycle can lead to a coma due to respiratory failure. Control of this situation would be possible by careful monitoring of arterial pO_2, pCO_2, and serum bicarbonate. The clinical conditions (prognosis, suffering, patient's wish, goals of care) will determine the choice between optimizing patient comfort versus maximizing respiratory function and biochemical control (Ventafridda et al. 1990b).

Respiratory failure, together with the metabolic abormalities already discussed, is a common scenario in the last days or hours of life for many terminal patients, but even in these cases the prevalence of respiratory failure as a cause of death is not known (Lawlor et al. 2000b). The only data available to us reports a 15% frequency of respiratory failure as the main cause of death in terminal cancer patients under hospice home-care (Groff 1993).

Pure metabolic changes due to systemic metabolic causes are probably more rare in palliative care than respiratory failure, but should not be discarded in cases with concurrent diabetes, hyponutrition or malabsorption, and renal failure. Diabetic ketoacidosis is the most common cause of encephalopathy of primarily metabolic origin (Posner and Plum 1967). Other rarer conditions can be found, e.g. cases of abnormal absorption of carbohydrates in short bowel syndrome combined with a dysmicrobic colonic flora (Gavazzi et al. 2001).

6.2.4 Cofactor deficiency

Nutritional reduced intake of vitamins is typical of patients with alcohol abuse, and it is not uncommon in the elderly or in patients with advanced cancer and anorexia. Thiamine (vitamin B1) deficiency is probably the most frequent vitamin deficiency and can manifest with an acute change of the state of consciousness, gross impairment of recent memory, and coma, for the endogenous reserve of this vitamin is easily depleted by relatively short-lived periods of insufficient intake. In the full-blown syndrome, dementia, abnormalities of eye movement, peripheral neuropathy, and hypotension are all present, but partial presentations with normal eye movements, modest peripheral neuropathy, and initial cognitive impairment or delirium are possible.

Thiamine has a key role in carbohydrate metabolism and its daily intake should be at least 1 mg, but intake increases when carbohydrates become the main source of energy. Thiamine bodily reserves are not abundant and are strictly dependent on alimentary intake. A number of factors can predispose to a relatively fast exhaustion of thiamine deposits: surgery followed or preceded by hyponutrition (Vidal et al. 2001); emesis associated with treatment with glucose IV solutions; and chemotherapy interfering with hepatic synthesis of thiamine. A significant association has been found between thiamine deficiency and neoplasms in a series of 31 paediatric patients (Vasconcelos et al. 1999). Early signs of thiamine deficiency occur after a week of thiamine deprivation.

For these reasons the role of thiamine deficiency has been investigated as an explanation of the increased risk of developing delirium in patients with poor general health, the elderly, or malnourished, but results have been not homogeneous (Barbato and Rodriguez 1994; O'Keeffe *et al.* 1994; Papersack *et al.* 1999). The addition of thiamine to the therapeutic regimen of a confused patient with poor general condition can be empirically recommended (1000 mg/day to start).

Another vitamin that is often neglected but has been associated with mental changes in hyponutrition and in alcoholic encephalopathy is nicotinic acid (vitamin PP; protects against pellagra; Serdaru *et al.* 1988). It could be supplemented in 250 mg tablets once a day in cases of severely reduced food intake and obscure encephalopathy (Checkley *et al.* 1939).

Vitamin B_{12} deficiency causes anaemia, polyneuropathy, spinal cord degeneration, and encephalopathy (Buchman *et al.* 1999). Cases of encephalopathy without anaemia have been described (Lindenbaum *et al.* 1988). Patients with gastric disease and malabsorption are at risk of vitamin B_{12} deficiency.

6.2.5 Electrolyte and water imbalances

In the medically ill, water balance can be easily affected because of insufficient attention to input and output of fluids. Particular attention must be paid to renal function, especially when IV fluids or diuretic therapy are instituted. Hyponatraemia is the most common condition. It is frequently an effect of the syndrome of inappropriate antidiuretic hormone secretion (SIADH), which is a complication of many drugs (morphine, cyclophosphamide, vincristine) and brain lesions. When hyponatraemia develops rapidly, brain oedema and change in neuronal membrane excitability cause encephalopathy ranging from delirium with asterixis and multifocal myoclonus, to coma and seizures. Figure 6.1 shows the relationship between sodium plasma levels and brain dysfunction found in an early study by Arieff *et al.* (1976).

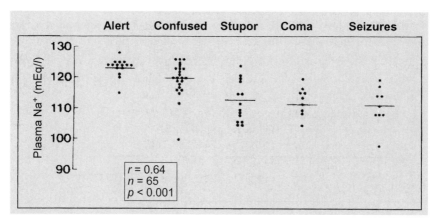

Fig. 6.1 This figure shows the relationship of sodium plasma levels and level of consciousness. A relationship between severity of clinical findings and hyponatraemia is quite evident, but also a wide degree of overlapping of laboratory values across very different clinical conditions. Reproduced with permission from: Arieff AL, Llach F, Massry SG: Neurological manifestations and morbidity of hyponatremia: correlation with brain water and electrolytes. *Medicine* (1976); 55: 121–9.

In patients with advanced cancer, it is very common to find that sodium levels are slightly or moderately below normal limits (between 130 and 120 mEq/l). The role of this finding in the pathophysiology of other complications—the so-called 'deterioration of general condition'—that we commonly see in the clinical picture of palliative care patients is not known. All electrolytes should be checked including magnesium. In rare cases even hypophosphataemia is a possibility (Hall *et al.* 1994).

Electrolyte abnormalities are, however, always to be considered in acute changes of mental status. Rare causes can be sought in particular conditions, but sodium, potassium, calcium, and magnesium should never be left out of a diagnostic screening (Hall *et al.* 1994). Hypercalcaemia is frequently associated with bone metastases or is a result of paraneoplastic secretion of endocrine active substances. When serum calcium levels are above 12 mg/dl, cognition can be impaired. Hypoalbuminaemia is frequently found in advanced cases, where the fraction of calcium ions bound to albumin is decreased; therefore it is important to calculate the actual calcaemia by correcting it for hypoalbuminaemia.

6.3 Toxic causes of delirium

6.3.1 Anticholinergic drugs

Since ancient times it has been known that anticholinergic drugs have the ability to cause delirium Belladonna alkaloids were described as deliriogenic by Theofrastus as long ago as the fourth century BC. Experimental human studies on anticholinerigic delirium were summarized in Chapter 2 (see Itil and Fink 1968) and show that drugs such as scopolamine, ditran, and atropine can cause delirium depending on dosage. Lower doses (e.g. scopolamine, 0.3–0.8 mg) usually produce somnolence, higher doses (atropine, $\geq$ 5 mg; scopolamine, 1 mg) produce agitated florid delirium, while paradoxical effects of low doses have also been demonstrated. The following observations are relevant to understanding the toxic CNS effect of these drugs.

- Attention and cognition are diminished by the administration of anticholinergics.
- Pharmacokinetics changes in the elderly and in children enhance the bioavailability of these drugs.
- In the ageing or demented brain the anticholinergic system is already compromised as part of the pathogenesis of global cognitive deficit.
- The elderly and children are more susceptible to delirium when comparable lower doses of these drugs are administered.
- Serum anticholinergic activity has been studied as one of the factors that might explain different clinical conditions such as drug toxicity and postoperative delirium.
- A list of the drugs in which CNS toxicity is believed to be related to their anticholinergic activity is given in Table 6.3.

True anticholinergic delirium should be reversible with physostigmine. The use of physostigmine is restricted to cases of proven anticholinergic toxicity (even though cases of miscellaneous deliria are reported to respond to cholinergic stimulation)

Table 6.3 Drugs with anticholinergic activity

Protoytpical anticholinergics

  Belladonna alkaloids

  Atropine

  Scopolamine

Tricyclic antidepressants

Marzine

Diphenidramine

Promethazine

Biperidene

Trihexyphenidyl

Chlorpromazine

Hyoscine butylbromide

Robinul

Hypnotics

  Barbiturates

  Chloral hydrate

  Paraldehyde

  Bromides

  Benzodiazepines

Antibiotics

Antimalarial

Antituberculous

Antiviral

Antifungal

Anticonvulsants

Antiparkinsonian

  Amantadine

---

because of the risk of inducing cholinergic toxic effects by using physostigmine. Anticholinergic toxicities should be associated with some other physical symptoms of cholinergic overactivity that are reported in Table 6.4. The recent introduction of cholinergic drugs for the therapy of dementia offers an interesting opportunity to test these drugs in some acute confusional states.

6.3.2 Opioids

Opioid therapy for pain, dyspnoea, and terminal sedation is a mainstay of palliative medicine. Delirium can be the result of some effects of opioids on the CNS (Stiefel

Table 6.4 Syndrome of anticholinergic toxicity

Dilated pupils with reduced light reactivity

Hot, dry skin and mucous membranes

Flushed face, peripheral vasodilatation

Blurred vision, impaired accommodation

Tachycardia

Urinary retention

Hypertension

Tachypnoea

Fever

and Morant 1991). To understand opioid-induced delirium, it is necessary to review the sedative activity of opioids and other toxic effects of opioids on the CNS (Lawlor 2002). Among the central side-effects of opioids, the modification of cognition and vigilance is the most important limitation in dose titration (Ripamonti and Bruera 1997). The subjective sensation of mental clouding and sedation ('foggy, obtunded' in patients' words) is the single most disliked component of opioid therapy and, in our experience, it is the most important reason to resist dose escalation, often before sedation or cognitive impairment is clinically evident to an external examiner. Subjective sedation is commonly related to sleepiness. Subjectively, patients feel as if they might easily fall asleep especially while reading or lying in bed in a quiet environment. Sleepiness can be considered objectively as the subject's propensity to fall asleep or, alternatively, as the subject's subjective sensation of sleepiness (Johns 1993). The two concepts do not necessarily overlap (Johnson *et al.* 1990). Opioid drugs induce sleepiness but have never been studied systematically in this regard by using a specific definition of sleepiness. While looking at the central side-effects of opioids it is therefore important to distinguish between subjective sedation, objective sedation, cognitive impairment, and delirium.

Patients' subjective sensation of opioid-induced sedation does not correlate with the impairment of cognitive performance as, at formal testing, patients report sedation while cognitive tests can still be performed efficiently (Caraceni *et al.* 1993). Opioid-sedation is dose-related and is a pharmacological phenomenon that shows dynamic and kinetic related changes. The only human data available on this subject comes from the EEG changes induced by potent opioids used for anaesthesia. In this setting opioids increase the power in the range of low (1–10 Hz) EEG frequencies, and specifically the percentage of delta rhythm (< 4 Hz; Scott *et al.* 1991). With this method the EEG slowing to the delta frequency was related to the drug plasma level. EEG sensitivity was also inversely related to age, showing a pharmacodynamic change due to ageing (Scott and Stanski 1987), demonstrating that the elderly brain is more sensitive to opioid effects. Slowing of EEG frequency is also a common finding in delirium as expected in a condition that shares with sedation a lowered level of consciousness. The relationship between these EEG changes and the clinical condition of chronic or acute opioid administration for pain is practically unknown. In the only study available, patients who were taking opioids alone for pain did not show cognitive failure or EEG changes, while patients taking benzodiazepines alone or in combination with opioids had both cognitive disturbances and EEG changes (Hendler *et al.* 1980).

In animal models, opioids changed the EEG organization of normal sleep of which the most constant finding was a reduction of rapid eye movement (REM) sleep. There was a similar finding in humans but in an experimental model that involved ex-addicts (Kay *et al.* 1969). These observations have never been reproduced in patients with opioid-induced delirium.

Cognitive performance is diminished when opioids are acutely given to normal volunteers (Zacny 1995) but in patients with pain the situation is more complex. Cognitive impairment has been documented after increasing dosage (Bruera *et al.* 1989, 1992*c*). It is reasonable to think that cognitive impairment is likely to occur when vigilance is compromised to an extent that the performance of complex tasks and thought are affected (Bruera *et al.* 1987). In chronic use a balance between the therapeutic analgesic effect and the sedative effect seems to occur, favouring a more functional cognitive situation that can be compatible with car-driving (Galski *et al.* 2000). When pain is controlled by adequate opioid dosing, the failure of cognitive performance is more related to the the pain and the underlying general conditions than to opioid therapy effects (Sjogren and Banning 1989; Sjogren *et al.* 2000). Tolerance to the sedative effects is also likely to develop in chronic dosing as has been demonstrated in studies on opioid addicts (Zacny 1995).

Objective sedation is, by definition, a reduced level of consciousness that can increase to the point of inducing sleep (morphine is named after the Greek god of sleep). A patient who has a significant degree of sedation and fails in keeping his attention on external stimuli and in performing cognitive tasks fulfils the clinical definition of delirium (Bruera *et al.* 1987). In our opinion it is therefore possible to talk of dose-related opioid-induced delirium of a somnolent form that can be readily induced in every patient depending on the dose employed. This type of effect is likely to be mediated via the interaction with opioid receptors, and be part of the opioid sedative properties discussed above. This effect can obviously be worsened by concomitant CNS depressive therapies or comorbidities often encountered in the advanced phases of terminal illnesses (Leipzig *et al.* 1987). The immediate predecessor of this condition could be sleepiness, when the arousal and attention are still sufficient to allow adequate cognitive performance.

The sedative effect of opioids and of morphine in particular has been associated with their inhibitory action on the cholinergic activating system. Peripheral anticholinergic effects of opioids are well known. As we discussed in Chapter 3, central cholinergic neuromodulation is essential for the regulation of arousal, the sleep–wakefulness cycle, and also respiratory function. Opioids have an inhibitory effect on cholinergic transmission at many CNS levels that are deemed relevant in controlling these functions. It is therefore possible that some central effects of opioids that are relevant to the syndrome of delirium—hallucination, disruption of the sleep–wakefulness cycle, diminished arousal and attention, and cognitive failure—are mediated at least in part through the cholinergic system. Recently, some clinicians who favour this hypothesis have tried to enhance cholinergic transmission with acetylcholinesterase (AChE) inhibitors in order to reduce sedation and delirium-like symptoms related to opioids (Slatkin *et al.* 2001).

A different set of opioid-induced CNS symptoms have been also reported—hallucinations, myoclonus, hyperalgesia, and seizures. These symptoms are found at times in isolation or can be part of the syndrome of delirium (Caraceni *et al.* 1994; Gregory *et al.* 1992). Drug-induced hallucinations or generalized myoclonus may be the only sign of encephalopathy due to opioid medication.

In one of our patients, delirium and visual hallucinations were present when 60 mg of oral morphine was prescribed daily, changing to visual hallucinations without delirium when the dose of morphine was reduced to 40 mg per day. In another patient, visual hallucinations occurred in a totally clear state of mind with 90 mg of oral morphine a day. In this last patient the same type of hallucinations was reported after switching the therapy to oral methadone and titrating the dose to 18 mg per day (Caraceni *et al.* 1994). (See also the cases reported by Jellema 1987 and Bruera *et al.* 1992*d*.) These cases demonstrate that delirium can manifest, in a paradoxical way, with or without associated hallucinations and myoclonus, with low to moderate doses of opioids. Some cases are facilitated by other concurrent toxic or metabolic factors (Bortolussi *et al.* 1994; Caraceni *et al.* 1994) but others, as shown by the examples, seem to reflect a true specific opioid toxicity.

Of the three cases of myoclonus reported by MacDonald *et al.* (1993) with high systemic opioid therapy (hydromorphone, IV infusions of 200 mg/h, 200 mg/h, and 65 mg/h), two were also delirious. At high levels of opioid administration, this type of excitatory toxicity seems to occur very often, provided that a a high enough dose can be reached without the onset of sedative or CNS depressive limiting effects. In some patients myoclonus evolved into generalized convulsions without other signs of encephalopathy or delirium in between (Hagen and Swanson 1997). Patients reporting myoclonus and eventually seizures have often reported generalized hyperalgesia and allodynia as well (Sjogren *et al.* 1993*b*). Myoclonus and hyperalgesia or their association seem to be the results of an excitatory CNS effect of opioid on some non-opioid neural circuits. With systemic administration, multifocal generalized myoclonus and total body hyperalgesia have been described (Sjogren *et al.* 1993*a*, *b*, 1994). Seizures can occur at very high doses (Bruera and Pereira 1997; Hagen and Swanson 1997) and delirium with hallucinations is also reported (Bruera and Pereira 1997; MacDonald *et al.* 1993; Sjogren *et al.* 1993*b*).

With the use of spinal opioids, both intrathecal and epidural, hyperalgesia and myoclonus can be seen with a segmental distribution without signs of encephalopathy (Cartwright *et al.* 1993; De Conno *et al.* 1991a; Glavina and Robertshaw 1988; Kloke *et al.* 1994). Different opioids have been associated with symptoms of CNS hyperexcitability, including morphine (Stiefel and Morant 1991), hydromorphone, sufentanyl (Bowdle and Rooke 1994), fentanyl (Steinberg *et al.* 1992), and methadone (Mercadante 1995).

The most credited pathophysiological mechanism for these effects implies a non-opioidergic disinhibition of glycinergic and/or GABAergic control systems that would bring about or cause an activation of the NMDA receptors. Hyperalgesia and seizures can be induced in animal models and are not reversed by naloxone (Frenk et al. 1984; Yaksh et al. 1986). Spinal cord neurons respond with paroxysmal depolarization to the application of opiates antagonizing postsynaptic glycine and GABA inhibition in a way that resembles the action of strychnine (Werz and MacDonald 1982). It is therefore possible that this peculiar non-opioid action is responsible, when high doses are employed or, for idiosyncratic reasons, for segmental or generalized myoclonus and hyperalgesia, hallucinations, delirium, and seizures depending on the neural system involved.

A more complete and complex view of the interaction of opioid and non-opioid systems has been reviewed by Frenk (1983; Van Praag et al. 1993), showing that some convulsive effects are also opioid-receptor mediated. This possibility is confirmed by at least one patient with encephalopathy with generalized myoclonus and hallucinations secondary to fentanyl overdosing who responded dramatically to naloxone (Bruera and Pereira 1997).

The role of morphine metabolites, morphine-3- and -6-glucuronides, in producing these effects is unsettled. Their accumulation in renal failure may be relevant to the development of toxicity (Sjogren et al. 1998) but it has been very difficult to define when and how morphine glucoronides have a role, if any, in the pharmacological effects of morphine in humans (Anderson et al. 2002; Lotsch et al. 1997; Morita et al. 2002; Teseo et al. 1995). Glare et al. (1990) have suggested that normorphine may also have a role to play. Other opioids such as fentanyl produce, as shown, similar effects and do not have known active metabolites. Meperidine on the other hand has more neuroexcitatory side-effects due to the accumulation of normeperidine (Szeto et al. 1977). Recently, a case was reported with anileridine associated with delirium (Moss 1995). However, oxycodone seems to be less often associated with toxic reaction (Maddocks et al. 1996). Meperidine and tramadol also have serotonergic effects that could justify some symptoms of toxicity mediated by serotonergic mechanisms.

The mechanisms underlying what is commonly seen in clinical practice are therefore likely to be multiple and still poorly understood. The contribution, for instance, of this type of excitatory toxicity to cases of terminal restlessness is unknown. The role of opiod- and non-opioid-mediated effects, concomitant drugs, or active opioid metabolites is still unknown. The presence of myoclonus, seizures, and other symptoms in such cases should be better documented (Potter et al. 1989).

Specific management recommendations for opioid-induced delirium are difficult to establish at the present state of knowledge. However, several guidelines can be tentatively offered to reduce the risk of this type of reaction (Cherny et al. 2001).

6.3.3   Serotonin syndrome

The availability and popularity of selective serotonin re-uptake inhibitors (SSRIs) for the treatment of depression has contributed to the slow epidemic diffusion of a previously rarely recognized toxic reaction due to overstimulation of serotonin receptors in the CNS (Gillman 1995, 1998, 1999; Sternbach 1991). This syndrome, originally described in 1960, has been reported more and more frequently in the last 10 years. It is characterized clinically by signs of encephalopathy (confusion, restlessness, myoclonus, hyperreflexia, rigidity, coma) and of autonomic instability (fever, dia-phoresis, diarrhoea, flushing, tachycardia, tachypnoea, blood pressure changes, mid-riasis, shivering, and tremor). It can be fatal or have a more benign course. It is usually seen after the addition of a serotonergic drug to a drug regimen already containing serotonin-enhancing drugs. Table 6.5 (Bodner *et al.* 1995; Bonin *et al.* 1999; Chambost *et al.* 2000; Daniels 1998; Gill *et al.* 1999; Hamilton and Malone 2000; Kesavan and Sobala 1999; Lee and Lee 1999; Margolese and Chouinard 2000; Perry 2000; Rosebush *et al.* 1999; Smith and Wenegrat 2000; Weiner 1999) reports the drugs and the combi-nations that have been associated with the syndrome. For the palliative care setting it is interesting to note that, in general, SSRIs are now more often found in the thera-peutic regimens of patients with advanced illness for their beneficial effects on mood and night-time sleep and that, in the complex polypharmacy so common in these patients, unexpected reactions can become less rare. Table 6.5 lists cases involving meperidine, tramadol, and dextrometorphan. These two last drugs at least are likely to be used in palliative care. Cases of delirium following the use of SSRIs have already been reported and may represent manifestations of partial serotonin syndrome or of a different toxic effect from the same drugs (Rothschild 1995).

Case report

A 72-year-old man, affected by a laryngeal carcinoma with local relapse and lung metastases, tracheostomy, and enteral nutrition via a percutaneous endoscopic gastrostomy (PEG) tube, had pain in his throat radiating bilaterally to both ears, insomnia, depression, cough, and dyspnoea due to the formation of mucous and necrotic material in the tracheostomy cannula. His drug regimen included: tramadol, 50 mg every 8 h; citalopram, 5 mg at night; ketorolac, 30 mg *pro re nata* (p.r.n.; 'as circumstances may require'); gabapentin, 200 mg every 8 h. When the tramadol dose was increased to 100 mg every 8 h, he developed generalized myoclonus, rigidity, diaphoresis, and delirium. Admitted to the hospital palliative care ward the therapeu-tic regimen was switched to morphine subcutaneous (SC) infusion alone (30 mg/day) with progressive recovery of the neurological status. The clinical symptoms fulfil the characteristics of the serotonin syndrome. The pathogenesis may involve a metabolic interaction of tramadol with citalopram or a pharmacodynamic potentiation of serotonergic effects by the combination of the two drugs.

6.3.4   Steroid-induced delirium

This is also commonly described as steroid psychosis. Since steroids are so commonly used in palliative care, it is worth bearing in mind that the possibility that corticos-teroid therapy is the direct cause of delirium should be considered with a dose equiv-alent to at least 40 mg of prednisone per day (see also the case report in Section 5.5). Usually at least a week or two of therapy are needed for psychiatric complications to develop (Stiefel *et al.* 1989). The symptoms can range from depression to mania and psychosis. The true incidence of mental changes related to steroid administration in palliative care is unknown. High doses are often reported to cause euphoria. One study, comparing cancer patients receiving high-dose dexamethasone (100 mg IV and

Table 6.5 Drugs and drug combinations associated with serotonin syndrome. (Modified from Bodner *et al.* (1995))

Drug	Combinations
Tryptopan	Fluoxetine
	Nonselective MAOIs
	Clomipramine
Fluoxetine	Carbamazepine
	Pentazocine
	MAOIs
	Moclobemide
	Nefazodone
	Tramadol
	Mirtazapine
Fluvoxamine	Alone
	Nefazodone
Venlafaxine	Alone
Paroxetine	Risperidone
	Moclobemide
Sertraline	Isocarboxazide
	Nortriptyline
	Tranylcypromine
	Erythromycin
	Buspirone
	Loxapine
Trazodone	Buspirone
	Nefazodone
Moclobemide	Citalopram
	Imipramine
Bromocriptine	L-Dopa
Meperidine	Iproniazid
	MAOIs
	Moclobemide
Phenelzine	3,4 Methylenedioxy-methamphetamine
Dextrometorphan	Nonselective MAOIs
Dothiepine	Alone

Modified with permission from Bodner, R.A., Lynch, T., Lewis, L. and Kahn, D., Serotonin syndrome, *Neurology*, 45 (1995) 219–23. Copyright 1995 American Academy of Neurology.

then a tapering schedule) for spinal cord compression with a group of patients not receiving steroids, found a higher incidence of depression and a tendency for greater incidence of delirium in patients treated with steroids (Breitbart *et al.* 1993).

Steroid withdrawal can also cause delirium together with other symptoms of hypocortisolism (Campbell and Schubert 1991). It is a useful precaution to taper slowly and discontinue steroids in any patient who does not need them for specific indications (Twycross 1992).

6.3.5   Miscellaneous drugs

A very extensive range of drugs is continuously reported in the literature because of the drugs' potential or actual association with delirium. Practically every drug with known CNS activity can potentially cause delirium with mechanisms that are only sometimes understood. In some cases anticholinergic properties are likely and are the first to be blamed. For most drugs however, mechanisms are unknown or hypothetical. Table 6.6 shows that old and new drugs continue to be reported as causes of delirium.

6.3.6   Drug interactions

The role of metabolic interactions as a cause of toxicity in palliative care is more and more likely as the number of drugs increases and the patient's general condition deteriorates (Bernard and Bruera 2000; Cheng *et al.* 2002). The induction or inhibition of hepatic enzyme metabolism is an important source of variability in drug effect and can lead to unexpected toxic reactions. The cytochrome P450 system is made of a family of more than 20 isoenzymes, among which CYP 2D6 and CYP 3A4 metabolize 80% of known drugs. The article by Bernard and Bruera (2000) reports on a number of examples of drugs of common use in palliative care that have high or moderate probability of interacting with the same metabolic pathways and of leading to unexpectedly high or low levels of a drug with the consequence of under- or overdosing (methadone, codeine, oxycodone, haloperidol, tricyclic antidepressants (TCAs), SSRIs, monoamine oxidase (MAO) inhibitors, benzodizepines, macrolides, azoles, rifampin, antifungals).

In particular, CYP 3A4 metabolizes fentanyl, alfentanyl methadone, alprazolam, midazolam, and dexamethasone and can be inhibited by most antifungal drugs, fluoxetine, and norfloxacin, while it is induced by dexamethasone, phenytoin, carbamazepine, phenobarbital, rifampicin, erythromycin, omeprazole, and cyclo-phosphamide. CYP 2D6 metabolizes codeine, oxycodone, tramadol, haloperidol, risperidone, fluoxetine, paroxetine, venlafaxine, and desimipramine. It is inhibited by cimetidine, desimipramine, fluoxetine, paroxetine, haloperidol, and sertraline and induced by carbamazepine, phenobarbital, and phenytoin.

These examples can be integrated with the available literature and may also explain cases of so-called serotonin syndromes as serotonergic drugs have significant interactions as already evident from the brief list provided (Bernard and Bruera 2000).

However the clinical role of drug interaction in producing specific effects may be very difficult to ascertain. Laboratory *in vitro* data may not be applicable to the clinical situation while *in vivo* other circumstances may be operating to change the effect that was expected on the basis of laboratory data (Bernard and Bruera 2000).

Table 6.6 Recent reports of drug toxicities manifesting with delirium

Drug	Reference
Fluoxetine	Leinonen et al. 1993
Mefloquine	Hall et al. 1994
Diphenydramine	Tejera et al. 1994; Agostini et al. 2001
Herbal medicine (loperamide, theales, valerian)	Khawaja et al. 1999
Amiodarone	Barry and Franklin 1999
Clarithromycin	Mermelstein 1998
Lithium neuroleptic combination	Normann et al. 1998
Clozapine	Wilkins-Ho and Hollander 1997; Szymanski et al. 1991
Risperidone	Tavcar and Dernovsek 1998
Diet pills (phentermine)	Bagri and Reddy 1998
Nizatidine	Galynker and Tendler 1997
Tacrine	Trzepacz et al. 1996
Omeprazole	Heckmann et al. 2000
Paroxetine–benztropine combination	Amstrong and Schweitzer 1997
Sertraline–haloperidol–benztropine combination	Byelry et al. 1996
Famotidine (6 cases)	Catalano et al. 1996
H2 receptor blockers	Nickell 1991
Ranitidine	Eisendrath and Ostroff 1990
Tacrine–ibuprofen interaction	Hooten and Pearlson 1996
Steroids	Stoudemine et al. 1996
Benzodiazepine–clozapine combination	Jackson et al. 1995
Mianserin	Bonne et al. 1995
Ciprofloxacin	McDermott et al. 1991
Ofloxacillin	Fennig and Mauas 1992
Cyclosporin	Steg and Garcia 1991
Ranitidine and cimetidine	Kim et al. 1996
Ethanol and niacin co-ingestion	Schwab and Bachhuber 1991
Zolpidem	Freudenreich and Menza 2000
Donepezil	Kawashima and Yamada 2002
Paclitaxel	Ziske et al. 2002
Ziconotide	Levin et al. 2002
Interleukin-2 and interferon	van Steijn et al. 2001

Case report

A patient affected by an advanced head and neck carcinoma presented with oral candidiasis, pain, and dysphagia. The patient received fentanyl transdermally (50 mg/h patch) and itroconazole 200 mg b.i.d, and, 24 hours after starting this therapy, developed an agitated delirium with myoclonus. All laboratory examinations and head CT scan were normal. The fentanyl patch was stopped and changed to oral methadone 7 mg t.i.d. without any change in neurological status in the following 48 hours. Methadone was also stopped and changed to morphine IV with resolution of the neurological symptoms. After a few days itroconazole was also discontinued and transdermal fentanyl reinstituted at the same dose (50 mg/h) without further complications (this case is reported courtesy of Dr Oscar Corli, personal communication). The most likely explanation involves the interaction of both fentanyl and methadone with itroconazole. Morphine, which is metabolized by glucoronization and does not interact with the P450 enzyme system (see list and literature), did not cause toxic effects and nor did fentanyl when administered alone.

6.4 Delirium and structural brain lesions

Structural brain lesions that can often cause delirium are vascular lesions and tumours. We can classify these lesions into two broad categories: lesions that cause widespread brain damage and focal lesions. All of these conditions, whether vascular, due to tumour, or to other causes, can produce reduced cerebral blood flow, raised intracranial pressure, and decreased brain metabolism.

6.4.1 Vascular causes of delirium

In the case of cerebrovascular disease, delirium can potentially be caused by focal or widespread cerebral damage (Table 6.7). Ischaemic stroke, without signs of intracranial hypertension, is the only condition where a precise focal aetiology of delirium can be explored and crucial brain areas for the development of this syndrome should manifest themselves.

The frequency of delirium in ischaemic strokes is uncertain. Two recent prospective studies found a prevalence of 24.3% (Henon *et al.* 1999) and 48% (Gustafson *et al.* 1991*b*), respectively, whereas cerebral hemorrhage is more frequently associated with delirium in up to 53% of cases (Dunne *et al.* 1986). Case reports associated some focal

Table 6.7 Cerebrovascular diseases that can be associated with delirium

Cerebral thrombosis or embolism

Cerebral haemorrhage

Subdural haematoma

Hypertensive encephalopathy

Cerebral vasculitis

Disseminated intravascular coagulation (DIC)

Other coagulopathies (e.g. Moscowitz syndrome)

ischaemic lesions with the onset of delirium. These lesions affected the right middle cerebral artery territory, left posterior cerebral artery territory, hippocampal area, lingula and fusiform gyrus, or thalamus (Lipowski 1990*b*; Trzepacz 1994*a*). Acute agitated deliria have been reported after an infarction of the right medial cerebral artery (Mesulam *et al.* 1976). In general, some observations suggest a higher frequency of delirium with right-sided lesions. On the basis of the attention deficit associated with these lesions, some authors have put forward the theory that delirium is primarily due to a disturbance of attention. With respect to these observations, most of the old case series do not offer a specific definition of delirium (Dunne *et al.* 1986).

In an article that used DSM-IV criteria for diagnosing delirium in stroke patients, the authors were able to define several important clinicopathological aspects associated with the onset of the syndrome (Henon *et al.* 1999). Pre-existing and concurrent morbid factors that were associated with delirium at univariate analysis were older age, alcohol consumption, previous cognitive decline, leukoaraiosis, more severe cerebral atrophy scores on CT scan, and metabolic or infectious disorders. The stroke location did not predict the onset of delirium, but a negative association with posterior fossa lesions was found. After logistic regression analyses the only factors that retained independent association with the presence of delirium were pre-existing cognitive impairment and metabolic or infectious disorders. When only the patients with previous cognitive impairment were considered, the presence of a right superficial lesion was independently associated with the onset of delirium. While in-hospital mortality was not affected by the presence of delirium, overall functional recovery and neurological outcome were worse for the patients who had delirium (Ferro *et al.* 2002; Henon *et al.* 1999; Sandberg *et al.* 2001).

If a strict clinical definition of delirium is used, a single brain lesion is very rarely sufficient to produce the full syndrome *per se*, and, more importantly, although some clinical observations suggest that at times a lesion of one brain area will produce delirium, there is no evidence that this type of lesion is invariably associated with delirium. Deficits in attention, language, and cognition that are commonly associated with focal brain lesions are not sufficient to cause delirium. Delirium can again be seen as a multifactorial syndrome that can also be precipitated by a focal brain lesion in predisposed patients or when concurrent precipitating factors are present. Right-sided lesions affecting attention and orientation are more likely to cause delirium when unfavourable underlying conditions are already operating.

The differential diagnosis of focal cerebral disorders causing selective failure of higher brain function versus delirium has already been discussed in Chapter 5.

Lesions in the hypothalamus have been associated with hypersomnia a condition that may largely overlap with the clinical definition of delirium (see later, Fig. 6.4).

Other cerebrovascular diseases, such as hypertensive encephalopathy, subdural haematoma, brain haemorrhage, multiple brain embolisms (Fig. 6.2), disseminated intravascular coagulation (DIC), and vasculitis (Table 6.6), can cause delirium via their interference with brain metabolism and function. In these cases, it is very difficult to say whether the pathogenetic mechanism has to do with the 'diffuse' cerebral hypometabolism or with the 'specific' failure of those hypothalamic and brainstem structures that are crucial for maintaining a normal state of consciousness.

6.4.2 Tumours

Altered mental status and psychiatric symptoms can be found in association with brain tumours, whether primary or metastatic, due to two main causes: the direct effect of the tumour on the brain or the effects of therapies. The clinical findings will be compatible with a diagnosis of delirium or dementia depending on the time course of the operating mechanism, potential reversibility, and the type of cognitive decline (see also Section 7.5). The differential diagnosis will not always be easy or clear-cut.

Brain tumours

Brain tumours often present with changes in cognition and personality, depressed mood, apathetic behaviour, memory failure, and disorientation to space and time. Clinical findings can develop subacutely but, at times, the onset is acute as in delirium. Attention can be affected and the level of consciousness as well. Findings will depend on the site and type of cerebral lesion. The principal mechanisms that cause mental changes and compromised consciousness due to the presence of intracranial tumour can be focal, due to compression (direct or due to oedema) on structures that are important for cognition and the regulation of consciousness level (the hypothalamus and the brainstem; Figs 6.3 and 6.4), or diffuse due to intracranial hypertension, hydrocephalus, or interference with brain metabolism and nutrition. The patient in Fig. 6.4 had a specific hypersomniac disorder that was characterized by easily falling

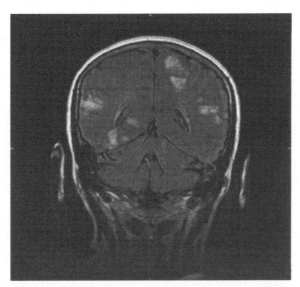

Fig. 6.2 Multiple ischaemic cortical areas are visible in this coronal MR image of the brain as white areas within the grey appearance of the normal brain tissue. This patient had metastatic colon carcinoma and multiple chemotherapy courses. Personality change and vigilance abnormalities were the first signs of brain ischaemia. The clinical picture progressed to coma and death. Multiple embolisms are likely to be the cause of such diffuse ischaemic disorder, probably due to a predisposing factor associated to the primary disease or therapy such as non-bacterial thrombotic endocarditis.

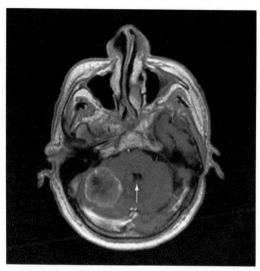

Fig. 6.3 Cerebellar metastases from small-cell lung cancer. The lesion is compressing the fourth ventricle and the underlying brainstem (arrow). The patient presented with somnolence, inattention, and delirium. In this case, compression on the ventricle could interfere with CSF circulation, or direct compression on the brainstem could be the cause of compromised consciousness.

asleep if not stimulated, even while talking to the examining physician, but with pre-served cognitive functions when fully awake. In view of this, it is very helpful to remember again the distinction between assessing the level of consciousness as opposed to the content of consciousness.

When tumour causes oedema and intracranial hypertension, fluctuations of intracranial pressure (plateau waves) can be responsible for unexpected, reversible, acute changes of mental status (Posner 1995). The association of headache and papilloedema greatly facilitate the diagnosis, but these findings can be absent.

Tumours can widely diffuse to the brain and cause global cognitive failure by miliariform or bulky metastatic lesions, or white matter diffuse infiltration such as in glioblastoma multiformis.

Case report

A 45-year-old woman presented with progressive difficulties of attention and mem-ory. Physical examination showed no focal neurological signs but short-term memory and calculation failure with slight constructional apraxia as shown by reproducing a simple design. Brain MRI with contrast (Fig. 6.5) showed a lesion of the corpus callo-sum. In this case the mild compromise of vigilance, slight disorientation with more pronounced and specific short-term memory deficit would make the diagnosis of delirium controversial. Cases like this not uncommonly progress with widespread white matter infiltration leading to profound dementia and other neurological impairment (aphasia, paralysis) before dying.

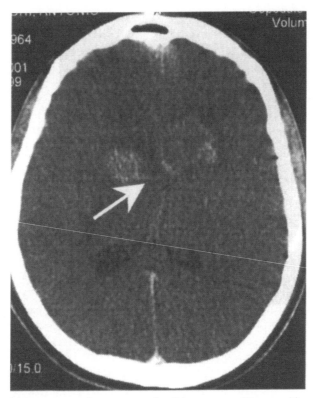

Fig. 6.4 Cerebral metastases from non-small-cell lung cancer. CT scan with contrast. Two sizeable lesions can be seen in the deep cerebral areas surrounded by oedema and compressing the thalamus and probably the underlying hypothalamus. A significant shift of the midline structures towards the right can be seen (arrow). A pronounced reduction of vigilance was the main symptom. The patient was oriented when awake but tended to go to sleep very easily if not stimulated.

Brain metastases

Brain parenchymal metastases and meningeal metastases from systemic cancer present with signs of altered cognition in about 50% of cases even before giving rise to other symptoms or focal signs (Formaglio and Caraceni 1998; Posner 1995; Wasserstrom *et al.* 1982). In the advanced phases of cancer, brain metastases are statistically associated with an increased risk of developing delirium, together with other clinical factors such as dyspnoea, anorexia, and low performance and clinical prediction of survival (Caraceni *et al.* 2000).

Case report

A 56-year-old man with metastatic melanoma presented with disorientation to space and time, low vigilance, and perseveration, without other focal signs. No metabolic,

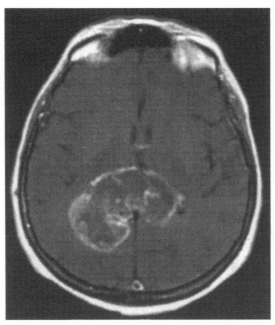

Fig. 6.5 Glioblastoma multiformis (MRI with gadolinium) presenting with memory impairment and slight mental changes (see text).

biochemical, or haematological abnormalities could be found. A CT scan of the head showed multiple brain metastases (at least 48 could be counted by the radiologist).

In another case, a 62-year-old woman with metastastic breast cancer was referred to the neurology unit because of depression and confusion. Her neurological examination was normal and her cognitive status examination showed only psychomotor slowing and apathy. This finding was reinforced by her husband's report of a major and sudden change in her mood and usually active behaviour. A CT scan with contrast showed multiple brain lesions with relevant brain oedema and frontal lobe involvement (Fig. 6.6).

Both cases show acute behavioural and cognitive symptoms. In the first case, the diagnosis of delirium is relatively straightforward. In the second case, it is more likely that the compromise of frontal lobe functions resulted in behavioural inhibition and loss of drive dominating the clinical picture.

Leptomeningeal metastases

Case studies show that microscopic meningeal infiltration can cause mental changes without focal signs and symptoms (Trachman *et al.* 1991; Weitzener *et al.* 1995). Seeding of malignant cells to the meninges can cause hydrocephalus (Fig. 6.7), but, before imaging can show cerebral ventricle dilatation, the CSF dynamics is often already altered and can by itself cause symptoms due to intracranial pressure changes (Grossman *et al.* 1982). Encephalopathy due to meningeal metastases can also be explained by tumour cell seeding to the meninges and interfering with CSF formation

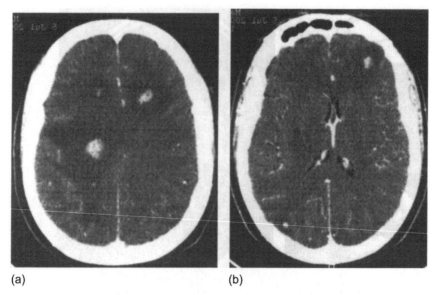

(a)   (b)

Fig. 6.6 Metastatic breast cancer. The patient presented with depression, behavioural changes, and psychomotor slowing. (a) The CT scan shows contrast-enhancing lesions with oedema and mass effect. (b) One lesion is located in the left frontal lobe and causes significant oedema.

and re-absorption, competing with the brain parenchyma for essential nutrients, and/or producing ischaemic damage by infiltrating the Virchow–Robin spaces.

The classic findings of papilloedema, severe headaches, or meningismus can be absent as in the case summarized in Fig. 6.7 (Grossman *et al.* 1982). As already mentioned in the case of brain tumour, fluctuations of intracranial pressure (plateau waves) can be responsible for unexpected, reversible, acute changes of mental status (Posner 1995).

Brain tumour therapy

Radiation is commonly employed to treat brain tumours and intracranial metastases. Other therapies such as chemotherapy are also used concurrently or in sequence and can contribute to brain toxicity. Side-effects of chemotherapy and remote effects of systemic cancer will be considered in Chapter 7. Whole-brain radiation is more frequently followed by cognitive sequelae than focal radiation. The cognitive failure due to radiation can be acute or subacute or delayed. Three main clinical variants can be seen (Posner 1995; Jennings 1995; Petterson and Rottemberg 1997).

- ◆ Early radiation encephalopathy can manifest as delirium within hours or days of treatment delivery and can be difficult to distinguish from symptoms of tumour progression. It is a transient phenomenon due to increased oedema that may fulfil the diagnosis of delirium.

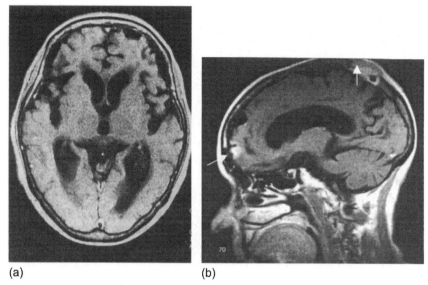

(a)   (b)

Fig. 6.7 (a) Meningeal metastases causing tetraventricular hydrocephalus. (b) The arrows show two contrast enhancement areas demonstrating a skull lesion (on the right) that invades the dura and is adjacent to the cortex and leptomeningeal covering and (on the left) a typical leptomeningeal lesion of the frontal lobe. The patient had a lung carcinoma and presented with delirium with disorientation to space and time, perseveration, and somnolence. Headache, meningismus, papilloedema, and focal signs were absent. CSF examination showed malignant cells.

♦ Early delayed encephalopathy can be seen, more often in children (the so-called somnolence syndrome), and occurs a few months after therapy, usually in patients with no apparent active tumour. Patients usually recover from it.

♦ Delayed encephalopathy is equivalent to radiation-induced dementia (De Angelis 1989). It is progressive, associated with cortical atrophy or white matter degeneration, and can occur years after radiation in patients cured of the initial tumour (Petterson and Rottemberg 1997).

Radiation toxicity can be enhanced by concurrent chemotherapy. Studies have focused on the late cognitive sequelae so important for the intellectual development of children treated for leukaemias and other tumours (Spunberg *et al.* 1981; Suc *et al.* 1990), but the risk of acute encephalopathy and, therefore, delirium is also increased by concomitant chemotherapy treatments (Gerritsen van der Hoop *et al.* 1990).

Chapter 7

Frequent clinical subtypes—
delirium in special populations

7.1 Delirium in HIV-infected patients

Delirium is a common psychiatric complication during the course of human immuno-deficiency virus (HIV) infection, with a prevalence of 30–40% of cases (Khouzam *et al.* 1998). Delirium prevalence tends to be higher among patients in more advanced stages of illness, in particular, in acquired immune deficiency syndrome (AIDS; Snyder *et al.* 1992). By analysing psychiatric comorbidity among hospitalized patients with HIV infection versus non-infected patients referred for psychiatric consultation, a prevalence of delirium of between 23% and 29% was found in the former group, in comparison with a 17–28% prevalence in the latter (Bialer *et al.* 1996; O'Dowd and McKegney 1990). The disorder, however, often remains underdiagnosed in AIDS patients (Lalonde *et al.* 1996).

In our experience, confusional states contributed to a minority of requests for psychiatric consultation in HIV-infected patients, with diagnosis of delirium made in only 5.2% of the cases (Grassi *et al.* 1995). These results were similar to a report in a multicentric Consultation–Liaison (C–L) Psychiatry Italian study (Grassi *et al.*, unpublished manuscript), where 5.8% of HIV-infected patients referred to C–L psychiatric services during a 1-year period were diagnosed as having delirium.

In a study of 137 AIDS patients residing at a skilled nursing facility, Uldall and Berghuis (1997) found that 46% patients met a diagnosis for delirium. Delirium was associated with medication changes, fever and infection, narcotics, benzodiazepines, anticholinergic/antihistamine and steroid medications. Delirium in AIDS patients can also develop as a consequence of antibiotic use (Salkind 2000). A recent study (Alciati *et al.* 2001) found that HIV-infected patients with cerebral opportunistic infections or metabolic encephalopathy were more likely to show disorders of consciousness, disorders of orientation, and disturbances of attention and memory associated with psychotic symptoms. The consequences of delirium in AIDS patients are multiple and severe. In a series of studies on the outcome of delirium in AIDS patients, Udall *et al.* (2000*a*, *b*) showed that patients with delirium were more likely to die during admission, had a longer hospital stay, or needed long-term care to a greater extent, if discharged, than non-delirious patients.

For these reasons, early identification of cognitive disorders, indicating possible prodromal symptoms of delirium, so that appropriate treatment can be initiated, is of the utmost importance in palliative care services dedicated to AIDS patients. Breitbart *et al.* (1996) carried out a randomized, double-blind trial aimed at evaluating the efficacy and the side-effects of haloperidol, chlorpromazine, and lorazepam in the treatment of delirium in 30 adult hospitalized AIDS patients. In this sophisticated study, the Delirium Rating Scale (DRS), the Mini-Mental State Examination (MMSE), and the Extrapyramidal Symptom Rating Scale (ESRS) were used to assess delirium and pharmacological side-effects. Each delirious patient was evaluated hourly with the DRS and the ESRS and, if the DRS score was still 13 or greater, the next dose of drug was administered.

The authors found that treatment with either haloperidol or chlorpromazine in relatively low doses produced a significant improvement in the symptoms of delirium, while lorazepam alone was ineffective and associated with treatment-limiting adverse effects. Cognitive function also improved significantly from baseline to day 2 in patients receiving chlorpromazine. The authors considered that the effects of HIV on subcortical structures of the brain (alterations in metabolism of the basal ganglia were observed in positron emission tomography (PET) scan studies) might produce an increased sensitivity to the effects of neuroleptic drugs, thus explaining the low doses needed to treat delirium in their study and, perhaps, the extremely low prevalence of extrapyramidal side-effects.

7.2   Delirium in primary psychiatric disorders

A recent area of research concerns the prevalence of delirium in patients with primary psychiatric disorders, especially in the elderly. Given the fact that patients with severe psychiatric illness share many of the risk factors for delirium, especially medications with anticholinergic properties (e.g. tricyclic antidepressants (TCAs), neuroleptics, anticholinergic drugs), delirium can be expected as a possible complication of psychiatric illness (Gill and Mayou 2000). The diagnosis of delirium can be complex among psychiatric patients due to the overlap of symptoms between delirium itself and acute mental illness. For this reason it has been reported that delirium is frequently underrecognized in mental health settings. Richtie *et al.* (1996) conducted a retrospective study of the charts of almost 200 patients admitted to a psychiatric unit. After excluding patients with alcohol or drug abuse, dementia, and those who developed delirium within 2 days of admission, the authors found a 14.6% prevalence of delirium following DSM-III-R criteria. The highest prevalence was found among individuals with a diagnosis of bipolar disorders (35.5%), schizoaffective disorders (15.8%), and schizophrenia or other psychoses (12.1%). Delirium developed after a mean of 3 weeks from admission and virtually doubled the length of hospital stay (92.2 days among delirious versus 50.7 days among non-delirious patients). Antiparkinsonian medication and old age were the most significant factors associated with the development of delirium, which was correctly recognized in only 48% of delirious patients. However, a different study carried out on 401 psychiatric admissions using a more specific methodology (the Delirium Symptom Interview, the Confusion Assessment Method, and the MMSE) found a 2.14% incidence of delirium (Patten *et al.* 1997). The risk factors for delirium included anticholinergic medications, electroconvulsive therapy, lithium–antipsychotic combination, high doses of low-potency neuroleptics, and nonpsychiatric medications capable of causing delirium.

In a study carried out by Huang *et al.* (1998), a diagnosis of delirium was made in 1.4% of psychiatric in-patients and was mostly related to the adverse effects of medication. However, in comparison with medical and surgical patients, the rate of mortality was lower among psychiatric patients in the short term (5.9%), but it increased during a 2-year follow-up period (39.4%).

See also the case reported in Chapter 5 highlighting the differential diagnosis of delirium in a patient with underlying psychosis admitted to a palliative care facility.

7.3 Postoperative delirium

Postoperative delirium is quite a common complication of surgery, especially invasive cardiac surgery, transplantation, and orthopaedic, ophthalmic, and urological surgery (Bitondo Dyer *et al.* 1995). Unlike other clinical types of delirium, however, postoperative delirium lacks a clear definition and operational criteria (van der Mast 1999) as well as well-designed prospective research (Winawer 2001). The term 'postoperative delirium' would seem to include either a temporal or an aetiological relationship between surgery and the occurrence of the disorder. Clinically, the notion that 'emergence' delirium (developing within the first 24 hours) should be separated from 'interval' delirium (developing after 24 hours or more of lucid consciousness) (Lipowski 1992) is considered artificial, although the term 'postoperative agitation' is still used and it is unclear whether it represents a specific condition (see below). Due to the number of different medical situations, types of surgery, population, pathophysiological mechanisms, and predisposing factors, postoperative delirium deserves to be further, and more specifically investigated.

A substantial underdiagnosis and underreporting of postoperative delirium has been shown. In only 12% of cases suffering from postoperative delirium, was it reported in the discharge documents (Glick *et al.* 1996).

Postoperative delirium usually develops during the first 4 days after surgery, with a peak on the first or second day, and should be distinguished from transient and emergent excitement or somnolence as a result of anaesthesia (O'Keeffe and Chonchubhair 1995). Immediate agitated reactions following anaesthesia are common and not well studied as they may actually be delirious episodes. Interestingly, this condition, usually described as postoperative agitation, is more frequent in children and with the use of volatile anaesthetics. Among anaesthetic gases, desflurane and sevoflurane seem to produce more postoperative agitation than halothane (Lapin *et al.* 1999; Welborn *et al.* 1996). Preoperative or perioperative medication with benzodiazepines and opioids reduces the degree and frequency of postoperative agitation (Galinkin *et al.* 2000; Lapin *et al.* 1999). No study that we know links the concept of postoperative agitation with the later-onset postoperative delirium.

Clinical features include the classic symptoms of delirium (e.g. impaired attention, hyperactivity or hypoactivity, progressive disturbance of thinking with a dream-like quality, illogical and incoherent speech, impaired capacity to judge, illusions, and vivid hallucinations), which tend to worsen at night. These symptoms are often associated with neurological symptoms such as asterixis, especially when metabolic alterations are present, multifocal myoclonus, and transient parietal signs such as apraxia, aphasia, and agraphia. Postoperative delirium tends to be of shorter duration than non-postoperative delirium in medical patients and usually disappears in a week (Manos and Wu 1997). However, it has been reported that it can last from one to several weeks, especially in the elderly (Parkh and Chung 1995).

As already indicated (see Section 3.1) the incidence of the disorder varies across the clinical context (e.g. orthopaedic or cardiosurgery units) as well as the type of population (e.g. elderly or severely physically ill patients).

An accurate evaluation of potential aetiologies is necessary and sometimes a specific cause can be found in previous or concurrent drug toxicity or withdrawal reaction as shown in cases of prolonged benzodiazepine use interrupted suddenly due to surgery (Madi and Langonnet 1988), or in other specific factors, such as thiamine deficiency (Vidal *et al.* 2001). More often, however, it is difficult to pinpoint a single specific cause and many cases are explained by a combination of preoperative risk factors and intra- and postoperative conditions (see Chapter 3).

A series of studies have confirmed that postoperative delirium is favoured by a series of factors. In a large study involving 1341 patients, 50 years of age and older, admitted for major elective non-cardiac surgery, Marcantonio *et al.* (1998) found a 9% incidence of delirium and showed that delirium was associated with greater intra-operative blood loss, more postoperative blood transfusions, and, especially, a post-operative haematocrit less than 30%. Pain also seems to be significantly associated with delirium. In a study of patients undergoing non-cardiac surgery Lynch *et al.* (1998) showed that, after controlling for known preoperative risk factors for delirium (i.e. age, alcohol abuse, cognitive function, physical function, serum chemistries, and type of surgery), higher pain scores at rest were associated with an increased risk of delirium over the first 3 postoperative days.

Among 105 elderly patients who underwent orthopaedic surgery for hip fracture or elective hip replacement, Galanakis *et al.* (2001) reported a postoperative delirium in 23.8% of the patients (40.5% hip fracture group; 14.7% hip joint replacement group). The authors showed that higher age, prior cognitive impairment as measured by the MMSE, depression, low educational level, and preoperative abnormal sodium were predictors of development of delirium. Furthermore, living in a nursing home, vision or hearing impairment, higher comorbidity, regular use of psychotropic drugs before admission, fracture on admission, and preoperative leukocytosis were also associated with delirium.

In a similar study, Duppils and Wikblad (2000), evaluated the occurrence of post-operative delirium in 225 elderly patients undergoing orthopaedic hip surgery (149 patients because of acute hip fracture and 76 for elective hip-replacement). A diag-nosis of delirium was made for 20% patients (24.3% in the hip-fracture group; 11.7% in the hip-replacement group). Predisposing factors were found to be older age, cog-nitive impairment, and pre-existing cerebrovascular or other brain diseases, while facilitating factors were communication and social isolation (e.g. impaired hearing and sight, reticence, and passivity). The use of psychopharmacological drugs was a precipitating factor.

Gupta *et al.* (2001) also indicated that certain clinical conditions, namely, obstructive sleep apnoea syndrome (OSAS), may be significantly associated with the onset of adverse postoperative outcomes, including delirium, among patients who underwent orthopaedic surgery (hip or knee replacement).

With regard to cardiac surgery, the incidence of delirium has been reported to range between 10% and 15%, although higher percentages have been found. The most significant predictors include old age, low level of albumin, poor physical condition, use of nifedipine, and a high ratio of the amino acid phenylalanine to the sum of isoleucine, leucine, valine, tyrosine, and tryptophan (van der Mast and Roest 1996).

A recent study confirmed that delirium affects the prognosis of elderly patients undergoing hip fracture repairs. In this study the Memorial Delirium Assessment Scale was useful for rating delirium severity and for accounting for subsyndromal delirum episodes that were associated with a worse recovery outcome than that of patients with mild delirum (Marcantonio *et al.* 2002).

In a recent study of 296 patients undergoing elective cardiac surgery, van der Mast *et al.* (2000) found no difference between delirious (13.5%) and non-delirious patients as far as preoperative cognitive function, history of psychiatric disorders, alcohol use, mood and functional status, type of surgery, intraoperative features, and medications used for anaesthesia are concerned. However, plasma tryptophan (Trp) and the ratio of Trp to other large neutral amino acids were reduced, while the ratio of phenylalanine was increased in delirious patients. The former result could produce decreased serotonergic function, while the latter could produce increased noradrenergic and dopaminergic function, causing an imbalance in cerebral neurotransmission. With regard to the role of noradrenaline (also called norepinephrine), Nakamura *et al.* (2001) measured the levels of plasma-free 3-methoxy-4-hydroxyphenyl (ethylene)glycol (pMHPG), a major metabolite of noradrenaline, in patients prior to surgery for cardiovascular diseases. The authors found that pMHPG levels before operation were higher in patients who subsequently developed postoperative delirium than in the patients who were non-delirious suggesting a hyperactivity of noradrenargic neurons as a possible risk factor of postoperative delirium.

The role of serotonin was evaluated by Bayindir *et al.* (2000) who analysed the effect of the 5-HT$_3$-receptor antagonist ondansetron (8 mg IV) in 35 patients with postcardiotomy delirium. The authors found that the use of ondansetron was effective and safe, leading them to hypothesize that impaired serotonin metabolism may play a role in postcardiotomy delirium. Although the multiple aetiology in postoperative delirium makes it difficult to understand the role of the several mechanisms involved, Stanford and Stanford (1999) have described a case that suggests that alterations of cerebral 5-HT induced by drugs (e.g. SSRIs and ondansetron) can play a major role in causing postoperative delirium. This report shares similarities with what we observed in a patient admitted to the hospital for surgery of colon cancer.

Case report

The patient, a 74-old-year woman, was admitted to the surgery department from the nursing home where she had lived for 5 years. The reason for admission was a colon cancer that had caused intestinal occlusion. She underwent surgery and morphine IV infusion was started to control her pain. After 2 days she developed symptoms characterized by severe agitation with disruptive behaviour, confusion, hallucinations, and pyrexia. A psychiatric consultation was immediately requested with the aim of transferring the patient to the acute psychiatric unit. Clinical evaluation confirmed a diagnosis of postoperative delirium due to multiple factors, including the patient's poor metabolic conditions, dehydration, and continuous use of opioids. By analysing the patient's chart, it was also noticed that she had used paroxetine 20 mg/day, which had been prescribed by the nursing house's physician 6 months earlier to treat the patient's depression. Paroxetine had been abruptly discontinued the day before surgery. The risk of SSRI discontinuation syndrome, especially for paroxetine, has been repeatedly shown (Black et al. 2000), and the possible interaction of opioids with serotonin and dopamine has been suggested (Stanford and Stanford 1999). Aetiological intervention (treatment of dehydration and metabolic imbalance), indications to the medical and nursing staff with regard to how to behaviourally treat the patient's confusional status, and the prescription of risperidone 2 mg/day were followed by recovery from delirium within 4 days.

In a study of elderly patients undergoing coronary artery bypass graft (CABG) surgery, Rolfson et al. (1999) found a 32% incidence of delirium, which was associated with a history of stroke, a longer duration of cardiopulmonary bypass, and, to a lesser degree, low postoperative cardiac output. In a recent prospective study of 500 patients undergoing elective surgery, Litaker et al. (2001) found, in those who developed delirium (11.4%), that factors significantly associated with delirium were age (70 years old or above), pre-existing cognitive impairment, greater preoperative functional limitations, and a history of prior delirium. Patients' perceptions that alcohol had affected their health and the use of narcotic analgesics just prior to admission were also significantly associated with delirium postoperatively.

The preoperative score by Marcantonio to predict the risk of postoperative delirium (Table 3.3) takes into account multivariate analysis of commonly identified risk factors.

It has to be said that risk factors for delirium vary according to the population examined as well as to the clinical context. Aldemir et al. (2001), for example, by studying 818 patients who had been hospitalized either for elective or emergency procedures, showed a prevalence of postoperative delirium of 10.9%. The authors found that delirium was *not* correlated with conditions such as hypertension, hypo/hyperpotassaemia, hypernatraemia, hypoalbuminaemia, hypo/hyperglycaemia, cardiac disease, emergency admission, age, length of stay in the intensive care unit, length of stay in hospital, and gender. In contrast, respiratory diseases, infections, fever, anaemia, hypotension, hypocalcaemia, hyponatraemia, uremia, elevated liver enzymes, hyperamylasaemia, hyperbilirubinaemia, and metabolic acidosis *were* predicting factors for delirium. In a study carried out by Dubois et al. (2001) on over 200 consecutive patients admitted to intensive care units, it was shown that, among the patients who developed delirium (19%), hypertension, smoking history, abnormal bilirubin level, epidural use, and morphine were statistically significantly associated with the disorder. Thus, the authors conclude that traditional factors associated with the development of delirium in patients on general wards may not be significant or applicable to critically ill patients.

The consequences of postoperative delirium are severe. Mortality is the most severe consequence with data showing an incidence of 4–40% among postsurgery patients who developed delirium (O'Keeffe 1994). Manos and Wu (1997) found a mortality over a 3.5-year period of 46.8% among patients who developed delirium and postoperative delirium. Medical complications, such as increased risk for infections due to a need for catheterization, increased falls with possible trauma, and bone fractures, are also important consequences of postoperative delirium. This can determine an increasing length of stay (LOS) in the hospital.

It is interesting to note that delirium is a predictor of poor functional recovery after hip fracture surgery in the elderly, independently of prefracture risk factors such as age and poor cognitive and functional status. Furthermore, hip fracture outcome is also worsened when patients present with delirium preoperatively (Dolan *et al.* 2000; Marcantonio *et al.* 2000).

As far as economic data is concerned, LOS is obviously associated with increased direct and indirect costs of care. Franco *et al.* (2001) have recently shown that both professional costs (i.e. those related to services provided by physicians and nursing) and technical costs (i.e. those related to non-medical services, such as number of medications, imaging, laboratory tests during admission) increased among 57 patients out of 500 (11.4%) who developed delirium during admission.

While it has been shown that about one-third of cases of delirium secondary to orthopaedic surgery go unrecognized by the staff (Gustafson *et al.* 1991*a*), it is likely that regular assessment of the patients' cognitive function, early diagnosis of confusional symptoms, and early treatment of underlying causes are the key factors for postoperative delirium prevention and management. Indeed, in a recent randomized controlled trial on hip fracture in the elderly, proactive geriatric consultation was proved to reduce the frequency of delirium from 50% to 32%, and severe delirious cases from 29% to 12% (Marcantonio *et al.* 2001).

7.4 Delirium in the elderly

The frequency of delirium in the elderly population and, above all in the cognitively impaired elderly patient, has led to the development of the specific interest of geriatricians in this syndrome (Carlson *et al.* 1999). Many different types of evidence concur to suggest that the process of ageing of the brain, the occurrence of dementia, and delirium must share some basic pathophysiological mechanisms.

Age and pre-existing cognitive impairment are independent risk factors for developing delirium as demonstrated by several well-conducted epidemiological studies (see Chapter 3 and tables therein). Age is still a risk factor when the population under study is over 65 years old. A failure of the cholinergic system, as a consequence of age, dementia, or acute events, is one of the core elements of these clinical conditions (Blass and Gibson 1999).

The differential diagnosis of delirium in the elderly with preceding and concurrent cognitive deficit and dementia is particularly challenging and already a subject of debate. The diagnostic criteria in use may not be specific enough to distinguish between fluctuations in cognition related to a chronic underlying, slowly evolving condition and superimposed acute events acting on an already compromised system. Geriatricians are very aware of the fact that, in many cases, the boundaries between these two conditions are fuzzy or may have no clinical impact on subsequent patient management (Lindesay 1999; MacDonald 1999).

According to EEG results and a phenomenological point of view, delirium in the course of dementia does not differ from delirium that is not associated with dementia. A quantitative analysis of the EEG can help in differentiating delirium from dementia in the elderly (Jacobson and Jerrier 2000; Jacobson et al. 1993a, b). Factor analysis of the Delirium Rating Scale showed that only subtle differences can be found between these two conditions and that the subtle differences due to dementia would require more study (Trzepacz et al. 1998). Delirium in the course of dementia seems to be of a longer duration than other types of deliria (Manos and Wu 1997).

The usefulness of a classification system obviously relies on its clinical impact. In the elderly the concept of 'acute confusional state' is still useful, especially when exogenous causes or potentially correctable risk factors are identified (Treloar and Macdonald 1997a, b). This can be difficult but not impossible (Inouye et al. 1999a). Recognizing an unexpected worsening in the cognitive performance of a demented patient can impact on the clinical management and be a guide to the diagnosis of many comorbidities, acute illnesses such as infection or miocardial infarction. This is even more important if it is recognized that the elderly, especially when cognitively impaired, are particularly prone to suffer from the toxic effects of drugs at doses that are usually thought safe for the general population (Tune et al. 1992).

The impact of the type of dementing illness on the likelihood of developing delirium and on its clinical aspects is unknown. Data on the demented population is preliminary and in part contradictory. In one study vascular dementias and late-onset Alzheimer's disease had a higher rate of delirium than early-onset Alzheimer disease and frontotemporal dementias (Robertsson et al. 1998). According to the authors, this observation could be due to the more widespread brain damage found in the more severe pathologies. Another study retrospectively correlated the presence of right hemisphere dysfunction with the risk of developing delirium (Mach et al. 1996), which would support the view of a particular role of the non-dominant hemisphere in the pathogenesis of delirium (Mesulam 1985). In a prospective study that distinguished the type of regional brain syndrome, but without considering right or left hemisphere functions, cases of delirium were more frequently associated with global brain dysfunction, more severe dementia, and older age, and were less frequent with predominant frontal lobe dysfunction, supporting the idea of delirium as a diffuse affection of cortical functions (Robertsson et al. 1999).

Postoperative delirium also has a particular impact in elderly populations that are at increased risk of hip fracture due to falls and osteoporosis. As we have already described, delirium whether present pre- or postoperatively, is a predictor of poor functional recovery after hip fracture surgery, independently of prefracture risk factors such as age and poor cognitive and functional status (Dolan et al. 2000; Marcantonio et al. 2000, 2002).

The recovery from delirium in the elderly is often slow and incomplete (Francis and Kapoor 1992), and the occurrence of delirium during hospitalization, independently from other factors including dementia, is a predictor of mortality and long-term poor functional and cognitive status (McCusker *et al.* 2001*b*, 2002).

Infections are another common offender in the elderly hospitalized populations. Both respiratory and urinary infections in the elderly, even with low-grade fever or no fever at all, often present with delirium. The sensitivity of the ageing or demented brain and other predisposing factors with the addition of a metabolic or infectious cause of relatively modest severity can be crucial for the onset of delirium. The strong association of urinary infections and delirium in the elderly can be explained by this line of reasoning (Manepalli *et al.* 1990). The situation is even more complex if we think that the use of antibiotics for the treatment of different infections can itself favour the onset of delirium among physically debilitated and vulnerable patients, as we have described in a case of hypoactive delirium secondary to the fluoroquinolone cyprofloxacin (Grassi *et al.* 2001*a*).

Case report

Mrs. T. was a 64-year-old woman affected by a severe chronic obstructive pulmonary disease (COPD) that required numerous hospital admissions. She lived alone, after the death of her husband 3 years earlier. Because of the worsening of her respiratory condition, she was readmitted to an internal medicine ward. The patient's home therapy was prednisone (12.5 mg), digoxin (0.125 mg), amiloride hydrochloride (5.7 mg) and hydrochlorothiazide (50 mg m.i.d.), ranitidine (300 mg m.i.d.), and inhalatory fluticasone propionate (500 mcg b.i.d). This therapy was maintained throughout hospitalization. Measurement of arterial blood gas showed a severe hypoxia (pO_2, 38 mm g) with hypercapnia (pCO_2, 66 mm g), which were normalized during the first few days of admission through proper cycles of O_2 therapy. Laboratory findings showed normal hepatorenal functions, no electrolyte imbalance, and no hypoglycaemia. The blood chemistry panel was normal, except for a mildly increased erythrocyte sedimentation rate (ESR) level (25 mm, 1 hour), as the only index of a possible inflammation process. In fact, chest X-ray showed a right basilar density, though there was no fever, for which ciprofloxacin therapy (250 mg t.i.d.) was added (fifth day of admission).

After 3 days, the patient became progressively depressed, inhibited, apathetic, and non-compliant with therapy and routine interventions. For these reasons, she was first assessed by a neurologist consultant who excluded CNS disorders and then referred to the C–L Psychiatric service for 'depression impairing cooperation and compliance'. At mental status examination the patient appeared extremely inhibited and apathetic with decreased reaction to internal and external stimuli. Reduced ability to maintain and shift attention and impairment in short-term memory, mild perception disturbances (misperceptions, illusions, and fragmented auditory hallucinations), and thought disorders (paranoid thinking) were the main symptoms. Vital signs and physical examination were unchanged from her baseline state. Data collected from family members indicated no previous history of psychiatric disorders. A diagnosis of hypoactive delirium was made. By considering the absence of mental disorders at admission, the lack of concomitant factors (e.g. substance withdrawal, neurological disorders) that could have explained her symptoms, and the absence of any metabolic disturbances, and the striking temporal relationship between the onset of psychiatric symptoms and fluoroquinolone use, ciprofloxacin was considered to be the most probable precipitant factor of the patient's delirium. Lorazepam 2 mg b.i.d. was started, in view of the literature indicating the possible inhibition of the binding of GABA to its receptor sites and the involvement of the benzodiazepine (BDZ)–GABA-receptor complex (Unseld *et al.*, 1990), and the efficacy of benzodiazepine in the treatment of delirium secondary to fluoroquinolones (Farrington *et al.* 1995). Orientation gradually improved, hallucinations and thought disorders disappeared, and the sleep–wake cycle was restored. Three days later her behaviour was nearly at baseline and her mental status returned to normality. She remained in the hospital for 2 weeks and, after discharge, a home-care assistance programme was set up. However, in a month, the patient's respiratory and cardiovascular conditions worsened and she was readmitted to the hospital where, because of multiple physical complications (cardiac insufficiency, respiratory infection), she died 10 days later.

In the future practice of palliative care, more and more elderly patients are likely to be seen and cognitive impairment has to be recognized in its manifold clinical aspects. A specific ability to manage risk factors, psychotropic drug administration, and complex cases will often be required.

7.5 Delirium in cancer

Delirium is very frequent in cancer patients as mentioned in Section 3.1. Metastatic aetiologies and brain radiation were discussed in Chapter 6, but cancer patients have many other risk and precipitating factors, partially in common with other severely ill patients, and partially specific to the disease. These are listed in Table 7.1.

Mental status change was the second most common reason for neurological consultation in cancer (Clouston *et al.* 1992). In a series of 140 consecutive patients, the most frequent diagnosis was toxic or metabolic encephalopathy in 64% and 53% of cases, respectively. A single aetiology could be found in 33% of cases, while multiple aetiologies were likely in 67% and a structural brain lesion was the only cause of confusion in 15% of cases (Tuma and DeAngelis 2000). See also the case described in Section 7.6.4.

Case report

The patient was a 75-year-old man. His past medical history showed that he had suffered from a subdural haematoma due to trauma and, more recently, underwent a right carotidectomy for thrombectomy. He worked as a technician with managerial experience and had a high educational level including good knowledge of English. He was diagnosed with a bronchogenic carcinoma, with a hilar mass infiltrating the D9 vertebral body and causing epidural compression at this site. He had severe thoracic pain and was transferred from a neurological facility to an oncology ward for radiation therapy and symptom control. Morphine infusion was started with a

Table 7.1 Causes of delirium in cancer patients

Secondary CNS tumour

  Brain metastases

  Meningeal metastases

Non-metastatic complications of cancer

  Metabolic encephalopathy due to hepatic, renal, or pulmonary failure

  Electrolyte abnormalities

  Glucose abnormalities

  Infections

  Haematological abnormalities

  Nutritional deficiency (thiamine, folic acid, vitamin B12 deficiency)

  Vasculitis

Paraneoplastic neurological syndrome

Toxicity of antineoplastic therapies

  Chemotherapy

    Chemotherapy drugs

    Methotrexate

    Cisplatin

    Vincristine

    Paclitaxel

    Procarbazine

    Asparaginase

    Cytosine arabinoside

    5-fluorouracil

    Ifosfamide

    Tamoxifen (rare)

    Thiotepa

    Etoposide (high doses)

    Nitrosourea (high doses or via arterial route)

  Radiation to brain

  Immunotherapy

Toxicity of other drugs

Other diseases not related to neoplasm with CNS involvement

Alcohol or drug abuse or withdrawal

patient-controlled anaesthesia (PCA) pump at an infusion rate of 1.5 mg/h and 10 mg p.r.n. bolus available as needed. Pain was well controlled with moderate somnolence; the infusion rate was reduced to 1 mg/h. At about 36 hours following the administration of morphine infusion, the patient became agitated in the night and started to hallucinate and to be violent. When examined, the patient was awake. Attention was compromised with perseveration and confabulation. The neurological examination showed many pathological reflexes: snout, palmomental, and grasping reflexes, and extensor plantar response on the left. He was asked to write a sentence (Fig. 7.1). The two sentences made sense ('Tomorrow I will go to school. Today is a humid day.'). Although the first one could reflect some disorientation, the man's mistakes are mainly represented by letter repetitions (perseveration).

Haloperidol was started at a dose of 4 mg/day. Morphine infusion was kept constant at 34 mg/daily. In the following 4 days delirium continued with nocturnal hallucinations and delusions. The patient reported that he saw a man with a threatening attitude printed on the wall, that the nurses wanted to kill him, and that during a night he was taken by the nurses to Piazza Castello (Piazza Castello 'the Castle Square' is a very popular downtown location in Milan). These episodes usually took place overnight. The patient, when questioned about them the following morning, although apparently vigilant and coherent, reported these experiences as real. He was disoriented for space, saying that he was still at the neurological hospital where he was initially admitted for spinal cord compression. He was also suspicious and believed that the nurses were not correctly administering the prescribed therapies.

Morphine infusion was stopped and substituted with a transdermal fentanyl patch (25 µg/h). Mental status recovered in 24 hours. The patient completed a course of radiation therapy and was discharged after a week without further neurological complications.

Laboratory examination showed mild hyponatraemia (129 mEq/l), and hypercalcaemia (11.7 mg/dl). CT scan of the head was compatible with normotensive hydrocephalus and cortical atrophy (Fig. 7.2).

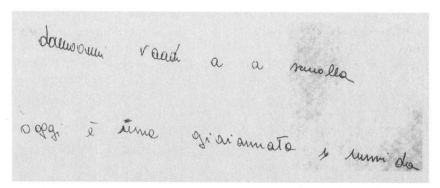

Fig. 7.1 Sample of spontaneous writing. There are evident perseverations and mistakes. The correct spelling of the phrases would be: (first line) domani [tomorrow] vado [I will go] a scuola [to school]; (second line) oggi [today] é [is] una [a] giornata umida [humid day]. Many 'a's are repeated (but also other letters) and 'giornata' is misspelled.

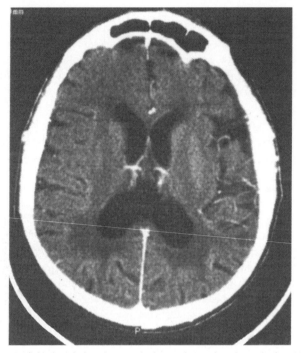

Fig. 7.2 CT scan of the head showing cortical atrophy and periventricular CSF reabsorption compatible with the diagnosis of normotensive hydrocephalus.

This case highlights several potentially important predisposing factors among which age, brain atrophy, and metabolic abnormalities may have facilitated a toxic effect from morphine administration. Fentanyl proved to have a more favourable therapeutic index in this case.

7.5.1 Paraneoplastic neurological diseases

The case of paraneoplastic neurological diseases is specific for the cancer population. These diseases will usually cause dementia but their onset and clinical course can be charaterized by acute mental symptoms and delirium. A paraneoplastic syndrome is a disease due to the presence of the tumour but not directly caused by it. The denomination 'remote effects of neoplasia' is also found (Dropcho 2002; Rosenfeld and Dalmau 2001; Voltz 2002). The definition excludes those indirect consequences of tumours that depend on metabolic, nutritional complications or are due to cachexia. Neurological paraneoplastic disease can involve the peripheral and the central nervous system, often preceding the diagnosis of cancer by a long time. These diseases are usually severe and have a rapidly progressive and invalidating course. Paraneoplastic syndromes are rare diseases and represent no more than 1% of all neurological complications of cancer (Posner 1995).

In many of these syndromes specific autoantibodies have been identified that react against antigens that are common to the nervous and tumour tissue (Posner 1995).

Neurological syndromes that can be paraneoplastic include the Lambert–Eaton myasthenic syndrome, encephalomyelitis, limbic encephalitis, dermato- and polymyositis, acute cerebellar degeneration, subacute sensory neuronopathy, and opsoclonus myoclonus in children.

Cognitive and psychiatric clinical presentation can occur in encephalomyelitis, limbic encephalitis, and opsoclonus myoclonus.

Limbic encephalitis can be found in association with microcytoma or testis carcinomas (but occasional associations can be found with many different tumours). The clinical findings can be of a subacute dementia, amnesia, personality changes, and psychotic features. The brain MRI can be normal or show an abormality of signal, and atrophy in the temporomesial cortical areas (Posner 1995; Voltz *et al.* 1999).

Encephalomyelitis is a syndrome of multilevel involvement of the central nervous system with complex clinical phenomenology. Altered mental status with delirium or dementia is frequent. The tumour most frequently associated is again microcytoma (Posner 1995).

Table 7.2 reports the most important paraneoplastic syndromes found in adult patients with their typical associated neoplasms and the autoantibodies most recently characterized. This field is in constant evolution and, although a role for autoimmunity is highly likely, pathophysiological mechanisms are still under research. Paraneoplastic syndromes should not be forgotten in the differential diagnosis of delirium in patients with cancer, while keeping in mind their rarity and their complex neurological presentations (Zeimer 2000).

Table 7.2 The principal neurological paraneoplastic syndromes found in adults with the most common associated tumours and the characteristic autoantibodies.* Delirium can be found in encephalomyelitis and in limbic encephalitis

Neurological syndrome	Neoplasm†	Antibody
Encephalomyelitis	SCLC	Anti-Hu
Cerebellar degeneration	Breast, ovary	Anti-Yo
	SCLC	Anti-Hu
	SCLC, others	Anti-CV2
	Hodgkin's lymphoma	Anti-Tr
	Breast	Anti-Ri
Limbic encephalitis	SCLC	Anti-Hu
	SCLC	Anti-CV2
	Testis	Anti-Ta
Subacute sensory neuronopathy	SCLC	Anti-Hu
Lambert-Eaton syndrome	SCLC	Anti-VGCC

* These associations are typical but miscellaneous cases can be found with different combinations of neoplasm and antibodies and, with practically any known neoplasm, unknown antibodies are often harboured in otherwise not explained cases.

† SCLC, Small cell lung cancer.

7.5.2 Chemotherapy toxicity

The role of chemotherapy in causing delirium is often overlooked. A list of the drugs that have been associated with encephalopathy can be found in Table 7.2 (see also case reports in Chapter 5 and Figs 5.2 and 5.3). In general, the use of high doses and intrathecal administration increases toxicity. Newer drug combinations and dosages may lead to unexpected toxicities. The whole field suffers from underreporting.

7.6 Terminal delirium

7.6.1 Cultural aspects

The study of delirium in advanced diseases and, in particular, in the terminal phases of incurable illness is one of the developments of palliative care influenced by the changes witnessed in the way of dying in our modern or post-modern society. Delirium was a common sign of impending death when infectious often epidemic, diseases were the first cause of death, frequently occurring at a very young age. The slowing of the dying process due to chronic progressive diseases, at a much older age than ever before has implied the possibility of new prevalent morbidities. Delirium is still very common as an immediately pre-agonic condition but is also characteristic of a prolonged dying process with alternating abnormalities of the state of consciousness at times with and at times without the potential for recovery. Nowadays, the demand to die without suffering is growing and embraces larger concepts than the simple relief of pain (Clark 1999).

Our hypothesis is that the mental suffering of dying is dramatically embodied, in the view of lay people, by the behaviours characteristic of delirium in the terminal phase. Palliative care is expected to take a very different approach to the abandonment of dying patients depicted in Thomas Mann's (1994, English translation) *Buddenbrooks: the decline of a family* when describing the death of the old Lady Buddenbrook. She dies of pneumonia after a considerable period of dyspnoea and suffering. The doctors would take no action to ease her subjective feelings and were strongly opposed to the request to give a sedative drug that might have worsened her respiratory condition. She finally develops delirium that is seen as a liberation by the family, and the writer, and dies without much help from official medicine.

Therapy today may mean dying without the perception of dying, without the perception of the mental impairment that precedes death. We are almost tempted to say 'dying without dying'. For many people, dying without noticing it would be the goal of good palliative care in the postmodern society. In more pragmatic words, the 'good death' that the contemporary palliative care patient expects from health-providers would be peaceful, without pain, and in absolutely normal mental health until the end, with the alternative of being unconscious when these requirements cannot be fulfilled. However, these are only hypotheses since the perceived qualities of a good death are unknown (Gordon and Peruselli 2001; Morrison *et al.* 2000).

Another issue of debate is the degree of medicalization and the real needs of conducting research in the palliative care context. Criticism has been raised about the possibility of applying traditional methods of research to the palliative care patient

(Rinck *et al.* 1997). Recently, the subject of conducting research on delirium in terminal patients raised a heated debate on the limitations of the medical approach to research in palliative care, which deserved more space and more in-depth discussion (Davis and Walsh 2001; Lawlor *et al.* 2001).

A very important question is, how is it possible to help people with the aids of palliative care to have a 'good death'? What is a 'good death'? Research instruments to study this approach are beginnig to be discussed but have not yet been applied to empirical situations, while the present difficulties in identifying outcome measures for assessing the result of palliative care are well recognized (Kornblith 2001; Morrison *et al.* 2000). Qualitative methods of research may be more appropriate and their use to study specific situations such as the impact of delirium at the end of life may be promising (Gordon and Peruselli 2001).

7.6.2 Clinical aspects

The hospice experience has contributed a number of important clinical observations on this subject. The term 'terminal restlessness' has been coined to describe a potentially specific condition of agitation and altered mental status that is often seen in hospices and that has been interpreted as the combination of a number of toxic and metabolic events (Burke 1997; Burke *et al.* 1991; Dunlop 1989). The proposed clinical characteristics of terminal restlessness are those of an 'agitated delirium in a dying patient frequently associated with impaired consciousness and multifocal myoclonus'. A more systematic description of this syndrome is lacking. In general, there are no phenomenological data on the clinical features of delirium at the end of life, but terminal restlessness has remained a term relatively specific to the hospice culture. In the most recent reports on a significant number of patients, agitated or hyperactive delira were found in a significant number of cases but no specific assessment of the deliria of the imminently dying was attempted (Lawlor *et al.* 1998). Earlier reports have suggested that the psychological content of deliria near to death is influenced by the unique existential meaning of the situation (Massie *et al.* 1983).

In our experience of the symptoms requiring sedation in the last 24–48 hours of life, we identified delirium with agitation as the main reason for sedation in 19% of the patients requiring sedation (Caraceni *et al.* 2002). In a small number of cases, agitation was a specific problem, clearly distinguished from hyperactive delirium. These patients had acute symptoms, due to rapid progression of the disease (often pain, dysphagia, and others), and extreme psychomotor agitation as a response to an unbearable physical and existential situation, but they were not clinically delirious.

The prevalence of delirium in patients undergoing palliative care was about 30% in two recent studies in the hospice and home-care populations with advanced incurable cancer (Caraceni *et al.* 2000; Minagawa *et al.* 1996) and 42% on admission in a specialized acute palliative care ward (Lawlor *et al.* 2000*b*). Terminal delirium, defined as delirium occurring at least 6 hours before death, occurred in 88% of 52 patients dying in hospital, and cognitive failure has been reported in 83% of patients, occurring on average 16 days before death (Bruera *et al.* 1992*b*).

As mentioned in Chapter 3, we now have data on risk factors for the development of delirium in palliative care (Caraceni *et al.* 2000; Lawlor *et al.* 2000*b*), on the potentially reversible aetiological or precipitating factors (Lawlor *et al.* 2000*b*), and on its prognostic meaning (Caraceni *et al.* 2000; Lawlor *et al.* 2000*b*; Morita *et al.* 1999). Table 7.3 reports factors more frequently found in palliative care and therefore relatively specific for the high delirium risk of this population and the general risk factors also found in palliative care.

At the moment we lack studies focused on delirium in the imminently dying that can identify the role of predisposing and precipitating factors with more detail in the palliative care situation.

7.6.3 Assessment

The systematic assessment of cognitive functions is very important in palliative care, for many reasons. Although the high prevalence and incidence of delirium in the patients with terminal illnesses could be enough to recommend the routine use of some instruments for screening of cognitive function in patients admitted to palliative care programmes, we also see many more specific reasons for adopting a systematic assessment of mental status.

• The ageing population is an extremely significant proportion of the palliative care population. In these patients the frequency of dementia or other more subtle forms of cognitive failure is high. Thus, a differential diagnosis between delirium, dementia, or adjustment disorders is often required (Farrell and Ganzini 1995).

• Symptom assessment is particularly difficult in patients with delirium. In one study patients admitted to a palliative care ward received higher p.r.n. opioid doses for pain when delirious than after recovering from the episode. Pain was rated as more severe by the staff during the delirious episode than by the patient himself after delirium had cleared (Bruera *et al.* 1992*a*; Coyle *et al.* 1994).

• This difficulty in interpreting symptom severity can cause conflicts within the staff and with the family. A compromised communication between patient and family can contribute to a compromised communication between staff and family in the

Table 7.3 Factors facilitating delirium in palliative care

Factors more frequent in palliative care	General factors in common with other medical conditions
Opioids*	Age
Psychotropic medication*	Previous cognitive failure
Cachexia/anorexia[†]	Dehydration
Low performance[†]	Environmental factors
Respiratory failure	
Infections	
Brain or meningeal metastases[†]	
AIDS brain pathology	

* Lawlor *et al.* (2000*b*).
[†] Caraceni *et al.* (2000).

terminal phases of life. This in turn can have a serious effect on the therapeutic decision and can be a factor in family morbidity (see Chapter 10).

• One of the more baffling aspects of delirium is its symptom fluctuation and night worsening. For this reason, a codified assessment with written reports is essential. Nurse observation is a very valuable source of information that can be improved by specific education on delirium characteristics. Standardized assessment will improve communication that is often limited to poorly informative dialogue between staff members such as nurses, e.g. nurse Jude: 'I saw Mr Smith last night; he is confused'; nurse Angela: 'No dear, I saw Mr Smith this morning and he is not confused!'

• Early detection and well-conducted assessment will enable the staff to inform the family, encouraging communication and counselling on several critical issues (Borreani *et al.* 1997).

• Early detection of prodromal symptoms of delirium should help in preventing further worsening in reversible cases and has been proven useful as part of the strategy to reduce the risk of developing delirium in the elderly population (Inouye *et al.* 1999*a*).

• The whole process is aimed at understanding the dying process, easing suffering, and providing support for the family in a way that is proportionate to the actual clinical situation, being careful not to be caught unprepared and at the same time to not overemphasize excessive testing that could result in patient burden.

7.6.4   Aetiological factors

Multiple potential aetiological or precipitating factors are commonly found in palliative care with an average of 2.2 probable or possible causes attributed to 71 delirium episodes in a recent prospective study (Lawlor *et al.* 2000*b*). Similar observations can be found in older studies (Bruera *et al.* 1992*b*; Caraceni *et al.* 1994; Stiefel *et al.* 1992).

Reversibility is possible when delirium is not part of the failure of vital homeostatic mechanisms leading to death. This is suggested by recent findings showing that irreversibility is associated with hypoxia and respiratory failure and metabolic factors (Lawlor *et al.* 2000*b*) while reversibility is related to the contributing effects of drug toxicity and dehydration (Caraceni *et al.* 1994; Lawlor *et al.* 2000*b*). Strategies that may reduce the incidence of reversible deliria have been suggested to improve the management of palliative care patients (Bruera *et al.* 1995), but their true impact on symptom control outcome cannot be clarified without performing controlled clinical trials, which are hard to propose in palliative care.

While metabolic irreversible failures are often found as causes of both the delirium and the coma that precede many deaths in palliative care, the exact contribution of these conditions as causes of death in terminal patients is not well established. In our experience of patients with advanced terminal cancer admitted to a home-care programme, death could be attributed to metabolic failure in 56% of patients (Groff 1993). The complexity of the final events leading to death and the peculiarity of the home-care setting are such that, in a number of patients (17%), no specific cause could be attributed to the final clinical event. The case reported below shows how delirium can characterize the dying process in a modern palliative care unit, even though a specific cause cannot be found.

Case report

The patient was a 69-year-old university professor of chemistry still actively teaching before his recent clinical condition deteriorated. The patient was affected by a locally advanced carcinoma of the pancreas. He underwent prolonged chemotherapy with 5-fluorouracil (5-FU) and palliative local radiation. Abdominal and back pain were treated initially with oral morphine and then with subcutaneous morphine infusion. Worsening of pain suggested admission to an in-patient palliative care unit.

On admission the patient started to be delirious while on oral morphine and had a fluctuating course of delirium with phases of complete recovery (Memorial Delirium Assessment Scale (MDAS) score, 12/30); (see Section 8.2.3 and Appendix 6 for details of MDAS) and phases of severe delirium (MDAS score, 30/30) that lasted for 26 days before death.

His neurological examination never showed any focal sign but bilateral palmomental reflexes and grasping reflexes were present.

Delirium was partially controlled with haloperidol. Then the patient required prometazine, and, finally, profound sedation in the terminal phase.

During the course of his last 4 weeks of life, respiratory, renal, and cardiac functions were within normal limits with the exception of oliguria in the last 3-day phase. His temperature reached 38.5 °C on one occasion, but fever was remittent and usually of low grade. In the last days, his fever reached 39.5 °C.

Laboratory findings showed no specific abnormalities that could justify delirium, but a very significant increase of specific tumour marker levels (Ca19.9, 142,290), low albumin, and high alkaline phosphatase. An MRI with gadolinium of the brain showed cortical atrophy, in particular, at the level of the temporal lobes (Fig. 7.3).

Finally, a diagnosis could not be established as to the aetiology of delirium. Cortical brain atrophy could be due to a pre-existing beclouded or compensated dementia and could have facilitated the occurrence of delirium in association with the use of opioid analgesics and advanced cancer. The long-term 5-FU administration might have produced brain toxicity. Even paraneoplastic limbic encephalitis, although a rare event (specific tests were not felt necessary for the clinical situation), might explain irreversible cognitive decline.

The content and the subjective perception of terminal delirium, as already mentioned, are unknown. Extrapolating from other anecdotal reports, it is reasonable to conclude that the experience of delirium is usually unpleasant. The most authoritative opinion in this regard is that: 'Delirium itself is usually a highly disturbing experience that augments the sufferer's distress' (Lipowski 1990b). More specifically, it is likely that the content of delirium is influenced by the dramatic physical and emotional conditions associated with the disease progression: hospitalization; invasive therapies; painful procedures; fear of death; existential and spiritual concerns. All these are hypotheses awaiting for empirical confirmation. The possibility that premorbid

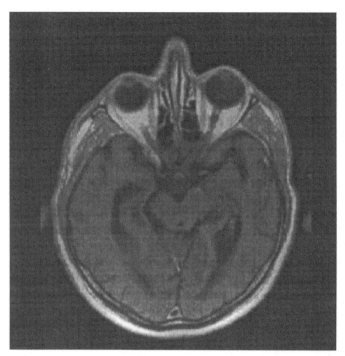

Fig. 7.3 Axial MRI view of the brain demonstrating some atrophy of the cortical mantle, in the temporal areas. See text for patient's case report.

psychologically distressful and significant past life events can be reactivated from unconscious processes within a delirium has been recognized for a long time (Wolf and Curran 1935), but how these mechanisms impact on the very special case of terminal delirium is certainly a question worth considering.

7.6.5   Management

There is little data on the specific management of delirium at the end of life. However, as already mentioned, a number of delirium episodes are reversible even in the advanced phases of disease. Therefore, general principles of aetiological screening need to be followed if the goal of care is to improve the patient's mental status.

Some authors suggest that a systematic approach to reduce a number of potential risk factors could be implemented in the palliative care setting, with the aim of reducing the prevalence of agitation and myoclonus characterizing the cognitive failure of terminal patients in hospice care experiences. The protocol that these authors suggest includes: intensive monitoring of cognitive functions, hydration, and opioid rotation to minimize toxicity due to uraemia and opioid toxicity (Bruera *et al.* 1995; Dunlop 1989). This approach recently created a controversy concerning the appropriateness of such an approach in the model of hospice care (Davis and Walsh 2001; Lawlor *et al.* 2001).

We have already mentioned that agitated terminal delirium is one of the situations that may require pharmacological sedation at the end of life (Cherny and Portenoy 1994; Stiefel *et al.* 1992). A discussion of the pharmacology of sedation can be found in Chapter 9.

The ethical implications of using sedation in the phases that precede death are beyond the scope of this chapter (Cherny and Portenoy 1994; Quill *et al.* 2000). In a multicentre international trial, the frequency of delirium as an indication for sedation varied from 14% to 60% of cases (Fainsinger *et al.* 2000*b*), while, in a Canadian series of patients who needed terminal sedation, this procedure was required in only 4% of cases and in most of them it was indicated because of delirium (Fainsinger *et al.* 2000*a*). In our experience delirium has been an indication for sedation in the terminal phase of cancer in 19% of the cases who required sedation (Caraceni *et al.* 2002). See also Section 9.3.

Acknowledgement: the authors are indebted to Bruno Bieucosiko, MD, and Michela Osti, MD, for their contribution to this chapter.

Chapter 8

Diagnostic assessment

Delirium is viewed as a medical emergency and the guidelines recommended for its immediate assessment and management usually come from the experience of emergency medicine. Certainly, the palliative care settings have different requirements but it is quite useful to recall some of these first-line recommendations, which retain their practical and mnemonic usefulness. One popular acronym, 'I WATCH DEATH', is reproduced in Table 8.1. In every care setting delirium can be an emergency depending on its severity and on the occurrence of agitation and aggressiveness in the individual cases.

8.1 Instrumental and laboratory findings

8.1.1 Diagnostic examinations

The onset of delirium should bring into play a series of diagnostic procedures that will be more or less aggressively pursued, depending on the clinical context. Table 8.2 summarizes one possible stepwise approach that can be followed to explore all the

Table 8.1 'I WATCH DEATH', a mnemonic for emergency assessment of the delirious patient

Infections
Withdrawal
Acute metabolic
Trauma
CNS pathology
Hypoxia
Deficiencies
Endocrinopathies
Acute vascular
Toxins or drugs
Heavy metals

Table 8.2 Screening of main aetiologies and diagnostic procedures

Toxic factors	Bedside drug screening for present and recent medications
	Urine or blood drug screening
Sepsis	Temperature
	Blood/urine and other cultures for infection screen
	Leukocyte count
	Urinalysis
	Red cell count
Glucose oxidative brain deficiency	Pulse oximetry
	Blood gases and acid-base balance
	Blood glucose
Electrolyte imbalances	Serum electrolytes (Na, K, Cl, Mg, Ca)
Renal failure	Urea, creatinine, creatinine clearance
Liver failure	Liver function tests
	Ammonia
CNS vascular, infectious or structural lesion	Screening for disseminated intravascular coagulation (DIC) and coagulation profile
	CSF examination: blood, glucose, proteins, lymphocytes leukocytes, malignant cells, culture
	Brain CT or MRI
Cofactor deficiency malnutrition	Vitamin B_{12} levels—administer vitamin B_1, 1g/day *
Endocrine dysfunction	Thyroid hormone and thyroid-stimulating hormone (TSH)
	Adrenal function
Seizures—nonconvulsive status	EEG
Paraneoplastic neurological disease	Determination of specific autoantibodies[†]

* The determination of vitamin B_1 levels is problematical. Our practice is to supplement B_1 to every elderly patient with poor nutritional status.

[†] See Chapter 7.

potentially correctable aetiologies. In our opinion, it is possible that, in many cases of the evolution of a quiet delirium as the terminal phase of metastatic cancer, none of these actions would be undertaken. It should be obvious that the role of any further investigation has to be weighted against the potential usefulness of the results to improve the patient's quality of life. As already discussed, in the severely ill population, it is often impossible to identify a single aetiology. A mean of two to three potential aetiological factors are common (Bruera *et al.* 1992*b*; Lawlor *et al.* 2000*b*; Tuma and DeAngelis 2000). See also the case reported in Section 7.5.

It is probably not fair to place the EEG in the penultimate position in Table 8.2. The EEG can be a source of very useful information in some cases of delirium and it is reasonably economical when compared to many of the other procedures.

8.1.2　Electroencephalography

As already mentioned, the EEG can be a sensitive and specific test for the diagnosis of delirium and, indeed, it was considered a candidate diagnostic criterion in the discussion that preceded the development of the DSM-IV (Tucker 1999). The relationship between consciousness level, EEG slowing, and the pathogenesis of delirium was originally described by Engel and Romano (1959). They clearly pointed out how the degree of slowing of the EEG corresponds to the degree of consciousness disturbance and parallels it, corresponding to the severity of the cause, reversibility of the disturbance, and the implementation of therapeutic interventions.

Traditional EEG combined with clinical findings can be used to diagnose delirium and differentiate it from functional psychoses (Brenner 1991; Trzepacz et al. 1988b) and from dementia (Jacobson et al. 1993a, b; Koponen et al. 1989), as well as to grade its severity and to follow up the patient's recovery. A grading system for the assessment of encephalopathies with altered level of consciousness was published by Young et al. (1992).

EEG findings that are typical of metabolic encephalopathy, and of many cases of drug toxicity parallel those seen with anaesthetic gases showing a progressive slowing of EEG frequency with increase in amplitude (see Fig. 5.3). Anaesthetic gases usually cause initial desynchronization and the appearance of fast activity in the beta frequencies followed by progressive slowing of the EEG. Fast activity of low voltage is also typically seen in alcohol withdrawal delirium. This is the only type of delirium in which fast activity is reported to dominate the EEG pattern.

In the case of toxic metabolic aetiologies, EEG slowing can be compounded with triphasic waves or epileptiform discharges (Bortone et al. 1998). Suppression of the EEG and burst suppression pattern is seen when coma occurs (Young et al. 1992, 1997).

In selected cases the EEG recording may be the only way to demonstrate the occurrence of non-convulsive status epilepticus (Towne et al. 2000b; Wengs et al. 1993; see also Fig. 5.2).

8.2　Clinical assessment tools

Although clinical evaluation according to the phenomenology of the symptoms and the nosographic criteria (DSM-IV-TR and ICD-10) is the gold standard for the diagnosis of delirium (see Chapter 1), many instruments have been developed for this purpose in clinical practice and in research. The importance of correctly examining the symptoms of delirium for epidemiological reasons (e.g. prevalence and incidence in specific palliative settings), research (e.g. evaluation of the severity of delirium, description of subtypes, aetiologies, and identification of new treatments), and clinical aims (e.g. development of the easiest methods of routine assessment) has been pointed out by a number of authors (Breitbart and Cohen 2000; Casarett and Inouye 2001).

Some concepts should be clarified when discussing the properties of methods for assessing delirium, since sound psychometric properties are necessary in order to have instruments that respect specific statistical constructs.

8.2.1 Validity of assessment tools

The first important consideration is *reliability,* which is a measure of the accuracy and consistency of a specified instrument. More specifically, *test–retest reliability* indicates the stability of the test scores over time, as indicated by the correlation between the scores obtained in two different assessments; *interrater reliability* evaluates the degree of agreement in test scores (total score or individual items) as obtained by different raters; *internal consistency reliability,* usually measured by the Cronbach alpha coefficient, refers to the relationship between the instrument items.

A second consideration is the *validity* of the instrument. *Content validity* indicates the extent to which the content of the items adequately explores the specified psychological area or function. *Criterion-related validity* refers to the relationship between the scores and a reference criterion (e.g. clinical diagnostic criteria) that represents the true state of the patient. More particularly, within criterion-related validity it is possible to distinguish the *sensitivity* (i.e. correct identification of true positive cases: true positives/(true positives + false negatives)), the *specificity* (i.e. correct identification of true negative cases: true negatives/(true negatives + false positives)). Sensitivity and specificity tend to vary according to the cut-off scores used on the instrument to classify the patients.

Related concepts are the *positive predictive accuracy* (i.e. the probability that a patient who is 'positive' on the test receives a diagnosis of delirium) and the *negative predictive accuracy* (i.e. the probability that a patient who is 'negative' on the test does not receive a diagnosis of delirium).

Lastly, *construct validity* refers to the accuracy of the instrument in measuring what it should measure, as indicated by high correlation with other instruments shown to measure the same construct (*convergent validity*) and low correlation with instruments shown to measure different constructs (*discriminant validity*).

Methods employed in clinical or research practice can be grouped in three broad categories: (1) general instruments for the evaluation of cognitive functions; (2) instruments specifically devised for the assessment of delirium; (3) other instruments. We will summarize here the most important tools for palliative care professionals, sending the interested reader to more detailed sources (Robertsson 1999; Smith *et al.* 1994; Trzepacz 1994*b*).

8.2.2 Instruments for the evaluation of cognitive functions

Among several instruments belonging to this category, the Mini-Mental State Examination (MMSE; see Appendix 1; Folstein *et al.* 1975) is one of the best known and uses tests for cognitive disturbances that can follow organic mental disorders, such as dementia, delirium, or other cognitive disorders (Tombaugh and McHugh 1992). It has been translated into several languages and is widely applied in clinical settings.

The MMSE (Appendix 1) consists of 11 questions that evaluate several parameters, including orientation to time and space, memory (instantaneous recall and short-term memory), attention and calculation (serial subtractions or reverse spelling), language, and constructional abilities. The score ranges from 0 to 30, with three cut-off scores used to evaluate cognitive functions: 24–30 indicates no impairment; 18–23 mild impairment; and 0–17 severe impairment. The influences of age and education have been introduced to adjust the score obtained by using the MMSE (Crum *et al.* 1993).

The psychometric properties of the MMSE have been examined in several studies. As far as delirium is concerned, however, the MMSE has been criticized on the following grounds.

- Certain symptoms of delirium are not examined by the instrument (e.g. perceptual and thought disorders).

- Specificity/sensitivity and positive/negative predictive values varied across studies, with high percentages of clinically delirious patients not being recognized by the MMSE (Smith *et al.* 1994). In our experience with delirious cancer patients, MMSE had a sensitivity of 38%, using the classic cut-off of 24 over 30 for normal subjects (Grassi *et al.* 2001*b*). See Yue *et al.* (1994) for the example of a delirious patient with a normal MMSE.

- Some tasks, such as writing a sentence and copying two intersecting pentagons, present difficulties of performance for severely delirious patients or in certain clinical settings (e.g. intensive care units).

The MMSE retains its importance because of its simplicity and popularity as a bed-side clinical tool. As is true of most instruments based on the assessment of orientation, short-term memory, calculation, and writing, the MMSE is particularly sensitive to attention deficit more than to other types of cognitive changes.

8.2.3 Instruments devised for the diagnosis and assessment of delirium

A number of instruments have been developed to assess delirium in clinical practice. They have different formats, such as algorithms, short interviews, and scales that assist clinicians in screening for the presence of delirium or in evaluating the severity of the disorder.

Confusion Assessment Method (CAM; Appendix 2)

The Confusion Assessment Method (CAM; Inouye *et al.* 1990) is an easy-to-administer instrument that has repeatedly been used as a tool for diagnosing delirium. The CAM consists of nine operationalized criteria from the DSM-III-R, with an *a priori* hypothesis (CAM algorithm) establishing the diagnosis of delirium according to four criteria: (1) acute onset and fluctuating course of symptoms; (2) inattention; and *either* (3) disorganized thinking; or (4) altered level of consciousness. The CAM algorithm has the highest predictive accuracy for all possible combinations of the nine features of delirium. When validated against psychiatric diagnosis and used by trained health professionals, the CAM shows good psychometric properties, with high levels of sensitivity (94–100%), specificity (90–95%), positive predictive value (91–94%), and negative predictive value (90–100%) (Farrell and Ganzini 1995; Inouye 1998; Inouye *et al.* 1990, 1999*a*; Zou *et al.* 1998). It can be administered in less than 5 minutes by clinicians, other than psychiatrists. and non-clinicians who, however, should have been trained in the method. The CAM was also shown to have convergent agreement with other mental status tests, including the MMSE, and high interobserver reliability (kappa, 0.81–1.0).

However, some reports have shown lower sensitivity, with values between 0.46 and 0.67, for the CAM when administered by a non-physician, in comparison with a physician, while specificity remained high (0.92–0.97) (Pompei *et al.* 1995; Rockwood *et al.* 1994). A recent study carried out in an emergency room showed that the coefficient of agreement between a trained non-physician and a geriatrician in the evaluation of delirium in 110 elderly patients using the CAM was good (0.91), with remarkably high levels of sensitivity (0.86), specificity (1.0), positive predictive value (0.97), and negative predictive value (1.0) (Monette *et al.* 2001).

A modified version of the CAM for use in intensive care unit patients (CAM-ICU; Appendix 3) was applied in a prospective cohort study and compared against the reference standard by a delirium expert who used delirium criteria from the DSM-IV. The CAM-ICU ratings showed high interrater reliability (kappa between 0.79 and 0.95) among the assessors (nurse and anesthaesthetist), with high sensitivity (95–100%) and specificity (89–93%) in comparison with DSM-IV diagnosis for patients who developed delirium (87%) (Ely *et al.* 2001a). In a study of 96 mechanically ventilated patients, the same author (Ely *et al.* 2001b) showed that, among the patients who developed delirium (83%), critical care nurses were able to detect the disorder, by using the CAM-ICU, with high sensitivity (93–100%) and specificity (98–100%) in comparison with DSM-IV diagnosis by delirium experts. Interrater reliability was also high ($\kappa = 0.96$). The CAM-ICU is different from the original CAM in the assessment of some items, such as inattention (which is rated as positive if the patient reports fewer than eight correct answers on either the visual or the auditory components of the Attention Screening Examination) and disorganized thinking (which is rated positive if the patient gives at least three incorrect answers to four predetermined questions and is unable to follow three simple commands).

Delirium Rating Scale (Appendix 4)

The Delirium Rating Scale (DRS; Trzepacz *et al.* 1988*a*) is one of the most frequently used instruments for the assessment of delirium. It is a 10-item symptom rating scale designed to identify delirium in the medically ill and to measure its severity. Items are not based on any particular DSM system and measure the clinical characteristics of delirium, namely, temporal onset of symptoms, perceptual disturbances (e.g. misperceptions, depersonalization, derealization), hallucinations, thought disorders (delusions), psychomotor behaviour, cognitive status, lability of mood, physical disorders, sleep–wake cycle disturbances, and variability of symptoms. The items are scored on different Lykert scales (most of them on a 0–3 scale). All available information from the patient interview, mental status examination, nursing observation, and family reports contributes to the DRS rating, which is based on a 24-hour period of observation The total DRS score is obtained by summing up the scores on the 10 items (range, 0–32). Although a cut-off score of 12 has been suggested to distinguish delirious from non delirious patients (Trzepacz and Dew 1995), a cut-off score of 10 has shown a sensitivity of 94% and a specificity of 82% (Rosen *et al.* 1994), while another study that used a less conservative cut-off of 7.5 showed a sensitivity of 90% and a specificity of 82% (Rockwood *et al.* 1996).

In our experience with the Italian version and validation of the DRS (Grassi *et al.* 2001*b*), 105 advanced cancer patients consecutively referred for cognitive disturbances were approached and a diagnosis of delirium was made in 62%. The DRS significantly differentiated delirious from non-delirious patients. Internal consistency was relatively high (Cronbach alpha, 0.70). Using the proposed cut-off score of 10, the DRS showed a sensitivity of 95% and a specificity of 61%, while, using the more conservative cut-off score of 12, sensitivity was 81% and specificity 76%. Factor analysis of the DRS showed the existence of three factors: the first comprising psychomotor behaviour, sleep–wake cycle, and cognitive status; the second consisting of psychotic items; and the third factor comprising other symptoms (temporal onset of symptoms, presence of causal physical disorder, lability of mood, and fluctuation of symptoms).

Delirium Rating Scale-Revised-98 (DRS-R-98; Appendix 5)

More recently, Trzepacz *et al.* (2001) have refined and revised the DRS, by developing the Delirium Rating Scale-Revised-98 (DRS-R-98). It consists of a 16-item clinician-rated scale with 13 severity items and 3 diagnostic items. It covers some areas also assessed by the DRS items (i.e. sleep–wake cycle disturbance, delusions, lability of affect, temporal onset of symptoms, fluctuation of symptoms, and physical disorder). Unlike in the DRS, perceptual disturbances and hallucinations are put together in the same category and psychomotor behaviour is separated into two categories that assess motor agitation and motor retardation. Cognitive status is separated into five specific items (i.e. orientation, attention, short-term memory, long-term memory, and visuospatial activity), and two further items assess language and thought process abnormalities. Each item is rated on a 0–3 Lykert scale. The sum of the first 13 items provides a severity score (range 0–39), while the last three (temporal onset of symptoms, fluctuation of symptoms, and physical disorder) can be used to help clinicians in differentiating delirium from other disorders or for research aims. They can be added to the first 13 to provide a total score (range 0–46). The DRS-R-98 is used for initial assessment and repeated measures. In addition to the examination of the patient, all available sources of information (e.g. family, nurses, chart reports) are used to rate the items.

The authors administered the DRS-R-98, the DRS, the Cognitive Test for Delirium, and the Clinical Global Impression scale to 68 patients with a diagnosis of delirium ($n = 24$), dementia ($n = 13$), depression ($n = 12$), schizophrenia ($n = 9$), and other disorders ($n = 10$). The DRS-R-98 significantly distinguished delirium from each of the other groups. Significant correlations were also found between DRS-R-98 and the other instruments. High levels of interrater reliability (0.98 for the DSR-R-98 total scale; 0.99 for the DRS-R-98 severity scale) and the internal consistency (Cronbach alpha, 0.90 for the DSR-R-98 total scale; 0.87 for the DRS-R-98 severity scale) were also found. Cut-off scores of 17.75 on the DSR-R-98 total scale resulted in 92% sensitivity and 95% specificity. Cut-off scores of 15.25 on the DSR-R-98 severity scale resulted in a sensitivity of 92% and a specificity of 93%. On the basis of these results, the authors point out that the DRS-R-98 is a valid measure of delirium severity over a broad range of symptoms and a useful diagnostic and assessment tool for longitudinal studies.

Memorial Delirium Assessment Scale (MDAS; Appendix 6)

The Memorial Delirium Assessment Scale (MDAS; Breitbart *et al.* 1997) was devised to assess delirium and to quantify the severity of the symptoms, when administered by experienced mental health professionals with minimal training. It is composed of 10 four-point (from 0 to 3) observer-rated items yielding a global score ranging from 0 to 30. The MDAS was developed to be consistent with the proposed DSM-IV diagnostic criteria for delirium, as well as earlier and alternative classification systems (e.g. DSM-III-R, ICD-9). Scale items explore arousal and level of consciousness, disorientation, short-term memory, digit span, attention, disorganized thinking, perceptual disturbances, delusions, psychomotor activity, and sleep–wake cycle disturbances. The MDAS integrates objective cognitive testing and evaluation of behavioural symptoms. It is rapid and easy to administer, requiring about 10 minutes for completion. It is also designed for repeated daily evaluation and to capture short-term fluctuations of symptoms and to document response to treatment. By using the suggested cut-off of 13 on the total score, the MDAS showed a sensitivity of 70.6% and a specificity of 93.7% in discriminating delirious from non-delirious patients in the cancer setting (Breitbart *et al.* 1997). The MDAS also accurately classified patients with different severity grades of delirium, in particular, those with moderate and severe delirium.

In the above-mentioned Italian study of 105 advanced cancer patients, the MDAS significantly differentiated delirious from non-delirious patients. The MDAS showed high levels of internal consistency (Cronbach alpha, 0.89). By using the cut-off of 13, the MDAS showed specificity 94% and sensitivity 68%. Factor analysis of the MDAS suggested the existence of two factors, one of which explained 51.1% of the variance and consisted of cognitive items, and the other that explained a further 11.5% of the variance and consisted of psychotic symptoms (disorganized thinking, perceptual disturbance, and delusions) (Grassi *et al.* 2001*b*).

In a study of 104 patients admitted to an acute palliative care unit, Lawlor *et al.* (2000*b*) assessed cognitive functions by using the MMSE, a standardized semistructured interview, and the MDAS. A DSM-IV diagnosis of delirium was made in 68% ($n = 71$) of the patients. Complete MDAS data were available for 56 patients. The authors found moderate to low correlations among the scale items. Two primary correlated factors emerged at the analysis of factor loadings: a global cognitive factor (factor I) and a neurobehavioural factor (factor II) with Cronbach's alpha coefficients indicating a relatively high level of correlation for items within each factor and a Cronbach's alpha for the MDAS (0.78), suggesting one general underlying factor. In a larger sample of complete MDAS ratings ($n = 330$), a cut-off score of 7 yielded the highest sensitivity (98%) and specificity (96%) for the diagnosis of delirium. The

MDAS score moderately correlated with the MMSE score ($r = -0.55$; Lawlor *et al.* 2000*c*).

Matsuoka *et al.* (2001), in a study of 37 elderly Japanese patients, confirmed the good internal consistency of the MDAS (Cronbach alpha, 0.92) and its moderate correlation with the MMSE ($r = -0.55$).

The MDAS was applied to postoperative delirium by Marcantonio *et al.* (2002). In this study it was used to differentiate the hypoactive from the hyperactive subtypes and showed a positive correlation between delirium severity and functional outcome.

Confusional State Evaluation (CSE; Appendix 7)

The Confusional State Evaluation (CSE; Robertsson *et al.* 1997) was developed to assess delirium with particular reference to the elderly. It consists of 22 items on a 5-point scale (0–4), with the possibility of rating each item on a half-point scale (e.g. 0–0.5–1–1.5–2). A group of 12 items measure the main clinical symptoms of delirium (disorientation to person, time, space, and situation; thought disturbance; memory disturbance; inability to concentrate; distractability; perseveration; impaired contact; paranoid delusions; hallucinations) and their sum yields the 'confusion score'. A group of seven items deals with frequent symptoms of delirium (irritability, emotional lability, wakefulness disturbance, increased or reduced psychomotor activity, mental uneasiness, and sleep–wake disorders). The last group of three items is comprised of the temporal characteristics of delirium (sudden impairment and/or fluctuations), the intensity of the current episode, and the frequency and the intensity of the episodes of delirium. The authors report the usefulness of the CSE in measuring the severity of symptoms and their changes over time. It can be administered in a maximum of 30 minutes by nurses, physicians, and psychologists. In a study of elderly patients with a DSM-III-R diagnosis of delirium, the CSE showed an acceptable level of internal validity. The correlation between the CSE and the MMSE was -0.87. A confusion score of less than 25 is considered to indicate mild delirium, between 25 and 35 to suggest moderate delirium, and over 35 to show severe delirium. The authors acknowledge the need for further validation studies, including studies on different diagnostic and age groups.

Cognitive Test for Delirium (CTD)

The Cognitive Test for Delirium (CTD) was developed to identify delirium in critically ill patients admitted to intensive care units (Hart *et al.* 1996). The main aims of the authors in devising the CTD were to have an instrument that would be brief and easy to administer, that would focus solely on cognitive functions, and that could accommodate the severe medical conditions of patients in intensive care (e.g. intubation, motor restriction). For this reason, the patient's responses to the CTD are nonverbal (pointing, nodding head, or raising hand). Following DSM-III-R-criteria, the CTD evaluates orientation, attention span, memory, comprehension/conceptual reasoning, and vigilance. Scores for each of these areas range from 0 to 6 and are added together, yielding a maximum total score of 30. The time for test administration is between 10 and 15 minutes. In a study of patients with delirium, dementia, depression, and schizophrenia, the CTD showed a sensitivity of 100% and a specificity of

95%. The authors indicate that, in almost half of ICU patients who completed the CTD, the MMSE could not be administered. More recently, the same authors (Hart *et al.* 1997) found that an abbreviated form of the CTD, consisting of two content scores (visual attention span and recognition memory for pictures), maintained a good reliability index and the ability to discriminate between delirium, dementia, depression, and schizophrenia.

Delirium Index

The Delirium Index (DI; McCusker *et al.* 1998) was developed to measure changes in the severity of symptoms of delirium over time. According to the authors, the DI was designed to be used in conjunction with the MMSE, the first five questions of which represent the basis of observation. The DI investigates seven symptoms of delirium, adapted from the CAM, namely, attention, disorganized thinking, level of consciousness, memory, perceptual disturbance, and motor activity. The symptoms are assessed through direct observation and questions at the patient's bedside, without any need for additional information from the family, the staff, or the patient's chart. Each symptom is rated on a 0–3 scale (from absent to severe), with a total score ranging from 0 to 21. It takes 5–10 minutes to complete and can be administered by research assistants and nurses. The authors used the DI in 27 delirious patients, showing a good agreement between psychiatrist's and research assistant's ratings (0.88) and a high correlation with the Delirium Rating Scale (0.84).

Delirium Symptom Interview

Among the structured interviews, the Delirium Symptom Interview (DSI; Albert *et al.* 1992) was designed for diagnosing the presence of symptoms of delirium. It consists of seven domains in a present–absent format according to the DSM-III criteria for delirium: disorientation, perceptual disturbances, disturbance of consciousness during the past 24 hours, disturbance of sleep, incoherent speech, level of psychomotor activity, and fluctuation of symptoms. Each item is evaluated through direct questions to the patients or judged by the interviewer. By consensus, it has been indicated that the diagnosis of delirium can be made if at least one of three critical items (i.e. disorientation, perceptual disturbances, disturbance of consciousness during the past 24 hours) scores positive. When compared with clinician-rated interviews, however, sensitivity was high (90%), while specificity was lower (80%). Interrater reliability showed kappa levels ranging from 0.90 to 0.93 for detecting one critical item. Although the DSI may be useful in epidemiological circumstances as trained lay interviewers can administer it, it is not easy to administer to severely ill patients who are unable to respond to questions (Trzepacz 1994*b*).

Delirium Writing Test (DWT)

The DWT (Aakerlund and Rosenberg 1994) has been used in a study of patients who underwent thoracotomy for lung cancer, with the rationale that writing ability was impaired in patients who developed delirium in comparison with patients who did not develop delirium. It consists of examining certain features, namely, reluctance to write, motor impairment because of tremor, clumsiness, and migrographia, and spatial disorders in writing, syntactical disorders, and spelling disorders, which were impaired in delirious patients (see Chapter 4 for more clinical detail). The authors indicate a high specificity/sensitivity of the instrument in detecting delirium in postoperative patients.

The usefulness of methods that assess dysgraphia in delirious patients has been confirmed in palliative care (Macleod and Whitehead 1997), while a recent study in psychiatry indicated that dysgraphia and constructional apraxia had predictive diagnostic value (Baranowski and Patten 2000), and, although sensitivity was low (33%), specificity was quite high (98%); see also Chapter 4.

Communication Capacity Scale (CS) and Agitation Distress Scale (ADS)

The CS and the ADS are two operational observer-rating scales that were recently developed by Morita *et al.* (2001) specifically to evaluate terminal delirium. The authors conducted a study in a palliative care setting in order to quantify patients' communication capacity and agitated behaviour in terminal delirium. They used, along with the CS and the ADS, the DRS and the MDAS on 30 terminally ill cancer patients with delirium. Both the CS and the ADS achieved high internal consistency (Cronbach's alpha, 0.91 and 0.96, respectively) and interrater reliability (Cohen's kappa values on each item of 0.72–1.00). The principal components analysis resulted in the emergence of only one component for each scale. The CS total score was associated with the MDAS ($r = 0.78$), and cognitive items from the MDAS and DRS ($r = 0.83$). The ADS total score was significantly correlated with the DRS ($r = 0.61$) and agitation items from the MDAS and DRS ($r = 0.61$).

Intensive Care Delirium Screening Checklist (ICDSC)

The ICDSC is a further instrument developed by Dubois *et al.* (2001) to assess delirium in patients admitted to intensive care units. The scale is completed using information collected during the previous 24 hours. It consists of 8 items evaluating the following parameters: altered level of consciousness, inattention, disorientation, hallucination, psychomotor agitation or retardation, inappropriate speech or mood, sleep–wake cycle disturbance, and symptom fluctuation. For each abnormal item a score of 1 is given. The authors showed a sensitivity of 99% when using a cut-off score of 4 on the ICDSC.

Other instruments

Other instruments focused on assessing delirium severity with the aim of being able to repeat assessments in a short time and therefore to follow the clinical course of the syndrome. One of these instruments is the Delirium Assessment Scale, which is based on observation of the patient, interviews with staff or relatives, and the DSM-III criteria (O'Keeffe 1994). Another tool is the Delirium Severity Scale, which is more focused on cognitive function assessment and consists of a modified version of cognitive tests such as the forward digit span and the similarities test from the Wechsler Adult Intelligence Scale and Wechsler Adult Memory Scale (Bettin *et al.* 1998). This scale showed sensitivity to change over a short period of time and in the authors' opinion has the advantage of not valuing anamnestic data for scoring as in the case of the DRS or MDAS (Bettin *et al.* 1998).

8.3 Conclusions

The diagnosis of delirium can be based on a variety of clinical procedures and instruments. It can be aided by the use of different assessment tools. These tools have some of the desirable characteristics of instruments aimed at diagnosing and evaluating delirium (Roth-Romer *et al.* 1997) but, in general, it is not advisable to use just one of them for both purposes at this time. Some instruments are clearly specifically designed for diagnosing the presence of delirium, whereas other instruments are used to describe symptoms and rate their severity. This distinction is not always so clear for some of the instruments described. For instance, while (see also appendixes) it is clear that the assessment of delirium severity and clinical features is feasible with the DRS and the MDAS, and that the CAM and the DSI are operational systems to make a diagnosis, attempts to combine these two characteristics by using cut-off points over the severity scores provided by DRS and MDAS have been made. In general, results were less than completely satisfactory (Breitbart *et al.* 1997; Grassi *et al.* 2001*b*; Rockwood *et al.* 1996). Other authors observed that, for instance, including the presence of a possible or definite precipitating physical disorder in a scale aimed at rating delirium severity may be inappropriate if severity has to be assessed on the basis of symptoms and signs (O'Keeffe 1994). It is our opinion that the diagnosis of delirium can be improved by a continuous perfecting of the application of diagnostic criteria but that clinical experience and decision should nevertheless be valued and incorporated in any diagnostic system. Severity scores will have fundamental importance in evaluation and screening procedures, if they are of a high enough sensitivity, but should not be a substitute for clinical diagnosis. The recent new version of the DRS is an attempt to combine in a single instrument a method for diagnosis and assessment. It is important to use this instrument to confirm the potential improvement that it represents.

The availability of different instruments is important in helping clinicians and researchers to choose a method that is adequate for their specific requirements. However, the continuous proliferation of instruments for the diagnosis and assessment of delirium does not *per se* serve the purpose of perfecting homogeneous guidelines and producing reproducible and comparable results across different international care settings.

Chapter 9

Management

The cornerstones of delirium management have varied little over the centuries, involving aetiological, environmental, nursing, and pharmacological interventions (Lipowski 1990b). The area that has received most attention from modern medicine is drug therapy with the introduction in the 1950s of major and minor tranquillizers (see below). Quite interestingly, pharmacological sedation has been considered helpful and necessary since the second century AD, when Areteus suggested the use of boiled poppy for this purpose (Adams 1861), and opium has been the most popular drug for this indication since the nineteenth century (Lipowski 1990b). Indeed, the current use of opioids in critical care and anaesthesia confirms their fortunate historical background. Some authors still recommend opioid-based regimens as the first-line therapy for agitated deliria (Adams 1988; Fernandez et al. 1989).

Current management guidelines are still largely empirical. Guidelines for management have been published by the American Psychiatric Association (APA; American Psychiatric Association 1999; Table 9.1 reports their general terms) but, due to the absolute rarity of controlled clinical trials, most recommendations are based on clinical experience rather than being evidence-based (Britton and Russell 2000; Cole et al. 1998; Meagher 2001). In cases with an underlying acute event that may allow for at least temporary recovery, management should consider supportive therapies to maintain vital functions and treat complications. Specific recommendations for the management of patients with delirum at the end of their life were released by a consensus

Table 9.1 General guidelines for management of delirium

Coordinate with other physicians caring for the patient
Identify the aetiology
Initiate intervention for acute conditions
Provide other disorder-specific treatment
Monitor and ensure safety
Assess and monitor psychiatric status
Assess individual and family psychological and social characteristics
Establish and maintain alliances
Educate patient and family regarding the illness
Provide postdelirium management

panel of the American Society of Internal Medicine (Casarett and Inouye 2001). One potentially difficult question may be posed when informed consent or patient competence is required for any reason (Auerswald et al. 1997). The response to these types of requests has been discussed only to a limited extent in the literature and may deserve more attention on ethical or medicolegal grounds.

9.1 Identifying the cause and other aetiologically oriented interventions

As already underlined in Chapters 6–8, the identification of a relevant aetiology should be part of any rational approach, even potentially when no action to remove the cause would be considered appropriate. Reversible causes, on the other hand, can be found in any population and can potentially be corrected (de Stoutz et al. 1995; Fainsinger et al. 1993; Grassi et al. 2001a; Lawlor et al. 2000b).

General principles of management in emergency medicine suggest providing treatment for potentially acute biochemical abnormality (such as hypoglycaemia), drug intoxication, and vitamin B_1 deficiency, factors that may be relatively rare in the palliative care setting or difficult to correct, as in the case of the toxicity of an opioid drug that is otherwise needed for pain control.

Recommendations based on the clinical experience of palliative medicine specialists and on systematic observation, but not on totally satifying scientific evidence, suggest that, besides all other procedures already reviewed in several parts of this book, moderate hydration is beneficial in dehydrated patients with complex pharmacological regimes to reduce the likelihood of accumulation of toxic drug or metabolite levels (Bruera et al. 1995).

In the case of opioid toxicity several observations support switching from one opioid to another in order to obtain a more favourable balance between analgesia and side-effects. The practice of switching (or 'rotating') opioids seemed useful in solving opioid-related delirium in several case series. It is our opinion that the most useful switching attempts imply changing from morphine or hydromorphone to methadone, fentanyl, or oxycodone (Cherny et al. 2001; Gagnon et al. 1999; Maddocks et al. 1996). General principles of managing opioid-induced delirium include: dose reduction, treatment with neuroleptics, switching to another opioid, switching the route of administration, providing hydration, stopping concurrent medications (Cherny et al. 2001).

9.2 Pharmacological management

Agitated delirium can be dangerous for the patient and the care-givers, and is a difficult experience for the family. A pharmacological symptomatic intervention is certainly justified. To implement an efficacious treatment regimen, continuous monitoring and frequent assessment are necessary as an integral part of treatment. Systematic recording of the patient's mental status can be facilitated by using one of the assessment tools described in Chapter 8 and is needed to account for fluctuations, partial recovery, and to reduce the impact of differing views among staff members and family, which may jeopardize therapeutic outcome. The aim of pharmacological management is to calm the patient, avoid dangerous behaviours, and control hallucinations and delusions that can have subjective negative content, while allowing aetiological and supportive therapies that can contribute to delirium resolution in the reversible cases. At times this aim can be obtained by relatively simple drug regimens, but more intensive approaches such as sedation or physical restraint in cases unresponsive to therapy may be needed.

Keeping in mind that better outcomes are related to better premorbid general conditions (Cole *et al.* 1998), in the cases associated with multiple medical problems and unfavourable prognosis, the aims of therapy are, in part at least, the same. In the palliative care of this particular condition, special attention should be paid to the assessment of symptoms unrelated to the altered mental state but concurrent with it (Bruera *et al.* 1992a), and to the benefit of improving the level of consciousness and awareness, which is always based on a case by case individual decision, where the knowledge of the patient's wishes should have an important role (Morita *et al.* 2000). Another related, but complicated issue is whether quiet somnolent patients suffering from hypoactive deliria would need or benefit from treatment at all (Platt *et al.* 1994; Stiefel and Bruera 1991). Conversely, the therapeutic recourse to sedation to control delirium and related suffering is often specific to the clinical situation of the terminal patient, although the frequency of this need varies across the experiences of different palliative care specialists (Fainsinger *et al.* 2000*a*, *b*). For the treatment of delirium recent guidelines have been published (American Psychiatric Association 1999) that make precise the necessary steps and drugs to use, in particular, neuroleptics (or antipsychotics), although other drugs have been proposed as adjuvant pharmacological treatment. Recent data relative to the use of neuroleptics for rapid tranquillization have drawn attention to the risk of severe side-effects and the need for new options (McAllister-Williams and Ferrier 2002).

9.2.1 Classic neuroleptics or antipsychotics

Neuroleptics are a broad class of different drugs discovered almost 50 years ago (chlorpromazine in 1950 and haloperidol shortly thereafter) that are characterized by a potent antipsychotic action and are, for that reason, routinely used in psychiatry and in medicine to treat psychotic symptoms present in several disorders (schizophrenia, affective disorders with psychotic features, and psychotic symptoms in organic mental disorders, such as dementia and delirium; Marder 1998). This class of drugs consists of several subclasses, namely, phenothiazines (e.g. chlorpromazine, thioridazine, fluphenazine), thioxanthenes (e.g. thiothixene, flupenthixol), butyrophenones (e.g. haloperidol, droperidol), and dibenzoxazepines (e.g. loxapine). Known as conventional or typical antipsychotics (to be distinguished from the most recent atypical antipsychotics—see Section 9.2.2), all these drugs share the property of blocking dopaminergic D_2 activity in different areas of the CNS. This action exerted in the mesolimbic pathway results in a block of positive psychotic symptoms (hallucinations, delusions), while the same action in the other areas is responsible for significant side-effects. More specifically, blockade of dopamine receptors in the nigrostriatal pathway results in extrapyramidal symptoms (parkinsonism after pure block, or dyskinesia as a consequence of upregulation of the system); blockade in the mesocortical pathway produces blunting of emotions and cognitive symptoms (known as negative symptoms); blockade in the tuberoinfundibular pathway causes an increase in prolactin secretion. Conventional antipsychotics also block: muscarinic receptors, resulting in generalized anticholinergic symptoms (e.g. blurred vision, dry mouth, constipation); histamine H_1 receptors, resulting in the onset of drowsiness and weight gain; and noradrenergic α_1 receptors, leading to orthostatic hypotension, drowsiness, and dizziness.

The use of neuroleptics in delirium is well established (Lipowski 1990*b*), given the need for both the reduction of psychotic symptoms and the amelioration of the cognitive filter, which is altered by the disorder and improvement of sleep. Sedation in the case of aggressive behaviour or agitation can also be an important effect of the use of antipsychotics. However, sedation is more appropriately described as a side-effect of neuroleptics and can be avoided, when not necessary, by accurately tailoring drug choice and dosage to the individual. This is not, however, always possible and the tranquillization or control of some cases of delirium and suffering can only be achieved through significant sedation.

Haloperidol

Haloperidol is pharmacologically a butyrophenone with etherocyclic structure. The use of haloperidol and neuroleptics in general to control delirium is supported by pharmacological rationale and by clinical experience. One controlled clinical trial (Breitbart *et al.* 1996) confirmed these empirical and theoretical assumptions by demonstrating that, while haloperidol and chlorpromazine were associated with the improvement of delirium symptoms, lorazepam worsened clinical symptoms.

Haloperidol has long been considered the first-line drug for this indication, with the exception of alcohol and benzodiazepine withdrawal delirium, because of its fewer vasomotor, cardiac, and central side-effects in comparison with all the other potentially useful drugs (Table 9.2). It is worth noting that haloperidol is today considered the drug of choice even in liver transplant patients for its favourable profile of side-effects (Trzepacz *et al.* 1993).

Table 9.2 Comparative profile of side-effects among several neuroleptics

Drug	Sedative	Hypotensive	Extrapyramidal	Anticholinergic
Haloperidol	+	+	++++	+
Droperidol	++	++	++++	++
Methotrimeprazine	++++	+++	++	+++
Promazine	++	++	+	++
Chlorpromazine	+++	+++	++	+++
Clozapine	++++	+	−	+++
Olanzapine	++	−	−	++
Risperidone	++	+++	+	+

Haloperidol has 60% bioavailability after oral administration and is metabolized by liver oxidative dealkylation. Absorption via the oral route is slow with plasma levels detectable after 60 to 90 minutes and peak levels not earlier than 4 hours. Intramuscular administration leads to peak plasma levels in 20–40 minutes, while, after IV injection, the action is rapid—within minutes—and concentration decay is rapid as well—within 1 hour in the distribution phase (Forsman and Ohman 1977; Settle and Ayd 1983). Its half-life ranges from 12 to 36 hours leading to sustained plasma levels long after repeated administration is discontinued.

Guidelines on haloperidol dosing in cases of agitated delirium are variable. Lipowski (1990b) suggests the use of oral administrations of 5 to 10 mg in the morning and at bedtime in mild to moderate cases, and IM injections of 5–10 mg every 30–60 minutes until tranquillization is achieved in severe cases. IM injections should be followed by oral maintenance doses equal to 1.5–2 times the parenteral dose. These guidelines apply to young patients without liver disease. In the elderly, aged 60 or older, dosing for rapid tranquillization should start with 0.5 mg IM every hour (Lipowski 1990b).

APA guidelines are not very detailed about dosing. For acute parenteral treatment, it is suggested to administer 1 to 2 mg for younger patients, and 0.25 to 0.5 mg for elderly patients, repeated every 2–4 hours as needed. Psychiatry textbooks are more detailed but fairly general. Usual doses, independently of route of administration, are: 0.5–1 mg for mild; 2–5 mg for moderate; and 5–10 mg for severe delirium with agitation. The dose should not be repeated before 30 minutes has elapsed, after which it can be repeated at 30 minute intervals until the clinical effect is achieved (Wise et al. 1999; Wise and Trzepacz 1996).

While the intravenous use of haloperidol is not approved in the UK and USA, a consensus exists on the usefulness and safety (e.g. lower incidence of extrapyramidal side-effects) of this type of administration for severe cases and in critically ill patients (Ayd 1987; Gelfand et al. 1992; Shapiro et al. 1995). Typical doses are reported to be 2–5 mg every 20–30 minutes until the clinical effect is reached (Gelfand et al. 1992).

Published experiences can help in choosing the initial dose and titration regimen. One study on the emergency control of agitated disruptive behaviour due mostly to alcohol intoxication and head trauma found that mean doses of 8.2 ± 4.5 mg given as 1.4 ± 0.75 IM doses per patient controlled agitation in 113 of 136 patients (Clinton et al. 1987).

In critical patients, very high doses of IV haloperidol have been used successfully to control agitation, doses ranging from more than 100 to 1000 mg in 24 hours (Levenson 1995; Riker et al. 1994; Wilt et al. 1993).

Lower doses are reported in two more cases of hyperactive delirium treated with IV infusion, one starting off with 6 mg/h, lowered after a few hours to 3 mg/h and the second one with 2 mg/h infusion (Dixon and Craven 1993).

A retrospective case series of delirious patients seen at a comprehensive cancer centre (Olofson et al. 1996) found that, in 54 cases of hyperactive delirium, the haloperidol doses employed were low in 61% of cases (mean, 2.5 mg/24 h), intermediate in 32% (mean, 15 mg/24h), and high in 7% (mean, 30 mg/24h).

Another study in the cancer patient population applied prospectively a 6-hour every-half-an-hour titration schedule (Table 9.3) using IM, IV, or oral haloperidol in

Table 9.3 Haloperidol: 30-minute titration schedule.* This schedule is given as one published example of titration with the understanding that it should be applied with judgement to individual cases[†]

Time	Haloperidol IV or IM dose (mg)
1	0.5
2	0.5
3	0.5
4	1
5	1
6	1
7	2
8	2
9	2
10	5
11	5
12	5

* Modified with permission from Akechi, T., Uchitomi, Y., Okamura, H., Fukue, M., Kagaya, A., Nishida, A., Oomori, N. and Yamawaki, S., Usage of haloperidol for delirium in cancer patients, *Supp Care Cancer*, 4 (1996) 390–2. Copyright 1996 Springer-Verlag.

[†] Doses are repeated evey 30 minutes according to clinical effects and increased every three doses if clinical effect requires it.

10 consecutive patients. The mean $\pm$ SD, dose of haloperidol on the first day was 6 ± 4.0 mg (range 0.5–11 mg) and the mean daily dose over the whole follow-up period until recovery was 5.4 ± 3.4 mg (range 0.5–10.5 mg). The dose needed on the first day of treatment was significantly related to the following average daily dose (Akechi *et al.* 1996). The most important general rule is that, without dose titration and tailoring to individual patient response, many cases are going to result in therapy failures.

These doses are profoundly different from the doses reached in another report on terminally ill AIDS patients, using a combined protocol of IV haloperidol and lorazepam with an average daily dose of haloperidol of 42 mg and lorazepam 7.5 mg (Fernandez *et al.* 1989).

It is important to recall that haloperidol may be insufficient to control symptoms of delirium. In one case series of consecutive patients with delirium and advanced cancer, only 60% could be managed by haloperidol alone—the others required various combinations of other neuroleptics (chlorpromazine, methotrimeprazine) or benzodiazepines (lorazepam, midazolam). In 26% of cases symptom control could be achieved only by sedation, which was implemented with midazolam (Stiefel *et al.* 1992), confirming the experience of several case reports (Fainsinger and Bruera 1992).

As mentioned in Chapter 6, haloperidol is also classified as a drug with high potential for metabolic interaction with many other drugs commonly used in palliative care (Bernard and Bruera 2000).

Droperidol

Droperidol is related to haloperidol but is available only for IM or IV use, and usually limited to hospital use. It has a short half-life (2–3 hours) and is usually reserved for anaesthesiological or intensive care use. It differs from haloperidol in its more rapid, potent, and sedative effects. It also has strong α_1-adrenergic blocking activity that results in significant hypotensive effects. Doses of 5–15 mg can be used and repeated every 4 to 6 hours if necessary. (van Leeuwen *et al.* 1977), but bolus injections are often followed by hypotension especially in critical patients (Frye *et al.* 1995). Two controlled clinical trials compared haloperidol with droperidol for the treatment of agitation One study compared 5 mg IM double-blind injections of haloperidol or droperidol in 27 agitated patients and found that, after 30 minutes, 81% of the patients treated with haloperidol needed another injection compared to only 36% of the patients treated with droperidol (Resnick and Burton 1984). In another study 5 mg of IM or IV droperidol were compared with the same dose of haloperidol when being used to control agitation and combativeness in patients admitted to an emergency room and requiring physical restraint (Thomas *et al.* 1992). Droperidol was more rapid in controlling agitation within 30 minutes of administration. There are no results available on the use of droperidol in patients with a diagnosis of delirium in palliative care. In a report of three intensive care unit cases, continuous IV infusions of 1, 8, and 20 mg/hour, respectively, caused a mean increase of QTc interval of 17% (Frye *et al.* 1995).

For these reasons and because of the risk of possible death (Haines *et al.* 2001), droperidol has been withdrawn in some countries and caution has been recommended in its use.

Chlorpromazine

The prototypical phenothiazine and the first neuroleptic medication to be discovered, available for oral and parenteral administration (IH, IV), the subcutaneous use is not recommended because it is an irritant. It has a half-life ranging from 16 to 30 hours. An oral dose of 100 mg is equivalent to 25–50 mg parenterally (oral bioavailability is $32 \pm 19\%$ and decreases after repeated administrations; mean half-life is 30 hours) and to 2–5 mg of parenteral haloperidol. Like thioridazine it has strong alpha-adrenergic blocking activity which explains the frequency of orthostatic hypotension and cardiovascular effects. For these reasons its use is not recommended especially in elderly, frail, and medically ill patients. Chlorpromazine has been used at times in advanced cancer patients for its more potent sedative effects (Stiefel *et al.* 1992). Phenothiazines have been implicated in exacerbating symptoms of restlessness and myoclonus in dying patients treated with high-dose opioids (Dunlop 1989; Potter *et al.* 1989). Phenothiazines lower the threshold for epileptic discharges. Chlorpromazine is sometimes indicated in this setting to control dyspnoea or other rarer symptoms such as hiccup (De Conno *et al.* 1991*b*).

Methotrimeprazine

This drug gained some popularity in palliative care because of its analgesic (Beaver *et al.* 1966; Lasagna and DeKornfeld 1961) and potent antiemetic properties suggesting its use in situations such as pain unrelieved by opioids or bowel obstruction (Baines 1993). Its half-life is 16 to 78 hours. It is available as a parenteral preparation in the USA (in Italy only the oral preparation is available). It has a powerful sedating effect and can be used in treating otherwise unresponsive agitation or for severely insomniac patients (Stiefel *et al.* 1992). In a recent review it was the preferred drug for sedation together with chlorpromazine after midazolam (Cowan and Walsh 2001).

9.2.2 Atypical neuroleptics

Atypical antipsychotics represent a class of new drugs characterized by a specific pharmacological property of serotonin$_{2A}$-dopamine$_2$ ($5HT_{2A}/D_2$) antagonism, which is absent among conventional antipsychotics. This property has significant clinical effects, principally little or no propensity to cause extrapyramidal side-effects, reduced capacity to elevate prolactin levels, and reduction of negative symptoms of schizophrenia (Owens and Riscj 1998; Stahl 2000). However, the receptor-binding profiles of the atypical antipsychotics vary consistently, with some (e.g. clozapine, olanzapine) interacting with multiple receptors, including noradrenergic (α_1 blockade), cholinergic (muscarinic blockade), histaminergic (antihistamine property), and serotonergic ($5HT_{2C}$, $5HT_3$, $5HT_6$, as well as $5HT_{2A}$), and others (e.g. risperidone, ziprasidone), with a predominant $5HT_{2A}$ selectivity (Goldstein 2000).

Clozapine

Clozapine is the first atypical antipsychotic drug, synthesized in the mid-1960s and used from the early 1970s. Its use was discontinued in many countries because of its side-effects (i.e. agranulocytosis). It was then re-evaluated and used in clinical practice. Its property of serotonin$_{2A}$–dopamine$_2$ ($5HT_{2A}/D_2$) antagonism at limbic rather than at striatal dopamine receptors explains the relative freedom from extrapyramidal side-effects. Clozapine is also an antagonist at adrenergic, cholinergic, histaminergic, and serotonergic receptors. Following a dosage of 100 mg b.i.d., the average steady-state peak plasma concentration occurs after about 2.5 hours (range, 1–6 hours). Clozapine is almost completely metabolized prior to excretion to inactive components or desmethyl metabolite which has only limited activity. The mean elimination half-life of clozapine after a single 75 mg dose is 8 hours (range, 4–12 hours). It is used mainly in psychiatry for the treatment of refractory schizophrenia. It has significant sedative properties, which justifies its use in treating aggressive and agitated patients and as a sleep adjuvant drug in patients with Parkinson's disease manifesting agitation, insomnia, or symptoms of delirium. Available in doses of 25 and 100 mg oral tablets, in the elderly it is better to start with the initial dose of a quarter of the 25 mg tablet. Its adverse cardiovascular effects (orthostatic hypotension, tachycardia, ECG repolarization changes), the possible onset of seizures, and, especially, the occurrence of clozapine-induced agranulocytosis (1–2%) limit the use of clozapine in patients with severe medical illness, especially if concomitant drugs are employed (e.g. chemotherapy). Furthermore, the relevant anticholinergic effects vindicate the observation of delirium favoured by clozapine administration (van der Molen-Eijgenraam *et al.* 2001; Wilkins-Ho and Hollander 1997).

Olanzapine

Olanzapine is structurally related to clozapine with high affinity binding to the serotonin $5HT_{2A/2C}$, dopamine D_{1-4}, muscarinic M_{1-5}, histamine H_1, and adrenergic α_1-adrenergic receptors. Antagonism of M_{1-5} receptors may explain its anticholinergic effects and antagonism of H_1 receptors and α_1 receptors may explain the somnolence and orthostatic hypotension, respectively, observed with this drug. Olanzapine is well absorbed after oral administration and reaches peak concentrations in about 6 hours. It is eliminated extensively by first-pass metabolism, with approximately 40% of the dose metabolized before reaching the systemic circulation. Its half-life ranges from 21 to 54 hours.

Olanzapine has been reported to be useful in delirium in a series of anecdotal cases (Passik and Cooper 1999; Sipahimalani and Masand 1998). Its mean half-life is 30 hours. Also devoid of extrapyramidal side-effects, it is much less likely than clozapine to decrease white blood cell counts. In a non-randomized comparison study of 22 patients, 11 treated with olanzapine and 11 with haloperidol for deliria of several aetiologes, the mean oral haloperidol dose was 5.1 ± 3.5 (SD) mg/day and the mean daily olanzapine dose was 8.2 ± 3.4 mg. Olanzapine was started at the dose of 5 mg q.h.s. (*quaque hora somni*, before going to sleep) and titrated upward as needed; the highest dose used was 15 mg/day. Patients tolerated olanzapine better than haloperidol. No side-effects were seen with olanzapine while three patients had extrapyramidal side-effects and two had excessive sedation with haloperidol (Sipahimalani and Masand 1998). Efficacy was assessed with the Delirium Rating Scale (DRS) and was similar for the two treatments. Olanzapine was also useful for treating a case of delirium that was complicated by the combined toxicity of many drugs including opioids and prochloperazine, in a patient with non-Hodgkin's lymphoma and secondary leukaemia. Delirium was not controlled with haloperidol and lorazepam and extrapyramidal symptoms were relevant. Olanzapine was given at 5 mg q.h.s. in the early evening and increased to 10 mg with 2.5 mg as needed doses available during the day (Passik and Cooper 1999). A non-controlled consecutive case series reports on the use of olanzapine in 79 patients with cancer and delirium. An initial mean oral dose of 3 mg (0.14 SD) was used in a single bed-time administration or b.i.d. and after a week daily mean dose reached 6.3 mg (0.52 SD). Most patients recovered. The worse results were seen in the elderly patients (> 70 year old), 70% of recovery compared with 90% of younger patients (Breitbart *et al.* 2002b).

Olanzapine is now also available also as a parenteral preparation and gave good results in the management of agitated demented patients when compared with lorazepam (Karena *et al.* 2002). It could be an interesting alternative for rapid tranquillization in cases where its efficacy and safety profile compare favourably with the standard treatment with haloperidol.

Risperidone

Risperidone is an atypical antipsychotic ($5HT_{2A}/D_2$ antagonism) with high affinity for α_1 and α_2 adrenergic, and H_1 histaminergic receptors and a low to moderate affinity for the $5HT_{1C}$, $5HT_{1D}$, and $5HT_{1A}$ receptors, weak affinity for the D_1 receptor, and no affinity for cholinergic muscarinic or β_1 and β_2 adrenergic receptors. Risperidone is well absorbed after oral administration and is extensively metabolized in the liver to a major active metabolite (9-hydroxyrisperidone), which is equieffective with risperidone in terms of receptor-binding activity. Mean peak plasma concentrations occur at about 1 hour, while a peak of 9-hydroxyrisperidone occurs at about 3 hours (17 hours in poor metabolizers). The apparent half-life of risperidone is 3 hours in extensive metabolizers and 20 hours in poor metabolizers, while the half-life of 9-hydroxyrisperidone is about 21 hours in extensive metabolizers and 30 hours in poor metabolizers. In clinical practice, it is widely accepted for treatment of agitation and aggression in elderly demented patients in doses ranging from 0.5 mg to 1.5–2 mg/day, and at low doses for a few cases of delirium (Ravona-Springer *et al.* 1998; Sipahimalani and Masand 1997). Doses of 3–4 mg/day can be reached. The existence of liquid formulation is important in clinical practice, when the use of tablets is difficult. A recent pharmacoepidemiological study estimated that risperidone can be associated with delirium in 1.6% of cases (Zarate *et al.* 1997).

Quetiapine

Quetiapine is a new atypical antipsychotic with serotonin ($5HT_{1A}$, $5HT_{2A}$, $5HT_6$, $5HT_7$), dopamine (D_2), histamine (H_1), and α_1 and α_2 noradrenergic blocker activity, without muscarinic properties. The antagonism of H_1 receptors may explain the somnolence observed with quetiapine, while antagonism of α_1 adrenergic receptors may explain the orthostatic hypotension secondary to its use. Rapidly and completely absorbed after oral administration, quetiapine reaches peak plasma concentrations in 1.5 hours and is extensively metabolized by the liver, with metabolites that are pharmacologically inactive. Quetiapine's short half-life (3–6 hours) facilitates rapid discontinuation in case of adverse or negative effects. Attention should be paid to elderly patients in whom oral clearance is reduced by 40% It is used in the treatment of delirium starting with low doses (e.g. 25 mg at night) and low increments according to clinical response (100–200 mg/day b.i.d. or t.i.d.). Recent clinical reports indicate the efficacy and safety of quetiapine in treating delirium (Schwartz and Masand 2000; Torres *et al.* 2001).

Ziprasidone

Ziprasidone is a very recent atypical antipsychotic with $5HT_{2A}/D_2$ blockade properties, associated with binding affinity for the D_3, $5HT2_A$, $5HT1_D$, and α_1-adrenergic receptors, and moderate affinity for the histamine H_1 receptor. It is also characterized by an agonism at the $5HT_{1A}$ receptor and a 5-HT and noradrenaline re-uptake blockade, which explains its anxiolytic and antidepressant properties. Antagonism at H_1 and α_1-adrenergic receptors is responsible for the somnolence and orthostatic hypotension side-effects. Ziprasidone is rapidly absorbed by oral administration (peak plasma concentrations in 6 to 8 hours) and its bioavailability is increased up to twofold by food. The half-life of the drug is estimated to be 7 hours. An intramuscular formulation, soon available, will be of help in several clinical situations, including palliative care, when oral administration is difficult or impossible. The dose for treatment of psychotic symptoms is in a range of 120–160 mg/day orally and 5–20 mg t.i.d. in IM injection. Ziprasidone has no extrapyramidal side-effects and little anticholinergic activity. A prolongation of QT interval has been reported, which suggests caution in its use in clinical practice, particularly in the elderly, patients using other drugs, and severely physically ill patients. Somnolence and dizziness are further side-effects of ziprasidone. There is only one case report, at the moment, that concerns the use of this drug in treating delirium. An oral dose of 100 mg per day (40mg/20mg/40mg) was considered effective in a patient with cryptococcal meningitis and electrolyte abnormalities for whom risperidone was stopped due to extrapyramidal side-effects (Leso and Schwartz 2002).

9.2.3 Side-effects of neuroleptics

Interactions with other drugs and disease conditions are relevant in some cases (Bernard and Bruera 2000). Drug interactions are briefly described in Section 6.3, which reviews opioid toxicity. Potentially significant interactions can be envisaged, for instance, when using haloperidol, which inhibits the CYP 2D6 isoenzyme, in combination with codeine or oxycodone, which are metabolized to active compounds by CYP 2D6. This interaction may explain the cases of patients not achieving significant analgesia notwithstanding incremental doses of oxycodone or codeine administered in combination with haloperidol (Gagnon *et al.* 1999). Also serotonin re-uptake inhibitors (SSRIs) and tricyclic antidepressants (TCAs) can interact with the metabolism of haloperidol. The role of drug interaction in modifying individual patient responses increases as the number of drug coadministered increases and is certainly complex. It is useful to recall that antidepressants (both TCAs and SSRIs), haloperidol, midazolam, opioids, steroids, anticonvulsants, some antibiotics, and antifungals can have significant interactions (Bernard and Bruera 2000).

The side-effects of neuroleptics are very similar. Differences between one drug and another are more quantitative than qualitative and can be categorized as having neurological side-effects and/or non-neurological and toxic effects, see also Table 9.2.

Neurological side-effects

Involvement of the extrapyramidal system is the most significant problem with the use of conventional antipsychotics, especially high-potency ones (e.g. haloperidol). These effects are directly due to the primary antidopaminergic action at the nigrostriatal pathway. Acute dykinesia or dystonic reaction can manifest as spasm of the buccofacial, neck, and back muscles, oculogyric crisis, and possibly laryngeal spasm and can be relieved by benztropine mesylate or biperiden.

Akathisia is also an early and quite common reaction characterized by a subjective need to move and often mistakenly interpreted as an exacerbation of psychotic symptoms or anxiety. Lowering the dose of antipsychotics or the use of β-adrenergic blocking drugs (e.g. propranolol) reduces the phenomenon. Parkinsonism is a gradual side-effect that mimics Parkinson's disease and is treated by re-equilibrating the acetylcholine–dopamine balance by administering anticholinergic drugs. However, both akathisia and parkinsonism are less problematic in short- to medium-term management of an acute episode of delirium and are less pronounced after parenteral haloperidol administration than after oral administration (Blitzstein and Brandt 1997; Menza *et al.* 1987). Other extrapyramidal side-effects, such as perioral tremor or 'rabbit syndrome' and tardive dyskinesias are long-term consequences of antipsychotics that rarely apply to the palliative care patient.

The neuroleptic malignant syndrome (NMS) is a rare and life-threatening complication of antipsychotic drugs. It is characterized by catatonia, stupor, fever, autonomic instability, elevated levels of white cells and creatinine phosphokinase, myoglobinuria, and delirium. It requires intensive care treatment. Administration of danthrolene and bromocriptine are considered beneficial.

Sedation is probably due to the anticholinergic effects of neuroleptics on muscarinic receptors. Phenothiazines are more sedating than haloperidol and also more often associated with paradoxical effects such as delirium itself. This is particularly true of thioridazine, clozapine (Szymanski et al. 1991; Wilkins-Ho and Hollander 1997), and olanzapine, but no drug is totally devoid of this risk (Tavcar and Dernovsek 1998).

The risk of seizures is more commonly associated with phenothiazines and is especially relevant in patients with other risks for seizure disorders, since the antipsychotics may lower the threshold for seizures. The use of phenothiazines in combination with opioids has been considered to explain the agitated delirious states with myoclonus seen by some palliative care specialists (Burke 1997).

Non-neurological side-effects

Adrenergic side-effects consist mainly of orthostatic hypotension and dizziness, due to α-adrenergic blockade. The least hypotensive drug is haloperidol (see Table 9.2). This effect is particularly important in cases with already compromised regulation of baroceptive reflexes, e.g. the elderly and patients already on most antihypertensive medications.

Peripheral anticholinergic effects are a significant problem with many neuroleptics, especially low-potency conventional antipsychotics (e.g. chlorpromazine, thioridazine). Blockade of muscarinic activity causes blurred vision, dry mouth, constipation, decreased bronchial secretion, decreased sweating, difficulty in urination, and tachycardia. Dry mouth, which is often very bothersome in the presence of the multiple symptoms and polypharmacy that often characterize palliative care, can sometimes be counteracted by using of pilocarpine in sublingual drops (Mercadante 1998). The central side-effects due to the anticholinergic properties of antipsychotics include impairment in concentration attention, and memory and, in the case of delirium, a worsening of the symptoms of confusion. Anticholinergic delirium can be a consequence of excessive doses of neuroleptics with anti-muscarinic properties.

Along with tachycardia, other cardiac effects should be considered. Arrhythmias and prolongation of the QT inteval have been observed with oral and parenteral use of haloperidol with both high- and low-dose regimens (DiSalvo and O'Gara 1995; Jackson et al. 1997; Sharma et al. 1998; Wilt et al. 1993). Torsades des pointes (TdP) have been seen in 4/1000 (Wilt et al. 1993) to 3.8% of patients receiving IV haloperidol and the relative risk increases with haloperidol doses ≥ 35 mg/day and with a QT interval ≥ 500 ms (Sharma et al. 1998). This should discourage the concurrent use of haloperidol with other drugs with similar effects of cardiac conductance and in patients with atrioventricular conduction blocks.

Sudden unexpected deaths have been reported with the use of other antipsychotics, however. TdP and prolongation of the QTc interval have been related to sudden death in patients treated with these drugs and caution has been suggested when using haloperidol, droperidol, thioridazine, pimozide, and sertindole, which seem to be more frequently associated with possible cardiac toxicity and death (Glassman and Bigger 2001; Haddad and Anderson 2002).

Liver toxicity has been described frequently as an asymptomatic increase of liver enzymes. Severe toxicity has been associated mainly with phenothiazines. For this reason several authors would not recommend the use of haloperidol in hepatic encephalopathy delirium but this opinion is controversial (Trzepacz *et al.* 1993).

Ocular disorders can consist in pigmentary changes in the lens and retina, and in pigmentary retinopathy, especially after long-term treatment, which is not the case in the treatment of delirium.

Endocrine side-effects deserve to be examined. Increased prolactin levels are related to dopamine receptor blockade at the tubero-infundibular pathway. Symptoms of hyperprolactinaemia (dysmenorrhoea, galactorrhoea, gynaecomastia, impotence) are quite frequent with conventional antipsychotics and risperidone as well. The combination of endocrine, anticholinergic, and anti-adrenergic effects may also determine problems with sexuality.

At the haematolgical level, blood dyscrasia and transient leukopenia have been reported while using antipsychotics, while the risk of agranulocytosis seems to be especially linked to clozapine use.

Dermatological side-effects, consisting of rash and photosensitization, are possible consequences of antipsychotic use, mainly phenothiazines. If this is the case, the drug should be stopped and substituted with a structurally different antipsychotic.

9.2.4   Benzodiazepines and other drugs

Benzodiazepines

The role of benzodiazepine (BZD) in the management of delirium has to be clearly defined. Indications for which BZD would be benefical in patients with delirium and severe medical illness could be anxiety, insomnia, agitation, or excitement associated with hyperactive deliria. On the other hand, benzodiazepines are likely to impair cognition, are frequent causes of delirium, especially in the elderly, and are therefore not recommended for delirium itself. As already mentioned, BZD worsened the symptoms of delirium in the only randomized controlled study on this syndrome (Breitbart *et al.* 1996). BZDs should therefore be considered second-line treatment when neuroleptics fail and when consciousness sedation is the aim of the therapy. Important exceptions to this are deliria due to alcohol and benzodiazepine withdrawal, where BZDs are the first-line treatment (Daeppen *et al.* 2002; Newman *et al.* 1995).

Some authors would recommend BZDs for patients with hepatic encephalopathy because of the risk of liver toxicity associated with the use of neuroleptics.

When BZDs are needed it is better to use drugs with short half-lives and no active metabolites. Lorazepam is our preferred drug. Its half-life is 14 ± 5 hours. It has a very high oral availability and reaches peak concentrations 1 hour after oral and sublingual administration. Low doses can be used sublingually (1 mg) or orally (1–2.5 mg) and higher doses IV starting with 1 to 2 mg.

Midazolam has been employed mainly in the palliative care of advanced patients. It has the advantage of being well absorbed after SC administration. It has very fast onset of action, short elimination half-life (1.9 ± 0.6 hours), and can also be used for short-term reversible sedation. Single IV doses can be used for the induction of sedation and can be repeated after a short time. Prolonged sedation can be more difficult requiring frequent dose adjustment after starting the infusion with 1 mg/h. Daily doses can range from 40 to 60 mg but higher doses are often administered as well (see below) (Bottomley and Hanks 1990; Burke 1997; Burke *et al.* 1991; Stiefel *et al.* 1992).

Antihistamines

Antihistamine have sedative properties. Some authors would prefer to use hydroxyzine to aid sleep in patients with delirium (Lipowski 1990*b*) because of the lower potential of this drug for toxic reactions compared with BZD. Antihistamines all have anticholinergic effects and their use has been associated with delirium (Agostini *et al.* 2001; Garza *et al.* 2000). Thus, in our experience we limit their use to patients for whom we want to emphasize sedation over other therapeutic options (see below).

Physostigmine

In anticholinergic delirium physostigmine can be used if anticholinergic toxicity is well proven and only with careful monitoring for the occurrence of side-effects due to cholinergic hyperstimulation. Physostigmine salicylate (1 to 2 mg) should be given slowly IV or IM and repeated after 15 minutes. Contraindications to its use include a history of heart disease, asthma, diabetes, peptic ulcer, or bladder or bowel obstructions. It needs to be given cautiously to avoid seizures and cardiac arrhythmia. In a study on the treatment of proven anticholinergic intoxications, physostigmine was superior to BZD in controlling agitation and reversing delirium (Burns *et al.* 2000). Interestingly, in this study BZDs were effective in controlling agitation in only 24% of cases (Burns *et al.* 2000).

Newer drugs and miscellaneous case reports

The introduction of cholinesterase inhibitors for the treatment of dementia has suggested their potential usefulness for ameliorating symptoms of delirium. Some clinical observations of the use of donepezil are interesting but preliminary (Fischer 2001; Kaufer *et al.* 1998; Slatkin *et al.* 2001; Wengel *et al.* 1998). These drugs act by making acetylcholine more available at CNS level. These observations therefore suggest the relevance of acetylcholine transmission failure as one hypothesis in the pathogenesis of delirium. Their generalizability in the management of the syndrome is unknown.

Mianserin, a second-generation antidepressant with antagonism to α_2-adrenergic presynaptic receptors (increase of noradrenergic activity), serotonergic 5-HT$_{2A/2C}$ receptors (anxiolytic properties), and histaminic H$_1$ (sedative properties), has been reported to be effective in the treatment of symptoms of delirium in 62 consecutive elderly patients, of whom 40% suffered from pre-existing dementia. Mianserin at doses of 10 to 30 mg q.h.s. at night was effective in controlling behavioural symptoms, improving night-time sleep and reducing hallucinations as measured by the DRS, but it did not improve cognition (Uchiyama et al. 1996). The authors speculate that mianserin could exert a beneficial effect in delirious elderly patients by means of antihistamine (anti-H_1) and antiserotonergic (anti 5-HT_2) actions while being devoid of the anticholinergic potential of traditional anthistamines (Uchiyama et al. 1996).

Ondansetron (8 mg IV) has been used to treat postcardiotomy delirium in an open trial on 35 consecutive patients admitted to an intensive care unit. Eighty per cent of patients were reported to improve after ondansetron (Bayindir et al. 2000). This observation may lend weight to studies advocating a role for the serotonergic system and amino acid metabolism in postoperative delirium, but more controlled observations are needed (van der Mast et al. 2000).

One case report (Mark et al. 1993) supported the use of pimozide in delirium due to hypercalcaemia not responding to conventional neuroleptic therapy, because of its high potency in blocking T-type Ca channels.

Carbamazepine was combined with buspirone in treating agitation associated with head trauma in a case report (Pourcher et al. 1994).

Drugs used in hypoactive deliria

As already mentioned, the pharmacological treatment of hypoactive deliria in palliative care has no straightforward answer. Some cases with clouded sensorium and somnolence, which may partially overlap with excessive sedation as a pharmacological side-effect, may benefit from psychostimulant therapy (Levenson 1992; Morita et al. 2000; Stiefel and Bruera 1991). Neuroleptic medication has also been shown to improve delirium in hypoactive cases (Platt et al. 1994). In our experience the patient with a moderate, quiet delirium who can still use oral medication should have a trial with oral haloperidol. Advanced cases with irreversible causes of delirium and/or actively dying would suggest abstention from treatment in most cases. In some cases (see Section 7.4), such as substance-induced delirium (namely fluoroquinolones), the possible mechanisms of inhibition of the binding of GABA to its receptor sites suggest the use of BDZ as the treatment of choice (Farrington et al. 1995; Unseld et al. 1990).

A relatively new drug, modafinil, whose primary indication is for narcolepsy, has been shown to improve vigilance in several other conditions (Holder et al. 2002; Nieves and Lang 2002). The mechanism of action of modafinil is different from the amphetamines' aspecific activation of noradrenergic pathways. Modafinil should act at the level of the hypothalamic cells containing hypocretin that are implicated in the promotion of normal wakefulness (Scammell et al. 2000; see also Section 2.6). The potential use of modafinil in palliative care has been recently underlined (Cox and Pappagallo 2001). We used it successfully in two cases of encephalopathy with hypersomnia due to antineoplastic treatment toxicity.

9. 3   Sedation

9.3.1   Definition

Terminal sedation is a term that has appeared recently in the medical literature and still awaits consensus among experts (Cowan and Walsh 2001; Morita *et al.* 2001). One could even question if terminal sedation, as a medical term, is a helpful concept at all. Definitions vary: 'the use of high dose sedatives to relieve extremes of physical distress' (Quill *et al.* 2000); 'sedation for intractable problems near the end of life' (Cowan and Walsh 2001); 'the intention of deliberately inducing and maintaining deep sleep, but not deliberately causing death in specific intractable circumstances' (Fainsinger *et al.* 1998).

9.3.2   Controversies—frequency and indications

There has been heated controversy over the last 10 years about the role of terminal sedation in controlling specific symptoms or complications characterizing the terminal phases of advanced illnesses, mainly focusing on the frequency of cases needing this type of intervention. One initial report by Ventafridda *et al.* (1990*a*) found that, in a home-care programme, 52% of patients had symptoms that were controllable only by means of sedation in the last weeks of life (median survival, 23 days). A total of 80 different symptom episodes (a patient could have more than one difficult symptom at one time) were treated with sedation, of which 11 episodes were due to delirium (Ventafridda *et al.* 1990*a*). The controversy was fuelled by a subsequent report by Fainsinger *et al.* (1991) in a study conducted at a palliative care unit, who showed that in over 100 consecutive admission the need to sedate patients with uncontrollable symptoms was reduced to 16%. The leading symptom requiring terminal sedation was delirium (10 of 16 patients). Several authors have reported frequencies in between these extremes (16 to 52%; see Fainsinger *et al.* 1998 for a review) and a recent multicentre trial also failed to give a homogeneous answer. In four geographically and culturally diverse centres of palliative care (three hospices and one hospital palliative care unit) the intent to sedate varied from 15% to 36%. Delirium was the main indication for sedation in 29% (Israel), 15% (Durban), 32% (Cape Town), and 60% (Madrid) of cases (Fainsinger *et al.* 2000*b*).

   The difficulties of defining such basic concepts as terminal sedation and level of consciousness, together with patient selection, due to referral bias and setting of care, certainly have an impact in explaining the wide variability in the data (Morita *et al.* 2001). Indeed, a more recent analysis of the home-care programme from the same centre that produced the highest rate of recourse to terminal sedation showed that only 21% of patients needed sedation, at the end of life, in over 299 consecutive cases (De Conno *et al.* 1996; Groff 1993).

   A recent literature review found that, in over 328 cases of terminal sedation, indications included agitation/restlessness in 26% of cases, confusion in 14%, and muscle twitching or myoclonus in 11% (Cowan and Walsh 2001).

   In our experience the use of sedation in patients with a very short prognosis was indicated by the occurrence of agitated deliria in 19% of the cases that were sedated (Caraceni *et al.* 2002).

Guidelines for implementing sedation for 'refractory' symptoms have also been published with a specific definition of what should be considered a refractory symptom (Cherny and Portenoy 1994; Cherny et al. 1994). This definition can be useful as an example of the complexities that we face when we propose to investigate the presence of refractory symptoms and the potential therapeutic response to them in a way that is valid and reproducible.

Drugs used for sedation also vary considerably across different studies. Cowan and Walsh (2001) found that most patient already have an opioid-based therapy and that the most popular drug to achieve sedation is midazolam, but 10 other drugs were also used including methotrimeprazine, chlorpromazine, haloperidol, amobarbital, thiopental, propofol, amobarbitone, and pentobarbital.

9.3.3 Drugs used in sedation

Midazolam

Midazolam is the most popular drug used, at the moment, for sedation in palliative care, as reported by Cowan and Walsh (2001). Midazolam is a benzodiazepine with a high solubility that allows SC administration and a short elimination half-life of about 3 hours. It is higly bound to plasma proteins ($>$ 90%). After IM administration its bioavailability varies from 40% to 100% and plasma peak concentrations are achieved in 20–30 minutes. It is metabolized by the liver P450 cytochrome system (isoenzyme CYP 3A4) to an active metabolite (hydroxyl-1-midazolam) that is responsible for 60–80% of the clinical effects. This metabolite is readily cleared from the bloodstream after glucuronization and renal excretion, and therefore does not prolong the clinical effects of the drug. In long-term sedation in the intensive care unit, a high individual variability of effects has been seen. Clearance is dependent on hepatic function, hepatic blood flow, and interaction with other drugs with hepatic metabolism. A more pronounced sedative effect is seen in the elderly and accumulation may occur in cases of hepatic and renal failure. A reduction of midazolam concentrations and effects has been documented with co-administration of carbamazepine, phenytoin, and rifampicin. Prolonged sedative effects were seen when midazolam was administered in combination with macrolid antibiotics, ketoconazole and itroconazole (Bolon et al. 2002).

Indications for the use of midazolam in palliative care, however, would greatly benefit from studies specifically documenting clinical end-points and effective doses. It has been reported that, in 23 patients requiring treatment for restlessness and agitation who were mostly (18 patients) already on diamorphine infusion for pain, SC midazolam was effective in resolving these symptoms in 22 cases where a starting dose of 10–20 mg/24 h, followed by dose titration, was used. The mean maximum dose achieved was 69 mg/24 h, but doses ranged from 5 to 200 mg per day (Bottomley and Hanks 1990). In one patient 120 mg/day midazolam infusion was not effective, and methotrimeprazine, 80 to 300 mg in a subcutaneous daily infusion, also failed to control the symptoms. No information was given as to the level of consciousness. General guidelines on the use of sedation included recommendations to use 2.5 to 10 mg SC midazolam injections 2 to 4 hourly to obtain rapid symptom control and 10–30 mg over 24 hour infusion thereafter (Burke 1997).

While it is likely that the use of SC midazolam offers adequate sedation in a number of patients (Bottomley and Hanks 1990), which also agrees with our experience, comparative studies giving specific indications for this practice are lacking. In our experience the SC route of infusion is often less effective than the IV route in maintaining control of the level of consciousness. This is particularly true when faced with very difficult acute situations such as dyspnoea or haemorrhage, where rapidity of clinical effect is fundamental. We also found that the IV route facilitated monitoring the level of consciousness and adapting pharmacological treatments to it.

Indications of the doses needed to obtain prolonged sedation with midazolam come from the experience of intensive care units, where it is also common practice to administer it together with opioids. If rapid sedation is needed, midazolam should be used at a starting dose of 0.07 mg/kg IV. In one case series of patients requiring mechanical ventilation, the mean dose for inducing sedation was 0.22 ± 0.07 mg/kg (Chamorro et al. 1996). Midazolam requires frequent dose adjustment after inducing sedation and its clinical effect may be prolonged after withdrawing it. In the same study, maintenance doses varied (mean 0.14 ± 0.10 mg/kg/h). After discontinuing continuous infusion, reversibility was achieved after 13.6 ± 16.4 h in patients without renal failure and after 44.6 ± 42.5 h in patients with renal failure, Two patients with combined hepatic and renal failure took 124 and 140 h, respectively, to awaken (Shelly et al. 1991).

The sedative effect of midazolam is obtained at plasma concentrations above 150 ng/ml. Moderate sedation has been associated with concentrations of 346 ± 208 ng/ml and deep sedation required mean concentrations of 661 ± 477 ng/ml, confirming a very high individual variability (Bolon et al. 2002).

Midazolam can fail, even at high doses. In this case it is suggested to add a barbiturate, propofol, or, according to our experience, an antihistamine (Cheng et al. 2002).

Lorazepam

Lorazepam (available in 4 mg vials) is an effective alternative to midazolam with the only drawback of requiring the use of the itravenous route for administration. Lorazepam has a longer half-life than midazolam (8–24 hours). It is independent from liver oxidative metabolism as it is glucoroconjugated by the liver and excreted by renal glomerular filtration. For this reason less variability of its sedative properties could be expected from metabolic changes or drug interactions. Lorazepam was compared with midazolam in achieving sedation in the ICU. The average half-life of lorazepam was 13.8 hours and midazolam 8.9 hours but lorazepam showed less variability than midazolam average dose of lorazepam was 1mg/hr compared with 15.5 mg/hr of midazolam for an average sedation period of about 7 days {Swart, 1999 #8867} . In another study sedation was conducted over a much shorter time period and {Barr, 2001 #8866} and lorazepam 0.91 mg/hr (mean) compared with 2.54 mg/hr of midazolam.

Propofol

Propofol is a drug commonly used in anaesthesia and intensive care that has occasionally been used in palliative care. Propofol is not related to the other general anaesthetic agents used for IV sedation. It is an oil and is manufactured as a 1% emulsion that can only be used via IV administration. Its effect is very fast. Distribution occurs with a half-life of 2–8 minutes. Its elimination half-life is 1–3 h. Propofol is metabolized by the liver by glucuronization and excreted in urine. Its clearance is higher than liver blood flow suggesting an extrahepatic metabolism. A dose of 2 mg/kg is used to induce anaesthesia. Blood pressure is reduced by 30% during propofol anaesthesia due to peripheral vasodilatation. No direct cardiac effects are known. Apnoea and pain at the site of injection also occur. Only four cases of sedation in terminal phases with propofol are reported in the literature (Cowan and Walsh 2001).

Propofol has been proposed for the treatment of delirium tremens in the intensive care management of cases refractory to benzodiazepines. In a case series of 4 patients, doses of 90, 80, 45, and 40 mg/kg/h were used at the highest rates of infusion to control agitation. These patients are, of course, all mechanically ventilated (McCowan and Marik 2000).

One case report of a patient with agitated delirium due to terminal hepatic failure was managed with propofol infusion by giving a 20 mg loading bolus IV followed by a 50 mg/h infusion that needed to be increased to 70 mg/h after 2 hours because of insufficient sedation. The overall infusion lasted 8 hours (Mercadante *et al.* 1995). Our opinion is that its use should seldom be considered appropriate in palliative care.

Other drugs

As clarified by reviewing the literature, a number of different drugs are used for sedation that are more or less appropriate for this task. In particular, the combination of opioids with benzodiazepines is potentially useful and we would favour at this stage a more consistent use of midazolam and lorazepam for this indication. The combination of opioids and neuroleptics is also common as a result of trying to control delirium with increasing doses of haloperidol or of the more sedative phenothiazines (Fainsinger and Bruera 1992; Stiefel *et al.* 1992).

The addition of an antihistamine to opioids and neuroleptics when sedation is required and not easily achieved is suggested by anaesthesiological esperience (Laborit's cocktail). In the absence of clearly defined guidelines, our suggestions, summarized in Table 9.4, rely on clinical experience. They are, therefore, general, and cannot be applied to individual cases without specific considerations. In our experience,

Table 9.4 Stepwise approach for the treatment of refractory delirium. Drugs and doses are indicative and should be adapted for each individual case

1	Haloperidol IV infusion can be titrated to produce effect within hours; the full effect can be appreciated after about 24 hours of infusion
2	Switch to more sedative neuroleptics such as chlorpromazine, 50 mg IV or IM every 8 h
3	Add antihistamine to an opioid and neuroleptic combination: promethazine 50 mg IV or IM every 8 h
4	If immediate effect is needed, start midazolam, 0.07 mg/kg IV, and titrate to effect. Continuous IV or SC infusion can be planned depending on the indication and context of care starting with 1 mg/h

delirium is not the most frequent indication for terminal sedation nor is it the most problematic if we consider that patients with delirium in very advanced phases of disease already have, by definition, significant failure of consciousness and cognition. On the other hand, patients with dyspnoea or haemorrhage as terminal complications may present with a preserved state of awareness. One significant case example is reported in Chapter 7.

9.3.4   Key issues in terminal sedation

Listing the key issues of terminal sedation may clarify the differences between cases that can be easily managed at home with SC infusion and cases that need more aggressive interventions and intensive monitoring:

- patient level of consciousness before sedation, performace status, and age;
- indication for sedation;
- level of suffering associated with the indication;
- rapidity of effect required;
- duration of sedation before death (very short interventions may last hours and just require the acute administration of a sedative drug);
- monitoring the level of consciousness (particularly important when sedation is prolonged over hours and days).

9.4   Non-pharmacological management

Psychiatric literature has repeatedly demonstrated the role of psychoeducational and behavioural interventions in increasing the efficacy of treatment of several psychiatric disorders, including mood disorders, schizophrenia, and chronic mental disorders. The active involvement of both the patients and the family in the educational process represents the key therapeutic ingredient and psychoeducational intervention is considered as part of the best practice guidelines and treatment recommendations (Dixon et al. 2001; Dowrick et al. 2000; Magliano et al. 2001; Miklowitz and Hooley 1998; Pollio et al. 2001).

In the case of delirium, it is important to recognize that the intervention should have specific characteristics, dependent on the patient's cognitive impairment and inability to sustain attention and to maintain a relationship with the staff. However, as already shown for patients with dementia (Boehm et al. 1995)or other cognitive disorders (Commissaris et al. 1996), behavioural and educational interventions should be considered an important part of the treatment for the patient and the family. In other words, although aetiological and psychopharmacological interventions are the hallmarks of the treatment of delirium, a more integrated approach should be available and routinely utilized in clinical settings (Cole 1999; Jacobson and Schreibman 1997; Rabins 1991). Only a few studies, however, have provided data on the importance and the efficacy of integrated treatment. In contrast, it has repeatedly been pointed out that the recognition of delirium is low among staff members and, consequently, the knowledge and skills in using pharmacological and non-pharmacological strategies are poor on hospital wards (American Psychiatric

Association 1999; Inouye *et al.* 2001). With respect to this, Inouye *et al.* (2001) have shown that the ability of nurses to recognize delirium in elderly patients was low (15–31% of true cases), especially for hypoactive delirium, patients aged 80 years or older, patients with vision impairment, and patients with dementia. On this basis the authors concluded that recognition of delirium could be enhanced by educating nurses about the features of delirium, cognitive assessment, and factors associated with poor recognition. Thus, training the staff on educational and behavioural interventions seems to be pivotal for a more appropriate management of delirious patients (Rockwood 1999).

With regard to this, Meagher *et al.* (1996) studied the use of eight basic nursing strategies in managing delirious patients. More specifically, the authors evaluated the following strategies: frequent observation (four-hourly or more); efforts by staff to re-orientate the patient to his surroundings; efforts made to avoid excessive staff changes; efforts to keep the patient in a single room; use of an individual night light; efforts to minimize environmental noise levels; specific requests for relatives or friends to visit the patient regularly as a way to re-orientate him; and an uncluttered nursing environment (no more than two non-orienting, non-vital objects in the vicinity of the bed; beds spaced an adequate distance apart). The authors also found that these behavioural strategies were not routinely used, with only four strategies implemented for fewer than half of the patients. Furthermore, nursing strategies were more frequently employed for patients with hyperactive delirium and more severe symptoms (agitation, mood lability, and disturbances of the sleep–wake cycle), and were associated more with difficulties in ward management rather than with the severity of the patients' cognitive disturbances.

Other studies carried out on elderly patients with delirium indicated that focusing attention on the environmental factors and supportive elements within the interpersonal relationships with the patients themselves are relevant to treatment (Cole *et al.* 1994; Simon *et al.* 1997). Similarly, studies on elderly hip fracture patients indicated that integrated intervention can in part favour prevention and, to a greater extent, treatment of delirium (Brännström 1999).

A recent report on delirious patients with hip fracture showed that certain factors, such as education of nursing staff, systematic cognitive screening, the consultative services of a delirium resource nurse, a geriatric nurse specialist, or a psychogeriatrician, and use of a scheduled pain protocol, improved the patients' cognitive functioning, decreased the duration of delirium, and decreased the postoperative length of hospital stay (Milisen *et al.* 2001). In line with these results, Marcantonio *et al.* (2001) indicated that proactive geriatric consultations using a targeted recommendations protocol to be followed by orthopaedics and repeated symptom evaluation, can reduce delirium by over one-third, and severe delirium by over a half in comparison with patients receiving the usual care.

From these data it is clear that awareness of the importance of delirium in palliative care and training of the staff are key elements for both prevention and treatment. A correct knowledge of the risk factors for delirium, the regular assessment of cognitive status, and the application of standardized protocols play a significant role. Once delirium has developed, the application of standardized procedures of behavioural and educational intervention is necessary to reduce the many consequences of the disorder and to help the family in dealing with the situation. On the basis of the literature and our own experience (Borreani *et al.* 1997; Inouye *et al.* 1999a), we will briefly present the most useful strategies to take into account in palliative care settings, by examining environmental and supportive strategies for the patient and for the family members (Tables 9.5–9.7).

9.4.1 Intervention for the patient

The role of environmental and social factors in precipitating or maintaining delirium has not been extensively examined, although it is clear that their contribution is important in clinical practice (Eriksson 1999) as now confirmed in clinical trial (McCusker *et al.* 2001*a*). The study by Inouye *et al.* demonstrated that an integrated preemptive environmental, nursing and cognitive intervention (systematic orientation, physiological hydration, non-pharmacological protocol for night-time sleep, attention to visual and hearing aids) can reduce the number of incident cases among elderly hospitalized patients (Inouye *et al.* 1999)(a). Another large randomized clinical trial, on the other hand, failed to demonstrate that early detection and targeted multidisciplinary care has an impact on delirium duration and recovery (Cole *et al.* 2002). Thus, integrated intervention for delirium should consider the significance of practical and relationship variables that we will summarize.

Manipulation of the environment

When possible, the patient should be transferred to a single room as contact with other patients, who are strangers to the patient and who are often themselves suffering from severe medical conditions, could represent a 'pathogenic' stimulus, increasing the vulnerability of the patient as far as his perception and thought processes are concerned. Furthermore, the noises heard on the often overcrowded medical or oncology wards (e.g. nursing activity, beeps, alarms, ringing bells, respirators, monitors) may be reduced if the patient is in his own room. Keeping the room quiet and well lit, with adequate light during the night-time, is useful for reducing the patient's confusion and decreasing frightening illusions. The availability of objects that are familiar to the patient (e.g. photographs, pictures, personal objects) is also of great help in giving a sense of reassurance and safety. Returning

Table 9.5 Manipulation of the environment

Quiet, non-noisy environment

Avoid over- and understimulation

Light (including night)

Provide clock and calendar

Make the environment familiar (photographs, personal objects, pictures)

Allow patient to have family members and well-known persons available

Allow patient to be familiar with at least one staff member per shift

Table 9.6 Supportive intervention for the patient

Maintaining the communication channels open

Active listening

Give meaning to symptoms

Evaluate the patient's emotions and the defences underlying the symptoms

Explain to patient what the staff is doing (procedures, interventions)

Table 9.7 Supportive intervention for the family

Elicit and respond to the family's concerns, problems, and needs

Identify and accept the family's emotional reactions (e.g. fear, anger, guilt, helplessness)

Understand the meanings underlying emotions and behaviour

Give clear information about the patient's symptoms and the necessary interventions

Involve family in the assistance plan

Involve other professionals or helping figures, when needed (e.g. volunteers)

Favour more adaptive strategies to cope with the situation

Improve communication between the family (or the key family member) and the individual members of the staff

Reduce attrition

Link the patient's 'bizarre' content of speech with possible previous experiences (e.g. work, interpersonal relationships)

aids (e.g. eyeglasses, hearing aids) to patients that normally need them is helpful in ameliorating the quality of sensory input and, consequently, in decreasing misinterpretation of the surroundings.

Orientation

Re-orienting the patients to time and space is a further helpful strategy. Re-orientation to time can consist in frequently repeating the date and the time to the patient and in providing the room with a calendar and a big clock. Re-orientation to space, context, and persons can consist in repeating where the patient is, why he is there, and the identity of the people assisting him, thus reinforcing the sense of control and familiarity with those who are present.

Giving information

Regular explanation of the procedures the staff are applying (e.g. blood examinations, pharmacological treatment and route, restraints when needed) and reassurance about what is happening is extremely important to increase the patient's sense of safety. When the symptoms of confusion decrease or delirium is cleared, information about what had happened (e.g. why the patient has restraints, what kind of symptoms the patient has had) and what could be expected in the following hours (e.g. fluctuations and possible returning of symptoms) is necessary to reduce the frequent distress that can follow delirium (MacKenzie and Popkin 1980) and to help the patient to understand his or her bizarre experiences and the frightening memories of the symptoms. We have recently showed that the experiences during intensive care admission, including sensations, factual memories, and emotional memories, are remembered by at least two-thirds of the patients, irrespective of the treatment (no sedation, morphine, morphine plus other sedatives; Capuzzo *et al.* 2001).

Company

Family members and close relatives or friends should be permitted to visit the patient and stay with him or her. Their presence can, in fact, reduce the feeling of abandonment and strangeness determined by unknown persons (e.g. other patients, family members visiting their own relatives in overcrowded wards). Staying with the patient, speaking to him or her, and touching him or her are important in that vocal and visual stimuli can favour the patient's awareness of his environment. Family members can also help the staff in facilitating and correcting the patient's reinterpretation of the surroundings, in re-orienting him or her to time and space, and giving him positive feedback as to what is happening. A balance between overstimulation (which could increase the patient's confusion) and understimulation (which could leave the patient in his or her poor conditions) should be found.

Staff

When possible, staff members who care continually for the patient should be maintained in their rotation scheme, so as to avoid the patient being attended by new, unknown, and unfamiliar professionals. Creating an atmosphere of trust is easier if the patient is familiar with at least one nurse per shift. This reduces the sense of strangeness and reinforces alliances and interpersonal relationships.

For these reasons, communication is extremely significant in the care of delirious patients. Communication channels should always be open. It is important to remember that the content of the patients' utterances always has a meaning and should not be dismissed as strange, incomprehensible, or bizarre. Attention should be paid to the patient's fears and worries and to possible illusions and hallucinations, reassuring him or her about the situation and his or her feelings and perceptions, and respecting his or her emotions. Challenging the patient about delusions is not helpful and can worsen the patient's trust in the staff. Patients should also be allowed to respond in their own time and non-verbal skills can be used to fill sudden communication gaps. Table 9.6 presents some of the significant goals of communicating with a patient with delirium.

It must also be remembered that delirium does not happen in a vacuum, but is a phase during a process of the illness of a patient with his or her own history and experience. Thus collecting data about the patient's life can be useful in interpreting the symptoms of delirium in a more comprehensive way, if and when it develops. The following case is an example of significant life elements, not known by the staff, that appeared during a confusional state and the knowledge of which could have been useful in the management of the disorder.

Case report

Ms P., a 49-year-old woman, was admitted to the oncology ward because of the worsening of her physical condition. She had been suffering from bone metastases secondary to breast cancer for several months. A few days after admission, the patient began to show sleep–wake disorders and, within the following day, a full-blown hyperactive delirium was present. Along with confusion, disorientation, and agitation, prominent thought disorders of a persecutory type and perception disorders were also evident. The patient was convinced she was in hell and screamed that the devil was threatening her from the top of her bed. The staff members were mistakenly perceived as enemies allied with the obscure 'forces of hell'. The patient seemed to live in a nightmare where a fight between her, as an angel, and the devil is taking place. Fragments of her past, especially her father's death, appeared during the short periods of awareness and return to a state of consciousness. The patient was referred for psychiatric consultation. Alcohol use and other possible causes of delirium were ruled out and a significant hypercalcaemia appeared to be the only possible cause of delirium. Her clinical situation improved in a few days after treatment of the metabolic disorder and a course of haloperidol, 3 mg/day. After a week the patient was discharged from the hospital and returned home. A home-care assistance programme was planned through the domiciliary oncology service.

During a scheduled home visit by the psychiatrist who saw her in the hospital, many aspects linked to the content of her delirium become clear and understandable. Her home was full of pictures of saints and holy images on all the walls of her bedroom. During a long and moving interview, the patient revealed dramatic experiences of her life, especially the death of her father, who committed suicide 15 years earlier after a diagnosis of an inoperable stomach cancer. A few years later, the patient's mother was diagnosed with breast cancer and the patient followed and assisted her during the course of the illness until her death, which happened 5 years later. The patient was profoundly shocked by this second death and gradually moved towards faith to give meaning to her destiny, including the sudden discovery of a malignant lump in her breast. 'It was like the ghosts of the past were returning with their bad forces in our home.' She joined a group of people called the 'Angels of Salvation' who met regularly and who used to sing together as a way to be in contact with God and the 'good' forces. As well as the clinical meaning of these thoughts and convictions, all these aspects of the patient's life were completely unknown to the doctors who had followed the patient in the 2 years she was seen for breast surgery, chemotherapy, and regular check-ups.

9.4.2   Intervention for the family

As stated in Section 9.4.1, the patient's family should be involved in different ways in order to provide the best possible treatment of delirium. For this reason, specific interventions should be targeted at family members, in order to reduce the frightening experience of caring for their loved one who, during fluctuations of delirium, is unable to communicate in a coherent and 'familial' way with his or her relatives (Fitzgerald and Parkes 1998). We will focus our attention in the next chapter on the complex problem of the psychosocial impact of terminal illness on the family and on the needs that should be addressed in palliative care, limiting ourselves here to the most important strategies to apply in the management of delirium, as summarized in Table 9.7.

Education and counselling

A number of factors can be recognized that suggest a role for counselling and education for the family of the delirious patient (Table 9.8) (Borreani *et al.* 1997). Education about the symptoms of delirium, especially disinhibition and agitation, hallucinations, and delusions, is extremely important for the family. This can alleviate the profound sense of helplessness, incredulity, and anxiety that family members can feel during delirium ('He doe not recognize me'; 'She seems like another person, someone whom I never knew'; 'His personality has changed'). The fear of a psychological death that will prevent the relative from having any further contact with their loved one is extremely frustrating and a source of desperation at not having had enough time to share. Furthermore, delirium can be interpreted as a sign of an impending death that has long been anticipated but not yet accepted. Helping the family to find possible sense in the patient's 'bizarre' behaviour, linking it with previous experiences (e.g. family life, social life, interpersonal relationships, work), can also be useful.

It is also important to explain the fluctuating nature of delirium, indicating that transitory phases of awareness, in which the patient is still in contact with reality, do not necessarily mean a recovery and that symptoms can recur.

The possible causes of delirium (e.g. metabolic imbalances, use of drugs) should also be clearly explained as well as treatment options. The fact that control of symptoms, such as pain, is important even if the drugs (e.g. opioids) could favour the onset of delirium should be honestly communicated to the family. This is particularly important in home-care assistance programmes, where the family can feel abandoned by the team and can develop ambivalent emotions about the use of pain-relieving drugs. Similarly, information about the pharmacological treatment of delirium (e.g. haloperidol) and possible side-effects should be given. Involvement of the family in

Table 9.8 Critical issues in counselling for the family of delirious patients

Communication barrier

Patient's awareness of physical and psychological suffering

Reversibility

Short-term prognosis

Fluctuations of cognitive functions

Role of opioid and other therapies in aetiology

Role and goal of sedation

Goals of care

* Reproduced with permission from Borreani, C., Caraceni, A. and Tamburini, M., The Role of Counselling for the Confused Patient and the Family. In: R. K. Portenoy and E. Bruera (Eds.), *Topics in palliative care*, Oxford University Press, New York, 1997, pp. 45–54.

the assistance plan is obviously in order, given the role of family members in staying with the patient, re-orienting him or her, and accepting the patient's confused speech.

In cases where the patient's clinical condition is rapidly deteriorating or where the reversibility of physiological functions can be achieved only at enormous costs in terms of suffering, the family should be informed and involved in the decision-making process. The patient's wishes and the family's opinion about deep sedation should be known and openly discussed. Similarly, the opposite situation, in which the family requests that their relative is 'put to sleep' should be evaluated and discussed in a sincere and open way.

Attention to the family's emotions and needs

Identifying and accepting family emotional reactions are fundamental. Allowing the family to express their doubts and feelings is necessary in order to reduce their burden in caring for their relative. Fear about the irreversibility of the clinical situation and death, anger towards the health-care system or the staff, guilt about their inability to sustain the situation, and hopelessness and helplessness about the possible loss are common reactions that should be addressed and accepted in a non-judgemental way. It is possible that these emotional reactions are sustained by behaviours that, at first glance, can be seen as inadequate and inappropriate (e.g. reducing visits to their relative, not asking the staff about the relative's clinical situation, isolation, or intrusion). In any case, the possible and multiple meanings underlying these behaviours should be scrutinized and understood. Attention and responses to practical needs can also help the family to find more adaptive coping mechanisms towards the situation. If good communication channels between the family (or the key family member) and the individual members of the staff are maintained, it is possible to identify and give priority to problems and concerns and to find possible solutions. Involving other figures and liaising with other professionals (e.g. hospital or community social workers, volunteer associations) who may provide assistance can give the family a sense of not being abandoned and model strategies for a better management of their loved one's situation.

During the terminal phases of illness, interventions that permit the family to express their feelings, to cry, and to grieve are the most significant part of assistance, as we will describe in the next chapter.

Chapter 10

Family issues

Your pallor / startled me. / One could read on your face / the abandonment of life and like clear water / your look meant the departing / from things human. You carried your pain inside / and did barely answer. / Then, with a brief nod, you quickly slipped away. / Leaving me with my grief. / Speechless.

Eugenio Montale from Diario Postumo, Mandadori, Milano 1996 [translation by Jody Fitzhardinge and Lorenzo Matteoli]

10.1　Introduction

As we discussed in the previous chapter, the family is extremely important in offering assistance in the management of delirium. Thus, the impact of the patient's disease on the family's psychosocial equilibrium and the roles of its members merits special attention, particularly in palliative medicine. The terminal phase of illness may be devastating for the family, and the emotional burden and concrete problems the family have to deal with can be immeasurable.

The impact of the terminal phase on family functioning, role reversals, and changes in interpersonal relationships make it even more evident that the illness is an event of the whole family ('family disease'; Northouse 1988). For that reason, family members are often referred to as 'second-order patients' (Lederberg 1998a) with their own needs, but at the same time they are also 'second-order therapists' in that they provide the majority of assistance and work with the staff in the care of their relative (Emanuel *et al*. 1999).

It is especially in home-care palliative programmes that the active involvement of the family in providing continuous assistance to their relative may often cause problems, given the ambiguity and conflict in being care-givers and care-recipients (Schachter 1992; Schachter and Coyle 1998). The diffusion of home-care programmes, the shift from a patient-focused to a patient/family-focused approach in health systems, and the development of community-based palliative-care services coordinated by family physicians represent further elements indicating the need for a holistic vision of terminal illness (Burge *et al*. 2001; Robinson and Stacy 1994; Steinmetz *et al*. 1993).

Thus, although very poorly covered in medical textbooks (Rabow *et al*. 2000), aspects concerning the family as a unit and the mixed emotional reactions during the palliative care process, before and after the loss of their loved one, should be given ethical and clinical consideration by health-care professionals (Kristjanson 1997; Kristjanson and Ashercraft 1994; McClement and Woodgate 1998).

It is apparent that the emotional aspects involving the family during palliative care vary greatly according to many significant variables, such as the identity of the dying person (e.g. child, adolescent, young wife, mother); his/her gender, age, and role; the context of care (e.g. hospital ward, hospice or palliative units, or patient's own home), as well as the cultural background and family rituals (Gatrad 1994; Kagawa-Singer and Blackhall 2001; Trill and Holland 1993), all of which influence the process of illness/death. It is beyond the scope of this chapter to examine these aspects in detail, for which we direct interested readers to more specific sources and texts (Baider *et al.* 2000; Rolland 1994). The focus here is on briefly reviewing the most significant psychological aspects evident in the family during the terminal phase of their relative's illness and after his/her death, and giving the reader elements that facilitate the analysis of the problem of delirium in a broader and more integrated framework.

10.2   The psychological impact of terminal illness on the family

Families are profoundly influenced by the hopeless disease progression of their relative. It is the conclusion of a long and difficult journey in the domains of suffering, adjustment, reframing expectations, illusions of recovery and fears of relapse, uncertainty, dilemmas, and, finally, the inevitability of the termination of one's own life. Understanding the continuity of this journey is paramount for a more precise awareness of the psychological impact of the terminal phase of illness on the family and, inextricably, on the patient and on the team caring for him/her (Cherny *et al.* 1994; Klagsbrun 1994).

To the same extent to which the patient is psychologically challenged by his or her own impending death (Kubler-Ross 1969; Vachon 1998), the family is also challenged by the devastating reality of the impending loss of their loved one. Their attempt to cope with this challenge is documented in this chapter (Leis *et al.* 1997).

Several factors must be considered as contributing to the family's psychosocial distress during the terminal phase. Although these factors are intimately connected and entwined, they can be classified as: (1) patient-related factors; (2) family-related factors; and (3) family/staff-related factors (Table 10.1).

10.2.1   Patient-related factors

Patient-related factors mainly comprise the problems determined by the progression of illness. Watching a loved one deteriorating and experiencing unbearable physical symptoms is a major source of suffering for the family. Pain is one of the most significant symptoms in advanced cancer patients (Vachon 1998). The meaning given to pain and the ability to recognize it are all elements that influence both the family's and the patient's perception of pain (Clipp and George 1992; Dar *et al.* 1992; Ferrell 1998). The management of pain can cause conflicts within the family. Wishing that their loved one does not suffer and, at the same time, coping with the fear of addiction or tolerance, oversedation, or death caused by analgesic drugs, is a very difficult situation to deal with for the family. Other symptoms are also important in the advanced phase of illness in determining emotional problems for the family. The patient's loss of

Table 10.1 Sources of distress for the family during the terminal phase of illness

Patients's domain

Physical issues (e.g. loss of mobility, pain, fatigue, constipation, nausea and vomiting, medication side-effects)

Psychological and psychiatric issues (e.g. fear of death, guilt, anger, requests for hastening death, psychiatric symptoms, e.g. cognitive deterioration, delirium, depression, anxiety)

Existential and spiritual issues (e.g. meaning of one's own life, fear of nothingness)

Family's domain

Psychosocial issues (e.g. impending bereavement; fear of separation, loss, and abandonment; anxiety, helplessness, and hopelessness; guilt; role changes; interpersonal relationships; conflicts)

Physical issues (e.g. fatigue; health behaviour, sleep–wake cycle disorders)

Practical issues (e.g. need for acquiring technical skills, economic strain, need for reorganization, work-related problems, changes in daily-life rythms, modifications of social relationships, dependency on others)

Health-care team domain

Psychosocial issues (e.g. communication with health staff members, ambiguity in the reciprocal roles, conflicts, burned-out staff)

Practical issues (e.g. organziational problems, relationship with the health-system organization, availability of resources)

mobility, for example, has been reported as a significant factor associated with family anxiety (Higginson and Priest 1996). Nausea and vomiting, constipation, dyspnoea, cough, and fatigue are other common physical symptoms that have an enormous impact on the family members providing care to the patient (Portenoy 2000).

Confronting the patient's concerns and emotional symptoms is also a very difficult task for the family. The patient's fears of physical deterioration and dependency, feelings of anger, hopelessness, and despair, existential and spiritual concerns (e.g. knowing that life had had a meaning, finding comfort in one's faith), and preoccupation with their own family (e.g. perceiving appreciation from the family, saying goodbye, knowing that the family will survive without them) are all sources of suffering that affect the family too (Greisinger *et al.* 1997). In fact, it has been shown that the patient's poor adjustment to illness is a factor favouring the increase of levels of distress in the family (Wellisch *et al.* 1989). Furthermore, the patient's level of depression, determined in large part by physical suffering and loss of mobility, has been related with high levels of depression in the family (Given *et al.* 1993; Kurtz *et al.* 1995). Family requests for help to the health-care system tend to exponentially increase at the worsening of the patient's clinical condition (Hileman *et al.* 1992; Lewis 1990).

Coping with the complex problems involved with cognitive deterioration is also a source of distress for the family (Breitbart *et al.* 2002a). As we discussed in the previous chapter, the several symptoms of delirium, such as the patient's inability to recognize relatives, the bizarre content of thoughts, the disturbance of perceptions and mood, the inability to control impulses, and the alterations in the sleep–wake cycle are extremely frightening for the family and can easily be interpreted as an anticipation of death (Lawlor *et al.* 2000*a*), with consequent intense feelings of impotence and the need for help from the health staff. In a study of family perception of palliative care services, it has been shown that expectations of the family members tend to be higher than the perception of the actual palliative care they receive in the families of delirious or unconscious patients, as compared with the families of conscious patients (Kristjanson *et al.* 1996).

10.2.2 Family-related factors

The quality of interpersonal relationships within the family, the level of communication between family members, adjustment to role changes, possible intrafamily conflicts, physical exhaustion or health problems, existential concerns (e.g. unfulfilled aspirations, unresolved guilt, searching for a meaning), lack of support from close or diffuse social resources (e.g. other relatives, friends, neighbours, associations), economic problems, and cultural variables represent further factors that intervene in determining family distress (Cherny *et al.* 1994; Sales *et al.* 1992; Spinetta 1984).

It is apparent that, within the family context, the nature of the relationships between members is an important variable in moulding the emotional response during the terminal phase of illness. As we will discuss (see Section 10.4), these are major issues influencing the impact of terminal illness on the family.

The level of communication between the family and the patient can become problematic in the advanced phases of illness. Hinton (1981) indicated that restricted communication among couples during the terminal phase of illness of one of them may be related to previous family patterns of communication antedating the illness or to the attempt to prevent emotional distress and to facilitate coping with the problems caused by the disease. The family tendency to hide the truth from the patient or to minimize the severity of his/her clinical situation is often an act made in order to protect the loved one from hopelessness and desperation. Even if this is understandable, it may cause problems in the relationship between the family and the patient as it becomes a major trap for the family (Faulkner 1998; Maguire 2000). The 'conspiracy of silence' and 'collusion', as it is sometimes interpreted, is a problem when the patient becomes aware of what is happening. At this time, the patient can feel a sense of betrayal and abandonment, with consequent distrust towards the family, which, in turn, can experience feelings of guilt, remorse, and futility. In other cases, the family and patient know what is happening but prefer not to openly discuss it, with the intention of not upsetting each other. However, the game 'I know that you know that I know' can influence the family relationships in a negative way, since the effort of not expressing one's own emotions has a high psychological cost, causing feelings of dishonesty, preventing the family from feeling really cohesive, and reducing the possibilities of discussing 'unfinished business'. In other cases, open communication is simply not possible because the patient has chosen to remain unaware of the situation leaving every decision to the family or the health staff.

10.2.3   Family–staff related factors

All the aspects described above are clearly entwined with the relationship between the family and the health-care team. This is a *de facto* 'second family', in touch with the 'primary (or true) family' at both a technical and a psychological level (Rolland 1994). In fact, being part of the treatment team causes the family to acquire complex technical skills (e.g. tube feeding, wound and skin care, use of oxygen, bowel and bladder management, use of drugs) and to share responsibilities with the health-care providers with regard to the medical condition of the patient (e.g. evaluating and 'objectively' reporting symptoms, such as pain, administering p.r.n. (*pro re nata* 'as circumstances may require') therapy; Grobe *et al.* 1981). Thus, significant sources of stress between family members and the team may emerge as a consequence of the overwhelming pressure and complexity of caring (Siegel *et al.* 1991). On the other hand, the staff themselves, as part of the care-giver system, have to deal with repeated confrontation with death and dying, with their own existential and emotional concerns (e.g. feelings of anxiety, anger, abandonment, hopelessness, or guilt), with overwhelming requests from the patient and the family, with possible conflicts between the single team members or between the team and the health-care organization (Feldstein and Buschman Gemma 1995; Graham *et al.* 1996; Lederberg 1998b; Ramirez *et al.* 1998; Vachon 1998; Yancik 1984a, b). This can in turn reverberate on the family increasing its level of distress.

10.2.4   Family psychosocial morbidity

For all these reasons, it is not surprising that a number of studies have tried to examine in more detail the extent and characteristics of psychosocial problems and psychological/psychiatric morbidity in families of terminally ill patients. In a study of 102 families taking care of patients with cancer, Kissane *et al.* (1994a) found that 35% of spouses and 28% of offspring showed symptoms of clinical depression ('cases') on the Beck Depression Inventory. About one-quarter of the family members were also 'cases' insofar as anxiety, phobia, and obsessive–compulsiveness were concerned. Harrison *et al.* (1995), studying 198 key relatives of cancer patients, found that 48% scored as possible cases on the General Health Questionnaire (GHQ), especially within the domain of anxiety/insomnia and somatic symptoms. In this study it was also shown that female family members were at a higher risk than males (63% versus 39%). In the above-mentioned experience at our institution, we found, in administering the GHQ-12 to the key family members, a high prevalence of psychological distress (69.8%), which was significantly associated with the number and intensity of problems determined by the care-giving situation (Grassi *et al.*, unpublished).

Thus, although the trajectory of care-giving during the terminal phase of illness is not a rigid process, but changes and fluctuates according to the changes and progress of the situation (Nijboer *et al.* 1998), being actively supported throughout the palliative care process is a major need for the family. Giving honest information about the patient's disease, including the prognosis, the way to control symptoms, the correct use of medications (dose, use, schedule-time, side-effects) and technical devices, and providing emotional support are important elements of palliative care that help the family to handle the difficult situation of their loved one's terminal illness (Cherny *et al.* 1994; Hinds 1985; Houts *et al.* 1991; Northouse 1988). In our own experience with family care-givers involved in a home-care assistance programme for terminally ill patients, we found that both the patients' physical symptoms, as well as the family's emotional burden were the most frequently reported concerns that the family would like to have addressed by the domiciliary health-care staff (Fig. 10.1).

Although some studies carried out in home settings have indicated that emotional support seemed less effective than the staff's active intervention aimed at reducing the patients's physical discomfort (De Conno *et al.* 1996; Peruselli *et al.* 1997), variations are possible according to the family structure and wishes. It has been shown, for instance, that some families express preference for home palliative programmes, which permits the family to be better connected with other relatives and friends and to search for and receive support (Beck-Friis and Strang 1993; Brown *et al.* 1990), while other families tend to gradually reduce their praise of home-care assistance as the disease progresses (Hinton 1994).

In any case, the physical, psychosocial, existential, and spiritual dimensions of the human experience should all be incorporated into the care of terminally ill patients and their family.

10.3   The assessment of family functioning

Assessment of family needs and evaluation of the main characteristics of family functioning are thus extremely important in palliative care (Hickey 1990; Osse *et al.* 2000). Although, during the process of illness/death, families switch their modes of functioning many times in order to adapt to the modifications imposed by the progression of illness, some central elements that characterize the family functioning should be considered and understood (Lipsitt and Lipsitt 1991; Rolland 1994; Wellisch 2000).

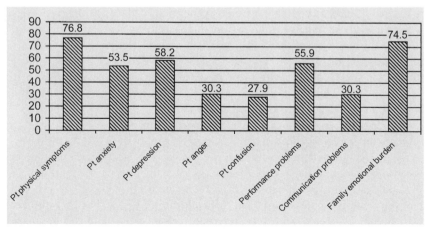

Fig. 10.1 Percentage of family members rating (moderate to extreme concern) about problems faced in home-care assistance.

The number of the family members who are present during the palliative care process and their respective roles are the first significant elements to take into account. Some families consist only of two members (e.g. an elderly couple); other are multi-generational families with many members. The capacity of the family to maintain its internal stability and, at the same time, to be flexible in the face of events that need new adaptations is another significant element to assess. The degree of closeness between members with respect given, at the same time, to the separateness and autonomy of each member is a key factor. Families in which the members are extremely dependent on each other or completely disengaged from family life are the opposite extremes of possible family functioning. The boundaries between the family members are also important. The rules, the roles, the rights, and obligations are points from which one can interpret how the members relate to each other (e.g. the relationship between the spouses, between parents and children, between grandparents and sons). Similarly, the family–community boundaries are important in describing to what degree the family has a clear sense of itself as a unit and, at the same time, is permeable to community systems (e.g. other families, neighbourhood, social or religious associations).

The time in which the illness develops and progresses has also to be considered in order to understand the family reactions. The development of the family (life cycle) is, in fact, characterized by different phases and the impact of illness is different according to the phases (e.g. a terminal illness in a spouse in a new family, rather than in a family consisting of two elderly people who have already experienced many losses, including retirement or departure of sons). According to Rolland (1994), the dimension of time is extremely important, since illness, individuals, and family development have in common the notion of periods or phases marked by different developmental tasks. Thus, the personal history of single members, the history of the family, and the history of the illness (its onset, course, and outcome) are all factors intervening in moulding the emotional reactions of the whole family (and of their individual members) to the terminal phase of illness.

Having a broad picture of the family's perception of the crisis imposed by the advanced phase of illness ('What is your understanding of what is happening?'; 'How is this situation affecting you?') and their main concerns ('What are your main concerns about your loved one's condition?'; 'What do you think could be helpful for you in dealing with these concerns?') can facilitate their relationship with the staff and lead to a gradual deepening of the investigation into the family as a unit (Welch-McCaffrey 1988; see also Table 10.2).

Examination of these elements provides helpful information that can guide the staff through the process of palliative care. With respect to this, Davies et al. (1994), transcribing individual and group interviews with families in a palliative care programme, has identified eight major themes that can be used as indicators of the functioning of the family as a unit. More specifically, the authors consider the following elements: (1) how the family integrates the past (e.g. remembering positive and negative events of the past, linking painful past experience to the present, and learning from the past rather than dwelling on the past, without integrating it with the present or learning from previous experiences); (2) how the family deals with feelings (e.g. ability to

Table 10.2 Assessing family functioning

Family history

1 Has the family already coped with difficult health situations, including life-threatening disease or death events?

2 Has the family had psychological or psychiatric needs in the past and what has been done for that? (Specify who, when and in what situation of family life.)

History of the disease

1 To what extent and in what way have the diagnosis and treatment modified the family roles?

2 What were the main crises during the 'journey' determined by the disease (diagnosis to treatment; recurrence to treatment; advanced phase to palliation)?

Communication and coping patterns

1 Is it possible for family members to speak openly among themselves about the illness and therapy and for the ill relative to speak openly with family members about the illness and therapy?

2 Are there members who are excluded from discussion about relevant aspects of the emotional or physical problems that the patient has? Who are they? For what reasons?

3 What are the main coping mechanisms of the family (or some members) with regard to the situation?

  ♦ minimization or, less often, denial of the reality of the disease as a way to reduce the devastating anxiety implicated in anticipated loss

  ♦ overprotection, with the often marked tendency to protect their loved one from information about his condition (collusion)

  ♦ overinvolvement and overidentification, causing both depression and anxiety in the family and search for miracle cures

  ♦ distancing, with delegation of every responsibility to the health system (hospital, staff)

4 What are the main family emotional reactions (e.g. anger, sadness, guilt, anxiety, hopelessness, coldness, detachment)?

Relationship with the staff

1 What are the relationships with the staff? Are the staff accepted in the family system? Does it cause conflicts, competition, distrust?

2 Is there a sharing of viewpoints regarding health staff recommendations and family expectations?

---

express a variety of feelings, including fear and vulnerability, rather than the tendency to express just a few feelings, especially the negative ones, such as anger, hurt, bitterness); (3) how the family solves its problems (e.g. identifying problems; considering multiple options; being open to suggestions; reaching consensus on a common plan of action rather than focusing on fault and guilt without finding solutions or withholding or inaccurately passing information to the other members, and feeling powerless in dealing with the problem); (4) how the family uses the resources (e.g. taking the initiative in searching for resources, utilizing them, and expressing satisfaction rather than not searching or finding or utilizing resources or expressing dissatisfaction with them); (5) how the family considers others (e.g. focusing attention on other family members and their needs rather than concentrating on one's own emotional needs); (6) how the family portrays the family identity (e.g. capacity to identify typical coping styles of the family as a unit, to consider the present situation as an opportunity for growth rather than describing one's own characteristics, giving a portrait of a fragmented family); (7) how the family fulfils roles (e.g. demonstrating flexibility in adapting to role change, sharing extra responsibilities willingly rather than showing rigidity in adaptation, considering care-giving a duty or obligation, criticizing care-giving provided by others); (8) how the family tolerates the differences among their members (e.g. tolerating different views from members of the family and persons outside the family, being willing to examine their own belief and value system rather than showing intolerance for different opinions, adhering rigidly to beliefs and value systems).

Starting from a different perspective and using their consolidated experience both in consultation psychiatry and palliative care, Kissane *et al.* (1994*b*) assessed the functioning of a group of 102 families (patients, spouses, and offspring) referred to a palliative care programme. According to the parameters of family cohesion, levels of conflict, and expressiveness of thoughts and feelings, the authors described five possible types of families. Of these, two were well functioning (supportive and conflict-resolving), two were dysfunctional (sullen and hostile), and one (ordinary) was intermediate between the two groups. Supportive families were characterized by high levels of intimacy between members and the capacity to share their distress and to provide mutual support. These familes were able to deal with the difficult process of care-giving, working together with the palliative care staff in a straightforward way. A conflict-resolving pattern was typical of families where the conflict, even if present, was faced and solved through the high level of cohesiveness between members and moderate, but significant, expressiveness. The most significant dysfunctional pattern was represented by hostile families. They showed the highest rate of conflict between members and the lowest levels of cohesion and expressiveness. Furthermore, psychiatric morbidity was the highest and social adjustment the poorest in this type of family. Working with these families was problematic since their distress reverberated throughout the treatment system, creating conflicts and emotional burden to the staff. Another dysfunctional pattern was represented by sullen families, in which members showed moderate levels of conflict, but tended to demonstrate poor cohesion and expressiveness and reported high levels of psychological morbidity, especially depression. The ordinary pattern had intermediate levels of conflicts, cohesion, and expressiveness but presented levels of psychological morbidity needing clinical attention. Identification of severe family conflicts is, however, not always helpful in resolving the situation, as indicated in the following example.

Case report

The patient, a 65-year-old man, was affected by prostate cancer with diffuse bone metastases. He had been bedridden for 3 months. He lived with his wife and

24-year-old daughter. An older son had married some years before and lived in another town, but not far away from his father's town. A palliative home-care programme planned to assist the patient was rapidly challenged by the increasing demands and requests from the family, especially from the patient's wife. She complained about the unavailability of the home-care service in terms of practical ('My husband is too heavy and I cannot move him for a proper washing') and emotional ('He is depressed and has a lot of trouble with pain, since pain killers do not work at all') needs. Dissatisfaction caused the sudden admission of the patient to different hospital wards, especially during the weekends, followed by equally sudden discharges for 'improper admission'. The tension between the family and the staff progressively increased with reciprocal accusations. The patient, caught in between, tried to negotiate, asking the staff to forgive his wife 'who is very anxious and depressed'. On the other hand, the tension between the daughter and her mother also increased to very high levels, with accusation from the former that 'I have always been hated by you, Mum. You are envious of the relationship I had with Dad, who was the only one who protected me when you interfered with all my relationships with my boyfriends, by following me, ruining my love affairs and never allowing my boyfriends to come home.' The intervention of the son to mediate the fight, which had extremely negative consequences on the patient, miserably failed. The inability to adjust to the role reversal in the family, the economic problems determined by the patient's disease, the never solved mother–daughter conflicts, and the impossibility for the patient, a strong man who was now stuck in a bed and completely dependent on his wife, to conduct his family seemed to be major problems for the family. Offers by Consultation–Liaison (C–L) Psychiatric Service to regularly meet the family and to help the wife and the daughter in clarifying their sense of what was happening also failed. In one of the biggest arguments between the two women, with open physical violence, the daughter, screaming, left the house, saying, 'I am sorry dad, your wife won') and slammed the door. She lived away from home for many months, while the wife concluded her relationship with the home-care programme, admitting her husband to a hospice unit.

In this case, the problems in previous family relationships emerged in all their force during the crisis determined by the progression of the illness. The inability of two family members (mother and daughter) to adapt to the changes in their roles and to face the pending loss of their relative is shown by the emphasis given to the old rivalry between them. The high level of criticism between the members was also projected on to the staff and only served to exacerbate the situation.

A continuous assessment of the levels of family functioning and adjustment in palliative care is important. First, as already mentioned, it gives vital information about the family system as a unit and about the best way to deal with the numerous and special tasks the palliative care staff have to deal with when assisting the patient, both from the medical and the psychological point of view. Secondly, it allows a better tailoring of the supportive and educational interventions directed to the family during the difficult or critical phases of terminal illness (e.g. pain management, onset of delirium, or other psychiatric disorders). Thirdly, it can demonstrate the need for referral of dysfunctional families to more specific psychiatric or psychological inteventions, as a way of reforming alliances with the staff and coping with the anticipation of loss. As a direct consequence of this, it represents a way to work through the subsequent phases, namely, bereavement, facilitating grief resolution, and promoting early intervention, when needed.

Given the importance for the family of these last two issues in palliative care, namely, anticipatory grief, on the one hand, and bereavement and grief, on the other, we will provide a short framework for this clinical area (Kissane and Bloch 1994). The definitions of the terminology used in this field are reported in Table 10.3.

10.4 Anticipatory grief

Ancipatory grief is commonly described as the experience (in the broad Latin meaning of *experiri*, 'to feel', but also 'to know through', 'to learn through', 'to try') that the family passes through before the death of their relative, involving the expectations of emotional pain and the life changes that the loss will bring about (Skinner Cook and Dworkin 1992). It represents a way for the family to rehearse or imagine in advance the loss of their loved one and to prepare themselves to work through the trauma of actual death, facilitating the adjustment to bereavement (Sweeting and Gilhooly 1990). The profound fears of the patient about his own pending death (e.g. fear of not having completed his plans, of abandoning his family to an unknown future, of being alone at the very moment of death, fears of nothingness) are intertwined with the family fears (e.g. fear of being left alone, desire for more intimacy and at the same time for letting their loved one go).

In palliative care, which usually lasts several months, the theme of anticipatory grief overlaps in part with what we have already discussed in examining the psychological impact of terminal illness on the family. However, certain aspects of this area merit closer scrutiny. In fact, anticipatory grief represents the opportunity to help families in their emotional preparation for the anticipated loss.

10.4.1 The concept and characteristics of anticipatory grief

With regard to the literature, it has to be said that different terms have been used to indicate the series of emotional events relating to the impending death of a loved one.

Table 10.3 The terminology regarding bereavement and grief

Bereavement refers to the loss of a person to whom one is attached

Grief indicates the cognitive, emotional, and behavioural reactions to bereavement

Grief work (or *grieving process*) indicates the psychological process of working through the loss over time

Mourning is the social expression of grief and it varies according to religion and culture

Anticipatory grief usually refers to the psychological and emotional experiences that precede bereavement

Complicated grief indicates the possible psychological complications of grief and the grieving process

---

Forewarning of loss, anticipatory loss, family emotional responses to terminal illness (or terminal response), anticipatory grief, or 'pre-mourning' phase (Evans 1994) are the most common terms used and indicate different theories and concepts in this area. In fact, some authors tend to confirm the existence of the anticipatory grief (Rando 1988), others tend to reject this concept, considering that there is a continuum between pre- and post-loss reactions (Bourke 1984), and others, complaining about the lack of data in this field, tend to criticize the oversimplification of terms and point out that a vast number of variables should be taken into consideration (Fulton and Gottesman 1989).

Several aspects of this problem deserve discussion. First, the family psychological reactions during anticipatory grief are different from those in response to grief, which, by definition, represents the psychological and emotional response to the actual death of a loved one (Parkes 1998c). The complex interplay of family emotional responses during anticipatory grief occurs in a context in which the patient is not dead and still has a role, although different from that of the past. Intensification of attachment is shown by a strong tendency to stay close to the loved one, and overprotection may be evident in the family during anticipatory grief, but not during grief (Parkes 1998a–c). In contrast to this view, Hays et al. (1994) found that the family's psychological symptoms in the weeks and months before their loved one's death were indistinguishable from the early emotional reactions after his/her death. More research is needed to clarify this.

A second issue concerns the concept of death itself. It has been indicated that death has multiple meanings and that, when linked to the concept of loss, it should be considered from different perspectives (Evans 1994). One such perspective is that of 'social death' (thus, a form of loss), which is largely anticipated during the process of the patient's illness. 'Social death' comprises the changes in and/or irreversibility of social roles, loss of identity, and loss of temporal boundaries (e.g. uncertainty about the future, disillusion, regret about lost opportunities and plans not yet achieved). Another perspective concerns clinical and psychological deaths, which are also evident in the palliative care process, and comprise both the worsening of the patient's physical condition (e.g. disfigurement, pain, fatigue, debilitation, cachexia) and psychological condition (e.g. modification of the patient's personality, onset of severe psychiatric disoders, including delirium and depression). Finally, biological death comprises the actual event of death, the transitional point from which grief begins.

A third topic is the nature of the interpersonal relationships between the family members and the individual psychological traits and coping abilities of each family member, including the patient. As we have seen in the different possible styles of family functioning, it is to be expected that the dynamics within the family influence the ways in which the loss of the relative is perceived and anticipated, making it clear that anticipatory grief is not an 'all or nothing' phenomenon. In this context, Zisook (2000) considers the difficulties for palliative care teams in dealing with possible distortions in the family's anticipation of loss, e.g. 'premature' grief. In this situation, withdrawal from the patient, as if he or she had died, before the actual event can provoke in him/her feelings of abandonment and loneliness, with evident negative consequences on the terminal phase of the patient's life.

A fourth problem concerns sociocultural and context variables that should not be dismissed in analysing the phenomenon of anticipatory grief. The culture to which a family belongs, both in broad (e.g. the values, norms, and rites of one's own culture) and in narrow terms (e.g. the values, norms, and rites of a single family), is an important variable to take into account. The interpersonal and practical resources available in the social milieu (e.g. social support systems, volunteer association, neighbourhood characteristics, church facilities) and their utilization should also be considered. Finally, the context in which palliative care is provided (e.g. hospice, hospital palliative care units, home) makes a difference in moulding the emotional reactions of the family, as we have already discussed.

Failure to consider these multiple aspects is in large part the origin of contradictory data in the literature as far as the role of anticipatory grief in working through the process of grief after the patient's death (Fulton *et al.* 1996; Fulton and Gottesman 1989).

10.4.2   The approach to anticipatory grief

In spite of all the problems we have discussed, the delicate phase of transition in anticipating the loss of the patient should be approached by the health-care staff with extreme attention. The specific needs of the family, their difficulties, and problems should be take into consideration and addressed in a proper way (Bates and the Psychological Work Group of the International Work Group on Death Dying and Bereavement 1993). It has been pointed out that maintaining honest and open communication with the family about the patient's clinical situation, giving information about the evolution of the disease, responding to the questions and doubts the family can have, reassuring them about the patient's symptom control and physical comfort, and encouraging family members to express their feelings are important objectives for the health staff (Ferrell 1998). Guilty feelings (e.g. 'We should have tried other options and therapies'; 'We have not done all we could for him'; 'I have horrible thoughts, hoping that all this can finish soon and wishing he would die'), fears (e.g. 'We are not able to cope with seeing him worsening and deteriorating day after day'; 'We are too weak and emotionally overwhelmed to help him'; 'Will we be able to meet his expectations?'), anger (e.g. 'What have we done to deserve this?'; 'How is it possible that medicine cannot do anything?'; 'The health system is the servant of the establishment and does not care about real people with real problems'), or denials (e.g. 'We don't think the situation is so severe'; 'There must have been some mistake; it is not possible that everything is going in a bad way') should be acknowledged, listened to, and understood (Faulkner and Maguire 1994; Maguire 2000). It is suggested that communication between family members should be encouraged (Twycross and Lichter 1998), although the way of doing this has to conform to the family and patient's own needs, wishes, values, religion, and culture. Staying close to their relative and sharing with him feelings, affection, and love may help to address unresolved conflicts, to forgive and be forgiven, to reciprocally thank, to say goodbye in the most appropriate way. It was recently found that family care-givers who have the opportunity to express their love through the care of a close member with terminal cancer can experience strong positive emotions (Grbich *et al.* 2001).

In the most advanced phases of illness, if the patient is delirious or unconscious, the family presence is important and communication, even if the patient seems unable to show any response, should be maintained. The family should be made to feel helpful and adequate in what they are doing and every effort and action should be reinforced and complimented, as a tangible sign of their personal and unique role in comforting their loved one. Through constant support it is possible that the family will be able to transcend and find meaning in their care-giving experience. In connection with this, it has been shown that, among family members of terminally ill patients, finding meaning involved 'being with' or 'doing for' their loved one, as death approached, and that this search for a meaning has positive consequences for the care-givers in the long run (Enyert and Burman 1999).

Attention to the family's own wishes and needs is also necessary (Bluglass 1991). Family members should be encouraged to take into consideration their own needs, correcting the misconception about being judged selfish or detached if they take some rest and reassuring them about the importance of recuperating energy in order to reduce the risk of their own psychological or physical breakdown. The family should also be respectfully encouraged to receive professional help if conflicts and emotional disruption emerge.

With respect to this, Kissane *et al.* (1998) developed a 6–8-session family intervention plan with the aim of reducing the level of distress in dysfunctional families during a palliative care programme. All the themes that emerged during the sessions (e.g. previous experiences with loss and bereavement, existential themes of suffering and death, difficulties in sharing intimacy and saying goodbye to their loved one, problems in receiving or utilizing care, conflicts among the family members) were reviewed and analysed. The aim of the intervention was to facilitate cohesiveness among members and to improve their communication and problem-solving skills, and, at the same time, to decrease family conflicts in order to improve the functioning of the family as a unit in caring for their relative.

Thus, attention to the psychological reactions of the family during anticipatory grief is a specific component of the palliative care programme, with the goal of providing support and recognizing both dysfunctional patterns and the possible onset of psychiatric symptoms as early as possible (Zeitlin 2001). This is illustrated in the following situation encountered in our practice.

Case report

The home palliative care staff had difficulties in dealing with the family problems emerging in the care of Mrs. A, a 65-year-old woman affected by diffuse bone metastases, secondary to breast cancer, who had been bedridden for 3 months. In fact, the relationship between the staff and Mrs. A's 68-year-old husband, Mr. P., had gradually worsened because of his increasing requests for home intervention ('my wife needs a home visit twice a day'), his dissatisfaction with and complaints about whatever the staff were doing, his inability to help his wife, and a diffuse sense of impotence and despair that prevented the man from leaving the home, since he wanted to be with his wife 'every minute of the day and night'. The couple lived alone and there was no support from relatives or friends. After a few weeks, the situation seemed unmanageable and the sense of failure and anger in the staff was increasing, with negative consequences on the quality of care provided to the patient.

After discussion of the situation in a meeting with the C–L psychiatric service, a domiciliary psychiatric visit was programmed. Mrs. A. seemed to be well adjusted to her situation and satisfied with the care she was receiving, but worried about the deterioration of her husband's psychological status. Mr. P., seated at his wife's bedside, showed high levels of anxiety and, only after several attempts, could he be persuaded to move to another room to speak more openly about his perception of the situation. At a mental status examination, Mr. P. appeared hypervigilant and anxiously attentive and, in a low voice, began to speak about his problems. He described the difficult situation at home, rapidly shifting his attention to his own physical condition, specifically his diabetes, which had affected him for 10 years and had caused several hospital admissions and medical complications, such as problems with sight and difficulty in ambulation. He was markedly preoccupied about the deterioration of his diabetes, his mood was depressed, and he felt desperate, worthless, and guilty about his inability to help his wife ('I am too tired and so weak that I cannot do anything at home') and hopeless about the future ('My wife will die and I also will die soon from my own disease'). Assessment of his personal history showed two previous episodes of major depression in the last 10 years. During the first one (concomitant with the diagnosis of diabetes), Mr. P. was followed by the Community Mental Health Service for a while through psychopharmacological intervention and supportive counselling. A diagnosis of a major depressive disorder, recurrent type was made, antidepressant therapy was prescribed, and a joint home-care programme with the Mental Health Service was planned for the following day.

In this case, the history of the family, including its previous and current functioning and the impact of the present illness, would have been of remarkable help to the palliative care team in making it possible for them to respond appropriately. The fact that the husband was affected by an important physical illness, i.e. diabetes, would have been seen as potentially having a significant impact on the couple, with a sense of vulnerability in the husband, a need for re-adjustment as far as the roles in the family were concerned, and, perhaps, economic problems. The onset of a depressive episode concomitant with the diagnosis of diabetes and of a recurrent episode some years later indicate, in fact, the high psychological vulnerability of the husband, which caused the need for psychiatric help. Thus, given these antecedents, it would have been predictable that the onset and progression of cancer in the wife might have had a severe impact on the husband himself, creating the basis for a new depressive episode.

10.5 Bereavement

At the actual death of the patient, the family begins the process of grieving. Grief is a human, universal, and healthy psychological response to the loss of a loved one. It has important aims, specifically those of gradually accepting the reality of the death, accommodating to the absence of the loved one, coming to terms with the changes that the loss has determined in the bereaved's life and world, and reorganizing one's own internal models. The main symptoms that emerge during grief are presented in Table 10.4.

These symptoms do not all occur at the same time, but follow the grief trajectory, which, although it is nonlinear and tends to vary from person to person, is usually conceptualized as a series of stages or phases. Several authors, including Kübler-Ross (1969), Worden (1991), and Parkes (Parkes 1998*b*), have proposed theoretical models that can be used in understanding the process of grief, as described in Table 10.5.

Although grief is a normal reaction to a human event, i.e. the loss of a loved one, this does not mean that support during the grieving is unnecessary. Usually bereaved persons are helped by other family members, close friends, and interpersonal and social resources, including religious affiliations, associations, or self-help groups, where they exist. However, it has been pointed out that it is important that clinicians and health professionals, both in general clinical practice (Casarett *et al.* 2001) and in palliative care (Katz and Chochinov 1998), are trained in helping persons who are experiencing grief after the death of a loved one.

Table 10.4 Common symptoms and phenomenology of normal grief

Feelings	Cognitive and perceptual symptoms
Shock	Disbelief
Numbness	Confusion
Yearning	Preoccupation
Anxiety	Sense of presence
Anger	Perceptual alterations (illusions, misinterpretations,
Sadness	possible hallucinations)
Guilt and self-reproach	**Behavioural symptoms**
Loneliness	Restless overactivity
Apathy	Searching and calling out
Helplessness	Sleep disturbances
Emancipation	Appetite disturbances
Relief	Social withdrawal
Physical symptoms	Sighing and crying
Hollowness in the stomach	Visiting places or carrying objects that remind the
Tightness in the chest and throat	survivor of the deceased
Breathlessness	Treasuring objects that belonged to the deceased
Lack of energy	Avoiding reminders of the deceased
Weakness	
Pain and muscle tension	

Table 10.5 Models of normal grief

Stage/phase/task	Description
Stages of grief (Kübler-Ross 1969)	
Denial	Shock and numbness about death; scanning the environment for sights or sounds of the deceased one
Bargaining	Hoping for the return of the loved one and making promises if it would happen
Anger	Frustration; anger towards fate and/or the doctors
Depression	Deep sadness and pain for the reality and irremediable nature of the death
Acceptance	Reorganization and return to living; retaining the memories without prolonged pain
Phases of grief (Parkes 1998b)	
Numbness and blunting	Shock; denial; feelings of unreality that can last hours or days
Pining and yearning	Intense pining; cry; separation anxiety; anger; irritability; self-reproach; loss of security and self-esteem
Disorganization and despair	Apathy and despair; isolation and disengagement from social life; feelings of mutilation
Reorganization and recovery	Gradual return to life; resurgence of interests; willingness to plan for the future
Tasks of grief (Worden 1991)	
To accept the reality of the loss	Confronting the reality of loss and overcoming a normal tendency to deny the event of death
To work through the pain of grief	Experiencing pain and feelings of depression, isolation, emptiness due to the loss of the loved one
To adjust to an environment in which the deceased is missing	Developing new skills to adjust to new roles, to a new sense of self, to a new sense of the world
To emotionally relocate the deceased and move on with life	Finding a place for the deceased in one's emotional life; thinking of the loved one with sadness, but not with overwhelming feelings of despair

As far as palliative care settings are concerned, data from the hospice experience indicate the importance of maintaining a relationship with the bereaved family and providing them with different kinds of support (e.g. practical, educational, counselling; Sheldon 1998). Parkes (1998b), warns us to avoid simplistic and schematic approaches to the complex but, at the same time, natural phenomenon of grief. Medicalization of what is part of life is not useful, whereas humanity, empathy, and compassion in the relationship with the bereaved are welcomed. Basically, actively listening to the person, allowing expression of the feelings that family members can or want to express (e.g. anger, guilt, anxiety, sadness, hopelessness, helplessness, fear of not being able to carry on their lives), reassuring them about the normality of these reactions, offering support, and maintaining follow-up are important for the bereaved family, who need to be accepted and not left alone in their suffering (Gregory 1994).

For these reasons, it has been strongly suggested that community palliative care teams improve their skills in evaluating the specific needs and in providing proper care during the bereavement follow-ups for families of deceased patients (Broomberg and Higginson 1996; Payne and Relf 1990). This seems well worth considering in order to provide the family with a continuity of care that involves community health-care systems, including general practitioners (GPs). In fact, although some studies have indicated that the family does not expect special action from their GP (Dangler et al. 1996), others have shown that almost 50% of families consider their GP's intervention to be helpful (Siegel et al. 1991). In a more recent evaluation of bereaved families, the majority would have appreciated a letter of sympathy from their GPs, and over half expressed some form of dissatisfaction either with their GP or with the hospital (Main 2000).

Given the significant changes in the health-care organization of palliative care services in many countries and the significant role of GPs in providing home care for patients with advanced illness (Robinson and Stacy 1994; Steinmetz et al. 1993), more effort and research are necessary to address the training needs of primary care physicians in assessing bereavement and in counselling families (Farber et al. 1999; Hermann et al. 1999). In this respect, it has been shown that most GPs tend to be worried about making clinical or diagnostic mistakes and report feelings of guilt about the death of their patients. However, they feel, at the same time, that it is their responsibility to make contacts with the bereaved families, complaining of a lack of specific bereavement strategies to help the family (Saunderson and Ridsdale 1999). Similarly, other studies have indicated that family physicians acknowledge that bereavement presents significant health risks to their patients and that the identification and treatment of bereaved patients is an important part of their role (Lemkau et al. 2000). Over the last few years, attention to this area has increased enormously, with the literature clearly indicating that GPs, and clinicians in general, need more specific training about the clinical and intervention implications for bereavement (Casarett et al. 2001; Charlton and Dolman 1995; Hermann et al. 1999; Woof and Carter 1997a, b).

Providing continuity of care during bereavement can also facilitate the evaluation of the grieving process over time and the referral of maladaptive situations that need intervention by specialist services. In fact, although literature is lacking in this area, it has been found that almost half of bereaved people meet the criteria for a psychiatric disorder during the first year of bereavement or show forms of maladaptive grief (Jacobs et al. 1990; Middleton et al. 1996), as we will describe in the next section.

10.6 Complicated grief

The problem of psychiatric morbidity and maladaptive reactions following bereavement has been the focus of intense research. Different definitions have been proposed to describe the possible psychiatric complications during bereavement, such as

abnormal grief, complicated bereavement, atypical grief, unresolved grief, and pathological grief (Katz and Chochinov 1998; Stroebe *et al.* 2000; Zeitlin 2001). This difference in terminology reflects, in part, disagreement about the different clinical
characteristics of complicated grief. For some authors, in line with the current
psychiatric nosological systems, depressive disorders should be considered the most
frequent and significant pathological evolution of grief (Bonanno and Kaltman
2001), while other authors emphasize the need to describe and classify complicated
grief in a more detailed way (Jacobs *et al.* 2000). As far as the former hypothesis, the
DSM-IV (American Psychiatric Association 1994) and its text revision (DSM-IV-TR;
American Psychiatric Association 2000) dedicate a short paragraph to bereavement,
which is included in the chapter 'Other conditions that may focus clinical attention.'
The DSM-IV-TR states:

> [the] duration and expression of normal bereavement varies considerably among differ-
> ent cultural groups. The diagnosis of Major Depressive Disorder is generally not given
> unless the symptoms are still present two months after the loss. However, the presence of
> certain symptoms that are not characteristic of normal grief reaction may be helpful in
> differentiating bereavement from Major Depressive Episode. These include (1) guilt about
> things other than actions taken or not taken by the survivor at the time of the death; (2)
> thoughts of death other than the survivor feeling that he or she would be better off dead
> or should have died with the deceased person; (3) morbid preoccupation with worthless-
> ness; (4) marked psychomotor retardation; (5) prolonged and marked functional impair-
> ment; and (6) hallucinatory experiences other than thinking that he or she hears the voice,
> or transiently sees the image of, the deceased person.

It is evident that psychiatric classifications tend to identify depressive disorders with
complicated grief. However, clinical experience indicates that grief can go unresolved
in different ways. Symptoms and/or behaviours, other than depression, can develop
and clearly indicate a poor grieving response that involves significant interference
with or impairment of the individual's functioning. Classification of complicated grief
is not homogeneous. Worden (1991) and Skinner Cook and Dworkin (1992) provide
similar outlines, describing four possible pathological forms: chronic grief; delayed
grief; masked grief; and exaggerated grief (with psychiatric features). The latter
authors also add avoidance of grief. Jacobs (1993) and Parkes (1998*b*) generally agree
to consider three pathological forms: traumatic loss; conflicted grief; and chronic
grief. Zisook (2000) has suggested separating the forms that exacerbate or favour the
onset of a medical or psychiatric condition (e.g. major depression, anxiety disorder)
from specific complications of grief, namely, absent, delayed, or inhibited grief, hyper-
trophied grief, and chronic grief. The characteristics of these disorders are indicated
in Table 10.6.

By using a more specifc methodological approach, over the last few years, psychiatric literature has confirmed that, within the realm of complicated grief, depressive
disorders secondary to bereavement should be separated from other clinical disturbances, which have their own phenomenological expression. Starting with the concept
of the traumatic nature that the death of loved one can have for the bereaved person,
Horowitz *et al.* (1997) conducted a 14-month follow-up study of 70 bereaved spouses.
They showed that symptoms of complicated grief did not overlap with those

Table 10.6 Possible forms of complicated grief

Psychiatric disorders following bereavement (exaggerated grief)

Major depression

Anxiety disorders

Eating disorders

Substance abuse disorders

Brief psychotic reactions

Avoidance of grief

Mummification with prolonged treasuring of objects and a tendency to leave everything (e.g. the person's room, personal objects, clothes) as immediately before death

Idealization of the qualities of the deceased person and magnification of the loss

Persistent anger or guilt response rather than acceptance of death

Chronic grief (or prolonged grief)

Excessive duration of grief response, with difficulty in speaking about the death without intense overwhelming grief several years after loss

Themes of loss coming out during daily conversation

Inability to resume one's own life and adjust to new roles

Delayed grief

Re-experience of excessive grief reactions secondary to new stressful events or losses and re-emergence of symptoms linked to the past loss

Inhibited grief (or masked grief)

Onset of physical complaints resembling the physical illness of the deceased ('facsimile' illness)

Physical symptoms (e.g. pain)

Behavioural problems (e.g. impulsive decisions, poor health care, promiscuity, acting out)

presented by subjects who received a diagnosis of major depression and, on this basis, they proposed diagnostic criteria for complicated grief (Horowitz *et al.* 1993; see Table 10.7).

In a series of studies of widowed subjects Prigerson and her group (1995, 1996) could distinguish symptoms indicating complicated grief (later called traumatic grief) and bereavement-related depression. The authors, in a longitudinal study of subjects interviewed at the time of their spouse's hospital admission and at 6, 13, and 25 months after the loved one's death, also found that traumatic grief at 6 months after the death predicted negative health outcomes (e.g. high blood pressure, suicidal ideation, changes in eating behaviour) in the survivor (Prigerson *et al.* 1997). In a recent consensus conference, possible criteria of traumatic grief have been proposed by the same group (Prigerson *et al.* 1999) as a guide to help clinicians in recognizing and treating bereaved individuals who do not adjust to the loss of their relative (Table 10.8).

Table 10.7 Proposed criteria for complicated grief disorder (Horowitz *et al.* 1997)

Event criterion/prolonged response criterion

Bereavement (loss of a spouse, other relative, or intimate partner) at least 14 months ago (12 months is avoided because of possible intense turbulence from a reaction on the anniversary)

Signs and symptoms criteria

In the last month, any three of the following seven symptoms have occurred with a severity that interferes with daily functioning

Intrusive thoughts

1   Unbidden memories or intrusive fantasies related to the lost relationship

2   Strong spells or pangs of severe emotion related to the lost relationship

3   Distressingly strong yearnings or wishes that the deceased were there

Signs of avoidance and failure to adapt

4   Feelings of being far too much alone or personally empty

5   Excessively staying away from people, places, or activities that remind the subject of the deceased

6   Unusual levels of sleep interference

7   Loss of interest in work, social, care-taking, or recreational activities to a maladaptive degree

10.6.1   Risk factors and consequences of complicated grief

An important aspect of complicated grief is the identification of its risk factors. From a research point of view, Kissane *et al.* (1996) carried out a study, the Melbourne Family Grief Study, involving 115 families that were followed for a year after bereavement. The authors showed that dysfunctional families, as described in Section 10.3 (i.e. sullen and hostile families), presented the highest psychosocial morbidity during bereavement. In the palliative care setting, Robinson *et al.* (1995) have confirmed the value of using a bereavement risk index in the course of the palliative care process to predict complicated grief after bereavement and Kissane *et al.* (1998) showed that family coping style (related to family functioning) was the most consistent correlate of bereavement outcome (grief, distress, depression, and social adjustment). Table 10.9 summarizes the most significant risk factors implicated in complicated grief that can be ascertained in the assessment of the family during the palliative care process.

The importance of identifying risk factors for complicated grief is evident in view of its negative consequences to the bereaved person, not only at the psychological level, but also in terms of physical health and quality of life. In fact, it has been shown that bereaved persons, especially those showing complicated grief, e.g. depressive disorders, are more prone to physical illness, especially cardiovascular diseases, and are at higher risk of death (Prigerson *et al.* 1997; Schaefer *et al.* 1995; Silverman *et al.* 2000; Stroebe and Stroebe 1993). The possible mechanisms include both neglect of the person's own health and possible psychobiological mechanisms, including reduction of

Table 10.8 Proposed criteria for traumatic grief (Prigerson *et al.* 1999)

Criterion A

1   Person has experienced the death of a significant other

2   Three of the four symptoms below are experienced at least sometimes

  ◆ Intrusive thoughts about the deceased

  ◆ Yearning for the deceased

  ◆ Searching for the deceased

  ◆ Loneliness as a result of death

Criterion B

In response to the death, four of the following eight symptoms experienced as mostly true:

1   Purposelessness or feeling of futility about the future

2   Subjective sense of numbness, detachment, or absence of emotional responsiveness

3   Difficulty acknowledging the death (e.g. disbelief)

4   Feeling that life is empty or meaningless

5   Feeling that a part of oneself has died

6   Shattered world view (e.g. lost sense of security, trust, control)

7   Assumption of symptoms or harmful behaviours of, or related to, the deceased person

8   Excessive irritability, bitterness, or anger related to the death

Criterion C

Duration of disturbance (symptoms lasted at least 2 months)

Criterion D

The disturbance causes clinically significant impairment in social, occupational, or other important areas of functioning

the immune system's defence mechanisms and neuroendocrine alterations (Biondi and Picardi 1996).

Taken together, all these factors indicate the need for more attention to the evaluation of responses to grief in palliative care settings in order to detect the onset of possible complications and to intervene with early and appropriate treatment (Stroebe *et al.* 2000). The following case illustrates this.

Case report

Ms. G., a 32-year-old woman, was admitted to the internal medicine department for physical complications and a facial trauma that occurred during alcohol intoxication. Her physical condition was very poor. She was suffering from a hepatic pre-cirrhosis state secondary to alcohol abuse with laboratory and clinical testing indicating the need for intensive treatment. Nevertheless, the patient tended to refuse every kind of medical intervention, including blood transfusion and oral and IV therapy and insistently asked to be discharged. She was then referred to the C–L Psychiatric Service to

Table 10.9 Risk factors for complicated grief (adapted from Worden 1991; Skinner Cook and Dworkin 1992; Sheldon 1998)

Historical variables
History of family dysfunction
History of multiple losses
Previous complicated grief
Previous psychiatric disturbances (e.g. depressive disorders, substance abuse)
Personality variables
Poor self-esteem and self-efficacy
Tendency to repress emotions
Tendency to physiological activation in facing stress rather than psychological activation
Relational variables
Ambivalent relationship with the deceased
Dependent relationship with the deceased
Conflicted relationship with the deceased
Circumstantial variables
Uncertainty of death (e.g. disppeared persons, catastrophes)
Sudden and unpredictable death
Untimely death of a young person
Stigmatized deaths (e.g. AIDS, suicide)
Culpable deaths
Social variables
Poor or inadequate support from social ties
Social reinforcement for secondary gains

evaluate the possibility of involuntary physical treatment for psychiatric reasons. She reluctantly accepted psychiatric evaluation 'only to be let to leave the hospital'. At the meeting with the psychiatrist, she was very upset, angry, and contradictive. She wanted to be discharged immediately or she would call the police to sue the hospital. She denied any problem, including drug use, and minimized her clinical conditions, including her three previous admissions to the general hospital within the last 2 months. Gently confronted with the real risk that she could die and the reasons why she was punishing herself so badly, a very sad scenario gradually emerged 'from the dark' ('I live only in the dark'). Ms. G. belonged to a very disruptive family, where the father had separated from the mother, even though he continued to live in the same apartment. Her father never cared for the family nor his two sons (the patient had an older brother, who was also an alcohol-abuser). The only affectionate bond was with her mother, a good and hard working woman, the 'victim of my father'. Unfortunately, Ms. G.'s mother developed a uterine cancer which, at the time of the diagnosis, had already spread and curative treatments were not possible. Ms. G.'s was repeatedly admitted to the hospital, because of the rapid worsening of her physical condition. During the last admission, Ms. G. was the only family member constantly present nearby her mother. Ms. G. was not ready to lose her mother. She did not believe that she should be alone by her mother's side, but no one else wanted to share with her 'this responsibility'. She did not accept that the only good bond could be destroyed like 'a broken dream over night'. During the last day of her mother's life, Ms. G. assisted her all day long. Her mother's abdominal pain, marginally controlled by drugs, and breathing problems, marginally controlled by an oxygen mask, were unbearable burdens for Ms. G. Her mother wanted to speak with her, but the oxygen mask prevented clear communication and, when the mask was taken off, breathing problems immediately worsened. The old lady whispered to her daughter, 'help me, take off this mask, it is unbearable.' Ms. G. obeyed and a few seconds later her mother died.

All this had happened 6 years before and since then Ms. G. had started to drink heavily, convinced that she had killed her mother. She felt that life had no meaning and no redemption. She said that she had never told this story before because no psychiatrist or psychologist ever saw her after bereavement.

It is evident that palliative care professionals have the opportunity to observe some problematic areas of family functioning and possible risk factors for psychological disorders that can emerge both in the anticipatory grief and bereavement phases. As recently indicated by the End-of-life Care Consensus Panel (Casarett and Inouye 2001), correct and repeated assessments, early and proper intervention, including psychological or psychiatric referral in case of complications, are the necessary elements that characterize a holistic process of care before and after the death of the patient (Table 10.10).

10.7 Conclusions

In this short review we have tried to show how the difficult voyage within the domain of palliative care involves all those (the patient, the family, and the staff) who are together protagonists of the life–death mystery. The different aspects that emerge during this phase should be taken into consideration when assisting terminally ill patients and their families. Thus, the confusional states that the patients may experience can be interpreted using a holistic perspective. This perspective should take account not only of biological and clinical aspects (i.e. the aetiology, the symptoms, the clinical subtypes, the treatment), but of the psychological and interpersonal aspects as well. From this point of view, delirium seems to represent an extreme attempt to chaotically maintain sense in a world that is collapsing and, at the same time, an expression of the loss of contact with a painful reality. Delirium is also the expression of something uncontrollable and terrible that transforms for the family the sense of coherence of their system. Giving a sense to this disorder, as a part of the trajectory of the advanced phase of illness, is a complex but important task, especially when suffering seems to be endless, pointless, and meaningless. Assisting the patient and the family (according to the Latin etymology of *adsistere*, 'to stay nearby', 'to stay still', but also 'to defend') in a clinical sense (according to the Greek etymology of κλινω, 'to stay' and 'to be

Table 10.10 Steps in the care of the family during anticipatory grief and bereavement (adapted from Caserett *et al.* 2001)

Anticipatory grief

- Assess family history and functioning
- Assess social support and coping resources
- Encourage open discussion*
- Facilitate emotional expression*
- Clarify plans for the future

Acute grief

- Be present
- Provide time and permission to grieve*
- Assess need for assistance and immediate plan
- Offer support and follow-up appointments

Early bereavement (< 1 month)

- Elicit concerns about the symptoms of grief
- Evaluate the characteristics of grief symptoms
- Reassure about the normality of grief reactions
- Re-assess social support resources
- Examine possible practical needs and problems

Late bereavement (> 1 month)

- Assess progress of mourning
- Identify symptoms indicating possible complicated grief
- Refer for counselling or specialist intervention when needed

* According to the family's own culture and values.

towards') thus has a precise significance for palliative care programmes. It means to give the patient and the family the hope that it is possible to accept being in a world of finitude and fallibility and to face our own mortality as the ultimate truth of our being in the world. It also provides a sense of authenticity in the relationship between the health professional and the patient/family systems. This way has been repeatedly pointed out by philosophical and psychiatric existential tradition in the past (Frankl 1984; Van Deurzen-Smith 1997) and it is equally valid today in the field of palliative medicine.

Acknowledgements

The authors are indebted to Professor Lea Baider, Hadassah University, Jerusalem, for her thoughtful comments and helpful suggestions on this chapter.

References

Aakerlund, L.P. and Rosenberg, J. (1994). Writing disturbances; an indicator for postoperative delirium. *Int. J. Psychiatry Med.* **24**, 245–57.

Adams, F. (1861). *The extant work of Aretaeus.* The Cappadocian, Sydenham Society, London.

Adams, F. (1988). Neuropsychiatric evaluation and treatment of delirium in cancer patients. *Adv. Psychosom. Med.* **18**, 26–36.

Adams, R.D. and Foley, J.M. (1953). The neurological disorder associated with liver disease. *Res. Publ. Assoc. Res. Nerv. Ment. Dis.* **32**, 198–237.

Agostini, J.V., Leo-Summers, L.S., and Inouye, S.K. (2001). Cognitive and other adverse side effects of diphenhydramine use in hospitalized older patients. *Arch. Intern. Med.* **161**, 2091–7.

Akechi, T., Uchitomi, Y., Okamura, H., Fukue, M., Kagaya, A., Nishida, A., Oomori, N., and Yamawaki, S. (1996). Usage of haloperidol for delirium in cancer patients. *Support Care Cancer* **4**, 390–2.

Akechi, T., Kugaya, A., Okamura, H., Nakano, T., Okuyama, T., Mikami, I., Sima, Y., Yamawaki, S., and Uchitomi, Y. (1999). Suicidal thoughts in cancer patients: clinical experience in psycho-oncology. *Psychiatry Clin. Neurosci.* **53**, 569–73.

Albert, M.S., Levkoff, S.E., Reilly, C.R., Lipzin, B., Pilgrim, D., Cleary, P., Evans, D., and Rowe, J.W. (1992). The delirium symptom interview: an interview for the detection of delirium symptoms in hospitalized patients, *J. Geriatr. Psychiatry Neurol.* **5**, 14–21.

Alciati, A., Fusi, A., D'Arminio Monforte, A., Coen, M., Ferri, A., and Mellado, C.M. (2001). New-onset delusions and hallucinations in patients infected with HIV. *J. Psychiatry Neurosci.* **26**, 229–34.

Aldemir, M., Ozen, S., Kara, I.H., Sir, A., and Bac, B. (2001). Predisposing factors for delirium in the surgical intensive care unit. *Crit. Care Med.* **5**, 265–70.

American Psychiatric Association (1980). *Diagnostic and statistical manual of mental disorders,* 3rd edn [DSM-III]. American Psychiatric Association, Washington, DC.

American Psychiatric Association (1987). *Diagnostic and statistical manual of mental disorders,* 3rd edn revised [DSM-III-R]. American Psychiatric Association, Washington, DC.

American Psychiatric Association (1994). *Diagnostic and statistical manual of mental disorders,* 4th edn [DSM-IV]. American Psychiatric Association, Washington DC.

American Psychiatric Association (1995). *Diagnostic and statistical manual of mental disorders,* 4th edn [DSM-IV-TM], Primary care version. American Psychiatric Press, Washington, DC.

American Psychiatric Association (1999). Practice guidelines for the treatment of patients with delirium. *Am. J. Psychiatry* **156**, 1–20.

American Psychiatric Association (2000). *Diagnostic and statistical manual of mental disorders,* 4th edn, text revision [DSM-IV-TR]. American Psychiatric Association, Washington, DC.

Amodio, P., Marchetti, P., Del Piccolo, F., Beghi, A., Comacchio, F., Carraro, P., Campo, G., Baruzzo, L., Marchiori, L., and Gatta, A. (1997). The effect of flumazenil on subclinical psychometric or neurophysiological alterations in cirrhotic patients: a double-blind placebo-controlled study. *Clin. Physiol.* **17**, 533–9.

Amstrong, S.C. and Schweitzer, S.M. (1997). Delirium associated with paroxetine and benztropine combination. *Am. J. Psychiatry* **154**, 581–2.

Anderson, G., Jensen, N.H., Christup, L., Hansen, S.H., and Sjogren, P. (2002). Pain, sedation and morphine metabolism in cancer patients during long-term treatment with sustained-release morphine. *Pall. Med.* **16**, 107–14.

Annese, M., Bacca, D., Francavilla, R., and Barbarini, G. (1998). Flumazenil for hepatic encephalopathy grade III and IVa in patients with cirrhosis: an Italian multicenter double-blind placebo-controlled, cross-over study. *Hepatology* **28**, 1338–9.

Arieff, A.L., Llach, F., and Massry, S.G. (1976). Neurological manifestations and morbidity of hyponatremia: correlation with brain water and electrolytes. *Medicine* **55**, 121–9.

Ashworth, M. and Gerada, C. (1997). ABC of mental health. Addiction and dependence-II. Alcohol. *Br. Med. J.* **315**, 358–60.

Auerswald, K., Charpentier, P., and Inouye, S. (1997). The informed consent process in older patients who developed delirium: a clinical epidemiologic study. *Am. J. Med.* **103**, 410–18.

Ayd, P.J. (1987). Intravenous haloperidol therapy. *Int. Drug Ther. Newslett.* **13**, 20–3.

Azorin, J.M., Dassa, D., Tramoni, V., Peretti, P., and Donnet, A. (1992). Confusione mentale. In *Encyclopedie médico-chirugicale psichiatrie*, 37124 A10, pp. 1–9. Elsevier, Paris.

Bagri, S. and Reddy, G. (1998). Delirium with manic symptoms induced by diet pills. *J. Clin. Psychiatry* **59**, 83.

Baider, L., Cooper, C.L., and De-Nour, A.K. (eds.) (2000). *Cancer and the family*, 2nd edn. Wiley, New York.

Baines, M. (1993). The pathophysiology and management of maliganant intestinal obstruction. In *Oxford textbook of palliative medicine* (ed. D. Doyle, G.W. Hanks, and N. MacDonald), pp. 311–16. Oxford University Press, Oxford.

Baranowski, S.L. and Patten, S.B. (2000). The predictive value of dysgraphia and constructional apraxia for delirium in psychiatric patients. *Can. J. Psychiatry* **45**, 75–8.

Barbaro, G., Di Lorenzo, G., Soldini, M., Marziali, M., Bellomo, G., Grisorio, B., Annese, M., Bacca, D., and Barbarini, G. (1998). Flumazenil for hepatic coma in patients with liver cirrhosis: an Italian multicentre double-blind, placebo-controlled, cross-over study. *Eur. J. Emerg. Med.* **5**, 213–18.

Barbato, M. and Rodriguez, P.J. (1994). Thiamine deficiency in patients admitted to a palliative care unit. *Pall. Med.* **8**, 320–4.

Barry, J. and Franklin, K. (1999). Amiodarone-induced delirium [letter]. *Am. J. Psychiatry* **156**, 1119.

Bates, T. and the Psychological Work Group of the International Work Group on Death, Dying and Bereavement (1993). A statement of assumptions and principles concerning psychological care of dying persons and their families. *J. Pall. Care* **9**, 29–32.

Bayindir, O., Akpinar, B., Can, E., Guden, M., Sonmez, B., and Demiroglu, C. (2000). The use of 5–HT-receptor antagonist ondansetron for the treatment of postcardiotomy delirium. *J. Cardiothorac. Vasc. Anaesthesia* **14**, 288–92.

Beaver, W., Wallenstein, S., Houde, R., and Rogers, A. (1966). A comparison of the analgesic effects of methotrimeprazine and morphine in patients with cancer. *Clin. Pharmacol. Ther.* **7**, 436–46.

Beck-Friis, B. and Strang, P. (1993). The family in hospital-based home care with special reference to terminally ill cancer patients. *J. Pall. Care* **9**, 5–13.

Berggren, D., Gustafson, Y., Erikson, B., Bucht, G., Hansson, L., Reiz, S., and Winblad, B. (1987). Postoperative confusion in elderly patients with femoral neck fractures. *Anesth. Analges.* **66**, 497–504.

Bernard, S.A. and Bruera, E. (2000). Drug interactions in palliative care. *J. Clin. Oncol.* **18**, 1780–99.

Berrios, G.E. (1981). Delirium and confusion in the 19th century. A conceptual history. *Br. J. Psychiatry* **139**, 439–49.

Bettin, K., Maletta, G., Dysken, M., Jilk, K., Weldon, D., Kuskowski, M., and Mach, J.J. (1998). Measuring delirium severity in older general hospital inpatients without dementia. The Delirium Severity Scale. *Am. J. Geriatr. Psychiatry* **6**, 296–307.

Bialer, P.A., Wallack , J.J., Prenzlauer, S.L., Bogdonoff, L., and Wilets, I. (1996). Psychiatric comorbidity among hospitalized AIDS patients vs. non-AIDS patients referred for psychiatric consultation. *Psychosomatics* **37**, 469–75.

Biondi, M. and Picardi, A. (1996). Clinical and biological aspects of bereavement and loss-induced depression: a reappraisal. *Psychother. Psychosom.* **65**, 229–45.

Bitondo Dyer, C., Ashton, C.M., and Teasdale, T.A. (1995). Postoperative delirium. A review of 80 primary data collection studies. *Arch. Intern. Med.* **155**, 461–5.

Black, K., Shea, C., Dursun, S., *et al.* (2000). Selective serotonin reuptake inhibitor discontinuation syndrome: proposed diagnostic criteria., *J. Psychiatry Neurosci.* **25**, 255–61.

Blass, J.P. and Gibson, G.E. (1999). Cerebrometabolic aspects of delirium in relationship to dementia. *Dement. Geriatr. Cogn. Disord.* **10**, 335–8.

Blitzstein, S. and Brandt, G. (1997). Extrapyramidal symptoms from intravenous haloperidol in the treatment of delirium [letter]. *Am. J. Psychiatry* **154**, 1474–5.

Bluglass, K. (1991). Care of the cancer patient's family. In *Cancer patient care: psychosocial treatment methods* (ed. M. Watson), pp. 159–89. BPS Books, Leicester.

Bodner, R.A., Lynch, T., Lewis, L., and Kahn, D. (1995). Serotonin syndrome. *Neurology* **45**, 219–23.

Boehm, S., Whall, A.L., Cosgrove, K.L., Locke, J.D., and Schlenk, E.A. (1995). Behavioral analysis and nursing interventions for reducing disruptive behaviors of patients with dementia. *Appl. Nurs. Res.* **8**, 118–22.

Bolon, M., Boulieu, R., Flamens, C., Paulus, S., and Bastien, O. (2002). Sedation par le midazolam en reanimation: aspects pharmacologiques and pharmacocinetiques. *Ann. Fr. Anesth. Reanim.* **21**, 478–92.

Bonanno, G.A. and Kaltman, S. (2001). The varieties of grief experience. *Clin. Psychol. Rev.* **21**, 705–34.

Bonin, B., Vandel, P., Vandel, S., Sechter, D., and Bizouard, P. (1999). Serotonin syndrome after sertraline, buspirone and loxapine? *Therapie* **54**, 269–71.

Bonne, O., Shalev, A.Y., and Bloch, M. (1995). Delirium associated with mianserin. *Eur. J. Neuropsychopharmacol.* **5**, 147–9.

Borreani, C., Caraceni, A. and Tamburini, M. (1997). The role of counselling for the confused patient and the family. In *Topics in palliative care* (ed. R.K. Portenoy and E. Bruera), pp. 45–54. Oxford University Press, New York.

Bortolussi, R., Fabiani, F., Savron, F., Testa, V., Lazzarini, R., Sorio, R., De Conno, F., and Caraceni, A. (1994). Acute morphine intoxication during high-dose recombinant interleukin-2 treatment for metastatic renal cell cancer. *Eur. J. Cancer* **30A**, 1905–7.

Bortone, E., Bettoni, L., Buzio, S., Giorgi, C., Melli, G., Mineo, F., and Mancia, D. (1998). Triphasic waves associated with acute naproxen overdose: a case report. *Clin. Electroencephalogr.* **29**, 142–5.

Bosisio, M., Caraceni, A., Grassi, L., Borreani, C., Mercadante, S., Luzzani, M., Maltoni, M., and Caraceni, A. (2002). Fenomenologia clinica del delirium nel paziente oncologico. *Riv. Ital. Cure Pall.* **4**, 17–30.

Bottomley, D. and Hanks, G. (1990). Subcutaneous midazolam infusion in palliative care. *J. Pain Symptom Manag.* **5**, 259–61.

Bourke, M. (1984). The continuum of pre- and post-bereavement grieving. *Br. J. Med. Psychol.* **57**, 121.

Bowdle, T.A. and Rooke, G.A. (1994). Postoperative myoclonus and rigidity after anesthesia with opioids. *Anesth. Analges.* **78**, 783–6.

Brännström, B. (1999). Care of the delirious patient. *Dement. Geriatr. Cogn. Dis.* **10**, 416–19.

Brauer, C., Morrison, R.S., Silberzweig, S.B., and Siu, A.L. (2000). The cause of delirium in patients with hip fracture. *Arch. Intern. Med.* **160**, 1856–60.

Breitbart, W. (1987). Suicide in the cancer patient. *Oncology* **1**, 49–54.

Breitbart, W. (1990). Cancer pain and suicide. In *Second International Congress on Cancer Pain*, Vol. 16 (ed. K.M. Foley, J.J. Bonica, and V. Ventafridda), pp. 399–412. Raven Press, New York.

Breitbart, W. and Cohen, K. (2000). Delirium in the terminally ill. In *Handbook of psychiatry in palliative medicine* (ed. H.M. Chochinov and W. Breitbart), pp. 75–90. Oxford University Press, New York.

Breitbart, W., Stiefel, F., Kornblith, A.B., and Pannullo, S. (1993). Neuropsychiatric disturbance in cancer patients with epidural spinal cord compression receiving high dose corticosteroids: a prospective comparison study. *Psychooncology* **2**, 233–45.

Breitbart, W., Marotta, R., Platt, M.M., Weisman, H., Derevenco, M., and Grau, C. (1996). A double-blind trial of haloperidol, chlorpromazine and lorazepam in the treatment of delirium in hospitalized AIDS patients. *Am. J. Psychiatry* **153**, 231–7.

Breitbart, W., Rosenfeld, B., Roth, A., Smith, M.J., Cohen, K., and Passik, S. (1997). The Memorial Delirium Assessment Scale. *J. Pain Symptom Manag.* **13**, 128–37.

Breitbart, W., Gibson, C. and Tremblay, A. (2002a). The delirium experience: delirium recall and delirium-related distress in hospitalized patients with cancer, their spouse/caregivers and nurses. *Psychosomatics* **43**, 183–94.

Breitbart, W., Tremblay, A., and Gibson, C. (2002b). An open trial of olanzapine for the treatment of delirium in hospitalized cancer patients. *Psychosomatics* **43**, 175–82.

Brenner, R.P. (1991). Utility of EEG in delirium: past views and current practice. *Int. Psychogeriatr.* **3**, 211–29.

Britton, A. and Russell, R. (2000). Multidisciplinary team interventions for delirium in patients with chronic cognitive impairment. *Cochrane Database of Systematic Reviews* (2), CD000395, 2000.

Broadhurst, C. and Wilson, K.W. (2001). Immunology of delirium new opportunities for treatment and research. *Br. J. Psychiatry* **174**, 288–9.

Brodal, A. (1981). *Neurological anatomy*, pp. 527–30, 756–8. Oxford University Press, Oxford.

Broomberg, M.H. and Higginson, I. (1996). Bereavement follow-up: what do palliative support teams actually do?. *J. Pall. Care* **12**, 12–17.

Brown, A.S. and Rosen, J. (1992). Lithium-induced delirium with therapeutic serum lithium levels: a case report, *J. Geriatr. Psychiatry Neurol.* **5**, 53–5.

Brown, P., Davies, B., and Martens, N. (1990). Families in supportive care—Part II: Palliative care at home: a viable care setting. *J. Pall. Care* **6**, 21–7.

Bruera, E. and Pereira, J. (1997). Acute neuropsychiatric findings in a patient receiving fentanyl for cancer pain. *Pain* **69**, 199–201.

Bruera, E., Chadwick, S., Weinlick, A., and MacDonald, N. (1987). Delirium and severe sedation in patient with terminal cancer. *Cancer Treat. Rep.* **71**, 787–8.

Bruera, E., Macmillan, K., Hanson, J., and MacDonald, R.N. (1989). The cognitive effects of the administration of narcotic analgesics in patients with cancer pain. *Pain* **39**, 13–16.

Bruera, E., Macmillan, K., Pither, J., and Mac, D.R. (1990). Effects of morphine on the dyspnea of terminal cancer patients. *J. Pain Symptom Manag.* **5**, 341–4.

Bruera, E., Fainsinger, R.L., Miller, M.J., and Kuehn, N. (1992*a*). The assessment of pain intensity in patients with cognitive failure: a preliminary report. *J. Pain Symptom Manag.* **7**, 267–70.

Bruera, E., Miller, L., McCallion, J., Macmillan, K., Krefting, L., and Hanson, J. (1992*b*). Cognitive failure in patients with terminal cancer: a prospective study. *J. Pain Symptom Manag.* **7**, 192–5.

Bruera, E., Miller, M.J., Macmillan, K., and Kuehn, N. (1992*c*). Neuropsychological effects of methylphenidate in patients receiving a continuous infusion of narcotics for cancer pain. *Pain* **48**, 163–6.

Bruera, E., Schoeller, T., and Montejo, G. (1992*d*). Organic hallucinosis in patients receiving high doses of opiates for cancer pain. *Pain* **48**, 387–99.

Bruera, E., Franco, J.J., Maltoni, M., Watanabe, S., and Suarez-Almazor, M. (1995). Changing pattern of agitated impaired mental status in patients with advanced cancer: association with cognitive monitoring, hydration and opioid rotation. *J. Pain Symptom Manage.* **10**, 287–91.

Bruera, E., Fainsinger, R.L., Schoeller, T., and Ripamonti, C. (1996). Rapid discontinuation of hypnotics in terminal cancer patients: a prospective study. *Ann. Oncol.* **7**, 855–6.

Buchman, N., Mendelsson, E., Lerner, V., and Kotler, M. (1999). Delirium associated with vitamin B12 deficiency after pneumonia. *Clin. Neuropharmacol.* **22**, 356–8.

Burge, F., McIntyre, P., Twohig, P., Cummings, I., Kaufman, D., Frager, G., and Pollett, A. (2001). Palliative care by family physicians in the 1990s. Resilience amid reform. *Can. Fam. Physician* **47**, 1989–95.

Burke, A.L. (1997). Palliative care: an update on 'terminal restlessness'. *Med. J. Aust.* **166**, 39–42.

Burke, A.L., Diamond, P.L., Hulbert, J., Yeatman, J., and Farr, E.A. (1991). Terminal restlessness—its management and the role of midazolam. *Med. J. Aust.* **155**, 485–7.

Burns, M.J., Linden, C.H., Graudins, A., Brown, R.M., and Fletcher, K.E. (2000). A comparison of physostigmine and benzodiazepines for the treatment of anticholinergic poisoning. *Ann. Emerg. Med.* **35**, 374–81.

Byelry, M.J., Christensen, R.C., and Evans, O.L. (1996). Delirium associated with a combination of sertraline, haloperidol, and benztropine. *Am. J. Psychiatry* **153**, 965–6.

Caltagirone, C. and Carlesino, G.A. (1990). Lo stato confusionale acuto. In *Manuale di neuropsicologia. Normalitá e patologia dei processi cognitivi* (ed. G. Denes and L. Pizzamiglio), pp. 1245–61. Zanichelli, Bologna.

Campbell, K.M. and Schubert, D.S. (1991). Delirium after cessation of glucocorticoid therapy. *Gen. Hosp. Psychiatry* **13**, 270–2.

Camus, V., Burtin, B., Simeone, I., Schwed, P., Gonthier, R., and Dubos, G. (2000). Factor analysis supports the evidence of existing hyperactive and hypoactive subtypes of delirium. *Int. J. Geriatr. Psychiatry* **15**, 313–16.

Capitani, E. (1985). Alterazioni neurologiche della coscienza e del sonno. In: P. Pinelli (Ed.), *Neurologia, Casa editrice ambrosiana*. Milano, pp. 79.

Capuzzo, M., Pinamonti, A., Cingolani, E., Grassi, L., Bianconi, M., Contu, P., Gritti, G., and Alvisi, R. (2001). Analgesia, sedation and memory of intensive care. *J. Crit. Care* **16**, 83–9.

Caraceni, A., Martini, C., Belli, F., Mascheroni, L., Rivoltini, L., Arienti, F., and Cascinelli, N. (1992). Neuropsychological and neurophysiological assessment of the central effects of interleukin-2 administration. *Eur. J. Cancer* **29A**, 1266–9.

Caraceni, A., Martini, C., Gamba, A., Pugnetti, L., Cattaneo, A., Biserni, P., De Conno, F., and Ventafridda, V. (1993). Cognitive effects of oral morphine administration in cancer pain. A neurophysiological evaluation. Seventh World Congress on Pain, p. 159, IASP Press, Seattle.

Caraceni, A., Martini, C., De Conno, F., and Ventafridda, V. (1994). Organic brain syndromes and opioid administration for cancer pain. *J. Pain Symptom Manag.* **9**, 527–33.

Caraceni, A., Scolari, S., and Simonetti, F. (1999). The role of the neurologist in oncology: a prospective study. *J. Neurol.* **246** (suppl. I), 68.

Caraceni, A., Nanni, O., Maltoni, M., Piva, L., Indelli, M., Arnoldi, E., Montanari, L., Amadori, D., De Conno, F., and an Italian multicentre study group on palliative care (2000). The impact of delirium on the short-term prognosis of advanced cancer patients. *Cancer* **89**, 1145–8.

Caraceni, A., Zecca, E., Martini, C., Gorni, G., Galbiati, A., and De Conno, F. (2002). Terminal sedation a retrospective survey of a three-year experience. Second Congress of the EAPC Research Network, Lyon, France.

Carlson, L.A., Gottfries, C.G., Winbland, B., Robertson, B. (Eds) (1999). Delirium in the elderly. Epidemiological, pathogenetic and treatment aspects. *Dement. Geriatr. Cogn. Dis.* **10**, 306–429.

Cartwright, P.D., Hesse, C., and Jackson, O. (1993). Myoclonic spams following intrathecal diamorphine. *J. Pain Symptom Manag.* **8**, 492–5.

Casarett, D. and Inouye, S. (2001). Diagnosis and management of delirium near the end of life. *Ann. Intern. Med.* **135**, 32–42.

Casarett, D., Kutner, J.S., and Abrahm, J., for the End-of-Life Care Consensus Panel (2001). Life after death: a practical approach to grief and bereavement. *Ann. Intern. Med.* **134**, 208–15.

Catalano, G., Catalano, M., and Alberts, V. (1996). Famotidine-associated delirium. A series of six cases. *Psychosomatics* **37**, 349–55.

Chambost, M., Liron, L., Peillon, D., and Combe, C. (2000). Serotonin syndrome during fluoxetine poisoning in a patient taking moclobemide. *Can. J. Anesth.* **47**, 246–50.

Chamorro, C., de Latorre, F.J., Montero, A., Sanchez-Izquierdo, J.A., Jareno, A., Moreno, J.A., Gonzalez, E., Barrios, M., Carpintero, J.L., Martin-Santos, F., Otero, B., and Ginestal, R. (1996). Comparative study of propofol versus midazolam in the sedation of critically ill patients: results of a prospective, randomized, multicenter trial [see comments]. *Crit. Care Med.* **24**, 932–9.

Chang, P.H. and Steinberg, M.B. (2001). Alcohol withdrawal. *Med. Clin. N. Am.* **85**, 1191–212.

Charlton, R. and Dolman, E. (1995). Bereavement: a protocol for primary care. *Br. J. Gen. Pract.* **45**, 427–30.

Chaslin, P. (1895). *La confusione mentale primitive.* Asselin et Houzeau, Paris.

Checkley, H., Sydenstricker, V., and Geeslin, L. (1939). Nicotinic acid in the treatment of atypical psychotic state. *J. Am. Med. Assoc.* **112**, 2107–10.

Chedru, F. and Geschwind, N. (1972*a*). Disorders of higher cortical functions in acute confusional states. *Cortex* **8**, 395–411.

Chedru, F. and Geschwind, N. (1972*b*). Writing disturbances in acute confusional states. *Neuropsychologia* **10**, 343–53.

Cheng, C., Roemer-Becuwe, C., and Pereira, J. (2002). When midazolam fails. *J. Pain Symptom Manag.* **23**, 256–65.

Cherny, N., Ripamonti, C., Pereira, J., Davis, C., Fallon, M., McQuay, H.J., Mercadante, S., Pasternak, G., and Ventafridda, V. (2001). Strategies to manage the adverse effects of oral morphine: an evidence-based report. *J. Clin. Oncol.* **19**, 2542–54.

Cherny, N.I. and Portenoy, R.K. (1994). Sedation in the teatment of refractory symptoms: guidelines for evaluation and treatment. *J. Pall. Care* **10**, 31–8.

Cherny, N.I., Coyle, N., and Foley, K.M. (1994). Suffering in the advanced cancer patient: a definition and taxonomy. *J. Pall. Care* **10**, 57–70.

Chochinov, H.V., Wilson, K.M., Enns, M., and Lander, S. (1994). Prevalence of depression in the terminally ill: effects of diagnostic criteria and symptom threshold judgements. *Am. J. Psychiatry* **151**, 537–40.

Chow, K.M., Wang, A.Y., Hui, A.C., Wong, T.Y., and Szeto, C.C. (2001). Nonconvulsive status epilepticus in peritoneal dialysis patients. *Am. J. Kidney Dis.* **38**, 400–5.

Clark, D. (1999). 'Total pain', disciplinary power and the body in the work of Cicely Saunders, 1958–1967. *Soc. Sci. Med.* **49**, 727–36.

Clinton, J.E., Sterner, S., Stelmachers, Z., and Ruiz, E. (1987). Haloperidol for sedation of disruptive emergency patients. *Ann. Emerg. Med.* **16**, 319–22.

Clipp, E.C. and George, L.K. (1992). Patients with cancer and their spouse caregivers. Perceptions of the illness experience. *Cancer* **69**, 1074–9.

Clouston, P.D., De Angelis, L., and Posner, J.B. (1992). The spectrum of neurological disease in patients with systemic cancer. *Ann. Neurol.* **31**, 268–73.

Cole, M.G. (1999). Delirium: effectiveness of systematic interventions. *Dement. Geriatr. Cogn. Dis.* **10**, 406–11.

Cole, M.G., Primeau, F.J., Bailey, R.F., Bonnycastle, M.J., Masciarelli, F., Engelsmann, F., Pepin, M.J., and Ducic, D. (1994). Systematic intervention for elderly inpatient with delirium: a randomized trial. *Can. Med. Assoc. J.* **151**, 965–70.

Cole, M.G., Primeau, F.J., and Elie, L.M. (1998). Delirium: prevention, treatment, and outcome studies. *J. Geriatr. Psychiatry Neurol.* **11**, 126–37.

Cole, M.G., McCusker, J., Bellavance, F., Primeau, F.J., Bailey, R.F., Bonnycastle, M.J., and Laplante, J. (2002). Systematic detection and multidisciplinary care of delirium in older medical inpatients: a randomized trial. *Can. Med. Assoc. J.* **167**, 753–9.

Commissaris, K., Verhey, F.R., and Jolles, J. (1996). A controlled study into the effects of psychoeducation for patients with cognitive disturbances. *J. Neuropsychiatry Clin. Neurosci.* **8**, 429–35.

Cowan, J.D. and Walsh, D. (2001). Terminal sedation in palliative medicine—definition and review of the literature. *Support Care Cancer* **9**, 403–7.

Cox, J.M. and Pappagallo, M. (2001). Modafinil: a gift to portmanteau. *Am. J. Hosp. Pall. Care* **18**, 408–10.

Coyle, N., Breitbart, W., Weaver, S., and Portenoy, R. (1994). Delirium as a contributing factor to 'crescendo' pain: three case reports. *J. Pain Symptom Manag.* **9**, 44–7.

Crammer, J. (2002). Subjective experience of a confusional state. *Br. J. Psychiatry* **180**, 71–5.

Craven, J.L. (1991). Cyclosporine-associated organic mental disorders in liver transplant recipients. *Psychosomatics* **32**, 94–102.

Crum, R.M., Anthony, J.C., Basset, S.S., and Folstein, M.F. (1993). Population-based norms for the Mini-Mental State Examination by age and educational level. *J. Am. Med. Assoc.* **269**, 2386–91.

Curyto, K.J., Johnson, J., TenHave, T., Mossey, J., Knott, K., and Katz, I.R. (2001). Survival of hospitalized patients with delirium: a prospective study. *Am. J. Geriatr. Psychiatry* **9**, 141–7.

Daeninck, P.J. and Bruera, E. (1999). Opioid use in cancer pain. Is a more liberal approach enhancing toxicity? *Acta Anaesthesiol. Scand.* **43**, 924–8.

Daeppen, J., Gache, P., Landry, U., Sekera, E., Schweizer, V., Gloor, S., and Yersin, B. (2002). Symptom-triggered vs fixed-schedule doses of benzodiazepine for alcohol withdrawal: a randomized treatment trial. *Arch. Intern. Med.* **27**, 1117–21.

Dangler, L.A., O'Donnell, J., Gingrich, C., and Bope, E.T. (1996). What do family members expect from the family physician of a deceased loved one? *Fam. Med.* **28**, 694–7.

Daniels, R.J. (1998). Serotonin syndrome due to venlafaxine overdose. *J. Accident Emerg. Med.* **15**, 333–4.

Dar, R., Beach, C.M., Barden, P.L., and Cleeland, C.S. (1992). Cancer pain in the marital system: a study of patients and their spouses. *J. Pain Symptom Manag.* **7**, 87–93.

Davies, B., Reimer, J.C., and Martens, N. (1994). Family functioning and its implications for palliative care. *J. Pall. Care* **10**, 29–36.

Davis, M.P. and Walsh, D. (2001). Clinical and ethical questions concerning delirium study on patients with advanced cancer. *Arch. Intern. Med.* **161**, 296–7.

De Angelis, L. (1989). Radiation-induced dementia inpatients cured of brain metastases. *Neurology* **39**, 789–96.

De Conno, F., Caraceni, A., Martini, C., Spoldi, E., Salvetti, M., and Ventafridda, V. (1991a). Hyperalgesia and myoclonus with intrathecal infusion of high-dose morphine. *Pain* **47**, 337–9.

De Conno, F., Spoldi, E., Caraceni, A., and Ventafridda, V. (1991b). Does pharmacological treatment affect the sensation of breathlessness in terminal cancer patients? *Pall. Med.* **5**, 237–43.

De Conno, F., Caraceni, A., Groff, L., Brunelli, C., Donati, I., Tamburini, M., and Ventafridda, V. (1996). Effect of home care on the place of death of advanced cancer patients. *Eur. J. Cancer* **32A**, 1142–7.

De Deyn, P.P., D'Hooge, R., Van Bogaert, P.P., and Marescau, B. (2001). Endogenous guanidino compounds as uremic neurotoxins. *Kidney Int.* **78** (suppl.), S77–83.

Denikoff, K., Rubinow, D.R., and Papa, M.Z. (1987). Neuropsychiatric effects of treatment with interleukin-2 and lymphocyte-activated killer cells. *Ann. Intern. Med.* **107**, 293–300.

Derogatis, L.R., Morrow, G.R., Fetting, J., Penman, D., Piasetsky, S., and Schmale, A.M. (1983). The prevalence of psychiatric disorders among cancer patients. *J. Am. Med. Assoc.* **249**, 751–7.

de Stoutz, N.D., Tapper, M., and Faisinger, R.L. (1995). Reversible delirium in terminally ill patients. *J. Pain Symptom Manag.* **10**, 249–53.

Deutsch, G. and Eisemberg, H.M. (1987). Frontal blood flow changes in recovery from coma. *J. Cereb. Blood Flow Metab.* **7**, 29–34.

Deutsche Lezak, M. (1995). *Neuropsychological assessment*, 3rd edn. Oxford University Press, New York.

Dilling, H. (2000). Classification. In *New Oxford textbook of psychiatry*, Vol. 1 (ed. M.G. Gelder, J.J.J. Lopez-Ibor, and N. Andreasen), pp. 109–33. Oxford University Press, New York.

DiSalvo, T.G. and O'Gara, P.T. (1995). Torsade de pointes caused by high dose intravenous haloperidol in cardiac patients. *Clin. Cardiol.* **18**, 285–90.

Dixon, D. and Craven, J. (1993). Continuous infusion of haloperidol. *Am. J. Psychiatry* **150**, 673.

Dixon, L., McFarlane, W.R., Lefley, H., Lucksted, A., Cohen, M., Falloon, I., Mueser, K., Miklowitz, D., Solomon, P., and Sondheimer, D. (2001). Evidence-based practices for services to families of people with psychiatric disabilities. *Psychiatr. Serv.* **52**, 903–10.

Dolan, M.M., Hawkes, W.G., Zimmerman, S.I., Morrison, R.S., Gruber-Baldini, A.L., Hebel, J.R., and Magaziner, J. (2000). Delirium on hospital admission in aged hip fracture patients: prediction of mortality and 2–year functional outcomes. *J. Gerontol.* **55**, M527–34.

Dowrick, C., Dunn, G., Ayuso-Mateos, J.L., Dalgard, O.S., Page, H., Lehtinen, V., Casey, P., Wilkinson, C., Vazquez-Barquero, J.L., and Wilkinson, G. (2000). Problem solving treatment and group psychoeducation for depression: multicentre randomised controlled trial. Outcomes of Depression International Network (ODIN) Group. *Br. Med. J.* **321**, 1450–4.

Dropcho, E. (2002). Remote neurologic manifestations of cancer. *Neurol. Clin.* **20**, 85–122.

Dubois, M.J., Bergeron, N., Dumont, M., Dial, S., and Skrobik, Y. (2001). Delirium in an intensive care unit: a study of risk factors. *Intens. Care Med.* **27**, 1297–304.

Duckett, S. and Scotto, M. (1992). An unusual case of sundown syndrome subsequent to a traumatic head injury. *Brain Inj.* **6**, 189–91.

Dulfano, M.J. and Ishikawa, S. (1965). Hyercapnia: mental changes and extrapulmonary complications. *Ann. Intern. Med.* **63**, 829–41.

Dunlop, R.J. (1989). Is terminal restlessness sometimes drug induced? *Pall. Med.* **3**, 65–6.

Dunne, J.W., Leedman, P.J., and Edis, R.H. (1986). Inobvious stroke: a cause of delirium and dementia. *Aust. NZ J. Med.* **16**, 771–8.

Duppils, G.S. and Wikblad, K. (2000). Acute confusional states in patients undergoing hip surgery. a prospective observation study. *Gerontology* **46**, 36–43.

Egbert, A.M., Parks, L.H., Short, L.M. and Burnett, M.L. (1990). Randomized trial of postoperative patient-controlled analgesia vs intramuscular narcotics in frail elderly men. *Arch. Intern. Med.* **150**, 1897–903.

Eidelman, L.A., Putterman, D., Putterman, C., and Sprung, C.L. (1996). The spectrum of septic encephalopathy. *J. Am. Med. Assoc.* **275**, 470–3.

Eisendrath, S.J. and Ostroff, J.W. (1990). Ranitidine-associated delirium. *Psychosomatics* **31**, 98–100.

Elble, R.J. (2000). Diagnostic criteria for essential tremor and differential diagnosis. *Neurology* **54**, S2–S6.

Ely, E.W., Inouye, S.K., Bernard, G.R, Gordon, S., Francis, J., Truman, B., Speroff, T., Gautam, S., Margolin, R., Hart, R.P., and Dittus, R. (2001*a*). Delirium in mechanically ventilated patients. Validity and reliability of the Confusion Assessment Method for the Intensive Care Unit (CAM-ICU). *J. Am. Med. Assoc.* **286**, 2703–10.

Ely, E.W., Margolin, R., Francis, J., May, L., Truman, B., Dittus, R., Speroff, T., Gautam, S., Bernard, G.R., and Inouye, S.K. (2001*b*). Evaluation of delirium in critically ill patients: validation of the Confusion Assessment Method for the Intensive Care Unit (CAM-ICU). *Crit. Care Med.* **29**, 1370–9.

Emanuel, E.J., Fairclough, D.L., Slutsman, J., Alpert, H., Baldwin, D., and Emanuel, L.L. (1999). Assistance from family members, friends, paid care givers, and volunteers in the care of the terminally ill patients. *New Engl. J. Med.* **341**, 956–63.

Engel, G.L. and Romano, J. (1959). Delirium a syndrome of cerebral insufficiency. *J. Chron. Dis.* **9**, 260–77.

Enyert, G. and Burman, M.E. (1999). A qualitative study of self-transcendence in caregivers of terminally ill patients. *Am. J. Hosp. Pall. Care* **16**, 455–62.

Eriksson, S. (1999). Social and environmental contributants to delirium in the elderly. *Dement. Geriatr. Cogn. Dis.* **10**, 350–2.

Erkinjutti, T., Wikstrom, J., Palo, J., and Autio, K. (1986). Dementia among medical inpatients. Evaluation of 2000 consecutive admissions. *Arch. Intern. Med.* **146**, 1923–6.

Erwin, W.E., Williams, D.B., and Speir, W.A. (1998). Delirium tremens. *South. Med. J.* **91**, 425–32.

Evans, A.J. (1994). Anticipatory grief: a theoretical challenge. *J. Pall. Med.* **8**, 159–65.

Ey, H., Bernard, P., and Brisset, C. (1989). *Manuel de psychiatrie*. Masson, Paris.

Factor, S.A., Molho, E.S., and Brown, D.L. (1998). Acute delirium after withdrawal of amantadine in Parkinson's disease. *Neurology* **50**, 1456–8.

Fahn, S., Marsden, C.D., and Van Woert, M.H. (1986). Definition and classification of myoclonus. In *Advances in neurology*, Vol. 43. *Myoclonus* (ed. S. Fahn, C.D. Marsden, and M. Van Woert), pp. 1–5. Raven Press, New York.

Fainsinger, R. and Bruera, E. (1992). Treatment of delirium in a terminally ill patient. *J. Pain Symptom Manag.* **7**, 54–6.

Fainsinger, R., Miller, M.J., Bruera, E., Hanson, J., and MacEachern, T. (1991). Symptom control during the last week of life on a palliative care unit. *J. Pall. Care* **7**, 5–11.

Fainsinger, R., Tapper, M., and Bruera, E. (1993) A perspective on the management of delirium in terminally ill patients on a palliative care unit. *J. Pall. Care* **9**, 4–8.

Fainsinger, R., Landman, W., Hoskings, M., and Bruera, E. (1998). Sedation for uncontrolled symptoms in a South African Hospice. *J. Pain Symptom Manag.* **16**, 145–52.

Fainsinger, R., De Moissac, D., Mancini, I., and Oneschuk, D. (2000*a*). Sedation for delirium and other symptoms in terminally ill patients in Edmonton. *J. Pall. Care* **16**, 5–10.

Fainsinger, R., Waller, A., Bercovici, M., Bengston, K., Landman, W., Hosking, M., Nunez-Olarte, J.M., and deMoissac, D. (2000*b*). A multicentre international study of sedation for uncontrolled symptoms in terminally ill patients. *Pall. Med.* **14**, 257–65.

Farber, I.J. (1959). Acute brain syndrome. (Clinical study of 122 patients). *Dis. Nerv. Syst.* **20**, 296–9.

Farber, S.J., Egnew, T.R., and Herman-Bertsch, J.L. (1999). Issues in end-of-life care: family practice faculty perceptions. *J. Fam. Pract.* **48**, 525–30.

Farberow, N.L., Schneiderman, E.S., and Leonard, C.V. (1963). *Suicide among general medical and surgical hospital patients with malignant neoplasms*, Vol. 9. US Veterans Administration, Washington, DC.

Farrell, K.R. and Ganzini, L. (1995). Misdiagnosing delirium as depression in medically ill elderly patients. *Arch. Intern. Med.* **155**, 2459–64.

Farrington, J., Stoudemire, A., and Tierney, J. (1995). The role of ciprofloxacin in a patient with delirium due to multiple etiologies. *Gen. Hosp. Psychiatry* **17**, 43–53.

Faulkner, A. (1998). ABC of palliative care: communication with patients, families, and other professionals. *Br. Med. J.* **316**, 130–2.

Faulkner, A. and Maguire, P. (1994). *Talking to cancer patients and their relatives*. Oxford University Press, Oxford.

Feldstein, M.A. and Buschman Gemma, P. (1995). Oncology nurses and chronic compounded grief. *Cancer Nurs.* **18**, 228–36.

Fenelon, G., Marie, S., and Guillard, A. (1993). Hallucinose musicale: 7 cas. *Rev. Neurol.* **149**, 8–9.

Fennig, S. and Mauas, L. (1992). Ofloxacin-induced delirium. *J. Clin. Psychiatry* **53**, 137–8.

Ferguson, J.A., Suelzer, C.J., Eckert, G.J., Zhou, X.H., and Dittus, R.S. (1996). Risk factors for delirium tremens development. *J. Gen. Intern. Med.* **11**, 410–14.

Fernandez, F., Levy, J.K., and Mansell, P.W. (1989). Management of delirium in terminally ill AIDS patients. *Int. J. Psychiatry Med.* **19**, 165–72.

Ferrell, B.R. (1998). The family. In *Oxford textbook of palliative medicine*, 2nd edn. (ed. D. Doyle, G.W.C. Hanks, and N. MacDonald), pp. 909–17. Oxford University Press, New York.

Ferro, J., Caeiro, L., and Verdelho, A. (2002). Delirium in acute stroke. *Curr. Opin. Neurol.* **15**, 51–5.

Fink, M. (1993). Post-ECT delirium. *Convuls. Ther.* **9**, 326–30.

Fischer, P. (2001). Successful treatment of nonanticholinergic delirium with a cholinesterase inhibitor. *J. Clin. Psychopharmacol.* **21**, 118.

Fitzgerald, R.G. and Parkes, C.M. (1998). Coping with loss: blindness and loss of other sensory and cognitive functions. *Br. Med. J.* **316**, 1160–3.

Flacker, J.M. and Lipsitz, L.A. (1999*a*). Neural mechanisms of delirium: current hypotheses and evolving concepts. *J. Gerontol. Biol. Sci.* **54A**, B239–B246.

Flacker, J.M. and Lipsitz, L.A. (1999*b*). Serum anticholinergic activity changes with acute illness in elderly medical patients. *J. Gerontol. MS* **54A**, M12–M16.

Flacker, J.M. and Wei, J.Y. (2001). Endogenous anticholinergic substances may exist during acute illness in elderly medical patiens. *J. Gerontol. A* **56**, M353–M355.

Folstein, M., Folstein, S., and McHugh, P. (1975). Mini-mental state. *J. Psychiatr. Res.* **12**, 189–98.

Formaglio, F. and Caraceni, A. (1998). Meningeal metastases: clinical aspects and diagnosis. *Ital. J. Neurol. Sci.* **19**, 133–49.

Forsman, A. and Ohman, R. (1977). Applied pharmacokinetics of haloperidol in man. *Curr. Ther. Res.* **21**, 396–411.

Fountain, A. (2001). Visual hallucinations: a prevalence study among hospice inpatients. *Pall. Med.* **15**, 19–25.

Francis, J. and Kapoor, W.N. (1992). Prognosis after hospital discharge of older medical patients with delirium. *J. Am. Geriatr. Soc.* **40**, 601–6.

Francis, J., Martin, D., and Kapoor, W.N. (1990). A prospective study of delirium in hospitalized elderly. *J. Am. Med. Assoc.* **263**, 1097–101.

Francis, J.F. (1999). Three millenia of delirium research: moving beyond echoes of the past. *J. Am. Geriatr. Soc.* **47**, 1382.

Franco, K., Litaker, D., Locala, J., and Bronson, D. (2001). The cost of delirium in surgical patients. *Psychosomatics* **42**, 68–73.

Frankl, V. (1984). *Man's search for meaning*. Simon & Schuster, New York.

Fredreriks, J.A.M. (2000). Inflammation of the mind. On the 300th anniversary of Gerard van Swieten. *J. History Neurosci.* **9**, 307–10.

Frenk, H. (1983). Pro-and anticonvulsant actions of morphine and the endogenous opioids: involvement and interaction of multiple opiate and non-opiate systems. *Brain Res.* **287**, 197–210.

Frenk, H., Watkins, L.R., Miller, J., and Mayer, D.J. (1984). Nonspecific convulsions are induced by morphine but not D-ala-methionine-enkephalinamide at cortical sites. *Brain Res.* **299**, 51–9.

Freudenreich, O. and Menza, M. (2000). Zolpidem-related delirium: a case report. *J. Clin. Psychiatry* **61**, 449–50.

Frye, M.A., Coudreaut, M.F., Hakeman, S.M., Shah, B.G., Strouse, T.B., and Skotzko, C.E. (1995). Continuous droperidol infusion for management of agitated delirium in an intensive care unit. *Psychosomatics* **36**, 301–5.

Fukutani, Y., Katsukawa, K., Matsubara, R., Kobayashi, K., Nakamura, I., and Yamaguchi, N. (1993). Delirium associated with Joseph disease. *J. Neurol. Neurosurg. Psychiatry* **56**, 1207–12.

Fulton, G., Madden, C., and Minichiello, V. (1996). The social construction of anticipatory grief. *Soc. Sci. Med.* **43**, 1349–58.

Fulton, R. and Gottesman, D.J. (1989). Anticipatory grief: a psychosocial concept reconsidered. *Br. J. Psychiatry* **137**, 45–54.

Gagnon, B., Bielech, M., Watanabe, S., Walker, P., Hanson, J., and Bruera, E. (1999). The use of intermittent subcutaneous injections of oxycodone for opioid rotation in patients with cancer pain. *Support Care Cancer* **7**, 265–70.

Gagnon, B., Lawlor, P.G., Mancini, I.L., Pereira, J.L., Hanson, J., and Bruera, E. (2001). The impact of delirium on the circadian distribution of breakthrough analgesia in advanced cancer patients. *J. Pain Symptom Manag.* **22**, 826–33.

Gagnon, P., Allard, P., Masse, B., and DeSerres, M. (2000). Delirium in terminal cancer: a prospective study using daily screening, early diagnosis and continuous monitoring. *J. Pain Symptom Manag.* **19**, 412–26.

Galanakis, P., Bickel, H., Gradinger, R., Von Gumppenberg, S., and Forstl, H. (2001). Acute confusional state in the elderly following hip surgery: incidence, risk factors and complications. *Int. J. Geriatr. Psychiatry* **16**, 349–55.

Galen (1978). *Galen on the affected parts.* Karger, Basel.

Galinkin, J.L., Fazi, L.M., Cuy, R.M., Chiavacci, R.M., Kurth, C.D., Shah, U.K., Jacobs, I.N., and Watcha, M.F. (2000). Use of intranasal fentanyl in children undergoing myringotomy and tube placement during halothane and sevoflurane anesthesia. *Anesthesiology* **93**, 1378–83.

Gallagher, R. (1998). Nicotine withdrawal as an etiologic factor in delirium. *J. Pain Symptom Manag.* **16**, 76–7.

Galski, T., Williams, B,. and Ehle, H.T. (2000). Effects of opioids on driving ability. *J. Pain Symptom Manag.* **19**, 200–8.

Galynker, I.I. and Tendler, D.S. (1997). Nizatidine-induced delirium. *J. Clin. Psychiatry* **58**, 327.

Garges, H.P., Varia, I., and Doraiswamy, P.M. (1998). Cardiac complications and delirium associated with valerian root withdrawal. *J. Am. Med. Assoc.* **280**, 1566–7.

Garza, M.B., Osterhoudt, K.C., and Rutstein, R. (2000). Central anticholinergic syndrome from orphenadrine in a 3 year old. *Pediatr. Emerg. Care*

Gatrad, A.R. (1994). Muslim customs surrounding death, bereavement, postmortem examinations, and organ transplants. *Br. Med. J.* **309**, 521–3.

Gavazzi, C., Stacchiotti, S., Cavalletti, R., and Lodi, R. (2001). Confusion after antibiotics. *Lancet* **357**, 1410.

Gelfand, S.B., Indelicato, J. and Benjamin, G. (1992). Using intravenous haloperidol to control delirium. *Psychopharmacology* **43**, 215.

Gerritsen van der Hoop, R., De Angelis, L., and Posner, J. (1990). Neurotoxicity of combined radiation and chemotherapy. In *Neurological adverse reaction to anticancer drugs* (ed. J. Hildebrand), pp. 45–53. Springer Verlag, Berlin.

Geschwind, N. (1982). Disorders of attention: a frontier in neuropsychology. *Phil. Trans. R. Soc. Lond.* **B298**, 173–85.

Giacino, J.P. (1997). Disorders of consciousness: differential diagnosis and neuropathologic features. *Sem. Neurol.* **17**, 105–11.

Gibson, G.E., Blass, J.P., Huang, H., and Freeman, G.B. (1991). The cellular basis of delirium and its relevance to age-related disorders including Alzheimer disease. *Int. Psychogeriatr.* **3**, 373–95.

Gijtenbeek, J.M.M., van den Bent, M.J., and Vecht, C.L. (1999). Cyclosporine neurotoxicity: a review. *J. Neurol.* **246** (5), 339–46.

Gil, R. (1989). *Neurologie pour le practicien.* Simep, Paris.

Gill, D. and Mayou, R. (2000). Delirium. In *New Oxford textbook of psychiatry*, Vol 1 (ed. M.G. Gelder, J.J.J. López-Ibor, and N. Andreasen), pp. 382–7. Oxford University Press, New York.

Gill, M., LoVecchio, F., and Selden, B. (1999). Serotonin syndrome in a child after a single dose of fluvoxamine. *Ann. Emerg. Med.* **33**, 457–9.

Gillman, P.K. (1995). Possible serotonin syndrome with moclobemide and pethidine. *Med. J. Aust.* **162**, 554.

Gillman, P.K. (1998). Serotonin syndrome: history and risk. *Fund. Clin. Pharmacol.* **12**, 482–91.

Gillman, P.K. (1999). The serotonin syndrome and its treatment. *J. Psychopharmacol.* **13**, 100–9.

Given, C.W., Stmmel, M., Given, B., Osuch, J., Kurtz, M.E., and Kurtz, J.C. (1993). The influence of cancer patients' symptoms and fucntional states on patients' depression and family caregivers' reaction and depression. *Health Psychol.* **12**, 277–85.

Glare, P., Walsh, T.D., and Pippenger, C.E. (1990). Normorphine, a neurotoxic metabolite? *Lancet* **335**, 725–6.

Glassman, A. and Bigger, J.J. (2001). Antipsychotic drugs: prolonged QTc interval, torsade des pointes, and sudden death. *Am. J. Psychiatry* **158**, 1774–82.

Glavina, M.J. and Robertshaw, R. (1988). Myoclonic spasms following intrathecal morphine. *Anaesthesia* **43**, 389–90.

Glick, R.E., Sanders, K.M., and Stern, T.A. (1996). Failure to record delirium as a complication of intraaortic balloon pump treatment: a retrospective study, *J. Geriatr. Psychiatry Neurol.* **9**, 97–9.

Goldstein, J.M. (2000). The new generation of antipsychotic drugs: how atypical are they? *Int. Neuropsychopharmacol.* **3**, 339–49.

Gordon, D. and Peruselli, C. (2001). *Narrazione e fine della vita. Nuove possibilità per valutare qualità della vita e della morte.* Franco Angeli, Milan.

Graham, J., Ramirez, A.J., Cull, A., Finlay, I., Hoy, A., and Richards, M.A. (1996). Job stress and satisfaction among palliative physicians. *Pall. Med.* **10**, 185–94.

Grassi, L., Pavanati, M., Bedetti, A., and Bicocchi, R. (1995). Analysis of psychiatric consultations in patients with HIV infection and related syndromes. *AIDS Care* **7**, S73–S77.

Grassi, L., Biancosino, B., Pavanati, M., Agostini, M., and Manfredini, R. (2001*a*). Depression or hypoactive delirium? A report of ciprofloxacin-induced mental disorder in a patient with chronic obstructive pulmonary disease. *Psychother. Psychosom.* **70**, 58–9.

Grassi, L., Caraceni, A., Beltrami, E., Zamorani, M., Maltoni, M., Monti, M., Luzzani, M., Mercadante, S., and De Conno, F. (2001*b*). Assessing delirium in cancer patients: the Italian versions of the Delirium Rating Scale and the Memorial Delirium Assessment Scale. *J. Pain Symptom Manag.* **21**, 59–68.

Grassi, L., Satriano, J., Biancosino, B., Rigatelli, M. and Gala, C. (unpublished manuscript). Psychiatric disorders in hospitalized HIV-infected patients referred to mental health services: an Italian multicentre investigation.

Grbich, C., Parker, D., and Maddocks, I. (2001). The emotions and coping strategies of caregivers of family members with a terminal cancer. *J. Pall. Care* **17**, 30–6.

Gregory, D. (1994). The myth of control: suffering in palliative care. *J. Pall. Care* **10**, 18–22.

Gregory, R.E., Grossman, S., and Sheidler, V.R. (1992). Grand mal seizures associated with high-dose intravenous morphine: incidence and possible etiologies. *Pain* **51**, 255–8.

Greiner, F.C. (1817). *Der Traum und das fieberhafte Irreseyn.* F.A. Brockhaus, Altenburg.

Greisinger, A.J., Lorimor, R.J., Aday, L.A., Winn, R.J., and Baile, W.F. (1997). Terminally ill cancer patients. Their most important concerns. *Cancer Pract.* **5**, 147–54.

Grobe, M.E., Ilstrup, D.M., and Ahman, D. (1981). Skills needed by family members to maintain the care of an advanced cancer patient. *Cancer Nurs.* **4**, 371–5.

Groeneweg, M., Gyr, K., Amrein, R., Scollo-Lavizzari, G., Williams, R., Yoo, J.Y., and Schalm, S.W. (1996). Effect of flumazenil on the electroencephalogram of patients with portosystemic encephalopathy. Results of a double-blind placebo-controlled multicenter trial. *Electroencephalogr. Clin. Neurophysiol.* **98**, 29–34.

Groff, L. (1993). *Risultati di un programma di assistenza domiciliare per pazienti oncologici in fase avanzata.* Faculty of Medicine and Surgery, Oncology Specialty School, Universitá degli Studi di Milano, Milan.

Grossman, S.A., Trump, D.L., Chen, D.C.P., Thomson, G., and Camargo, E.E. (1982). Cerebrospinal fluid abnormalities in patients with neoplastic meningitis. *Am. J. Med.* **73**, 641–7.

Gupta, R.M., Parvizi, J., Hanssen, A.D., and Gay, P.C. (2001). Obstructive sleep apnea syndrome. Postoperative complications in patients undergoing hip or knee replacement: a case-control study. *Mayo Clin. Proc.* **76**, 897–905.

Gustafson, Y., Brännström, B., Norberg, A., Bucht, G., and Winblad, B. (1991a). Underdiagnosis and poor documentation of acute confusional states in elderly hip fracture patients. *J. Am. Geriatr. Soc.* **39**, 760–5.

Gustafson, Y., Olsson, T., Eriksson, S., Asplund, K., and Bucht, G. (1991b). Acute confusional state in stroke patients. *Cerebrovasc. Dis.* **1**, 257–64.

Gyr, K., Meier, R., Haussler, J., Bouletreau, P., Fleig, W.E., Gatta, A., Holstege, A., Pomier-Layragues, G., Schalm, S.W., Groeneweg, M., Scollo-Lavizzari, G., Ventura, E., Zeneroli, M.L., Williams, R., and Yoo, Y.A. (1996). Evaluation of the efficacy and safety of flumazenil in the treatment of portal systemic encephalopathy: a double blind, randomised, placebo controlled multicentre study. *Gut* **39**, 319–24.

Haddad, P. and Anderson, I. (2002). Antipsychotic-related QTc prolongation, torsade de pointes and sudden death. *Drugs* **62**, 1649–71.

Hagen, N. and Swanson, R. (1997). Strychnine-like multifocal myoclonus and seizures in extremely high-dose opioid administration: treatment strategies. *J. Pain Symptom Manag.* **14**, 51–8.

Haines, J., Barclay, P., and Wauchob, T. (2001). Optimising management of delirium: Withdrawal of Droleptan (droperidol). *Br. Med. J.* **322**, 1603.

Hall, D.E., Kahan, B., and Snitzer, J. (1994). Delirium associated with hypophosphatemia in a patient with anorexia nervosa. *J. Adolesc. Health* **15**, 176–8.

Hall, W. and Zador, D. (1997). The alcohol withdrawal syndrome. *Lancet* **349**, 1897–900.

Hamilton, S. and Malone, K. (2000). Serotonin syndrome during treatment with paroxetine and risperidone. *J. Clin. Psychopharmacol.* **20**, 103–5.

Han, L., McCusker, J., Cole, M., Abrahamovicz, M., Primeau, F., and Elie, M. (2001). Use of medications with anticholinergic effect predicts clinical severity of delirium symptoms in older medical inpatients. *Arch. Intern. Med.* **161**, 1099–105.

Harrison, J., Haddad, P., and Maguire, P. (1995). The impact of cancer on key relatives: a comparison of relative and patient concerns. *Eur. J. Cancer* **31A**, 1736–40.

Hart, R., Levenson, J., Sessler, C., Best, A., Schwartz, S., and Rutherford, L. (1996). Validation of a cognitive test for delirium in medical ICU patients. *Psychosomatics* **37**, 533–46.

Hart, R., Best, A., Sessler, C., and Levenson, J.L. (1997). Abbreviated cognitive test for delirium. *J. Psychosom. Res.* **43**, 417–23.

Hays, J.C., Kasl, S.V., and Jacobs, S.C. (1994). The course of psychological distress following threatened and actual conjugal bereavement. *Psychol. Med.* **24**, 411–21.

Heckmann, J.G., Birklein, F., and Neundorfer, B. (2000). Omeprazole-induced delirium. *J. Neurol.* **247**, 56–7.

Hendler, N., Cimini, C., Long, T., and Long, D. (1980). Comparison of cognitive impairment due to benzodiazepines and to narcotics. *Am. J. Psychiatry* **137**, 828–30.

Henon, H., Lebert, F., Durieu, I., Godefroy, O., Lucas, C., Pasquier, F., and Leys, D. (1999). Confusional state in stroke. Relation to preexisting dementia, patient characteristics and outcome. *Stroke* **30**, 773–9.

Heritch, A.J., Capwell, R. and Roy-Byrne, P.P. (1987). A case of psychosis and delirium following withdrawal from triazolam. *J. Clin. Psychiatry* **48**, 168–9.

Hermann, I., Denekens, J., Van den Eynden, B., Van Royen, P., Verrept, H., and Maes, R. (1999). General practitioners caring for terminally ill patients resident in a hospice. *Support Care Cancer* **7**, 437–8.

Hickey, M. (1990). What are the needs of families of critically ill patients? A review of the literature since 1976. *Heart Lung* **19**, 401–15.

Higginson, I. and Priest, P. (1996). Predictors of family anxiety in the weeks before bereavement. *Soc. Sci. Med.* **43**, 1621–5.

Hileman, J.W., Lackey, N.R., and Hassanein, R.S. (1992). Identifying the needs of home caregivers of patients with cancer. *Oncol. Nurs. Forum* **19**, 771–7.

Hill, C.D., Risby, E., and Morgan, N. (1992). Cognitive deficits in delirium: assessment over time. *Psychopharmacol. Bull.* **28**, 401–7.

Hinds, C. (1985). The needs of families who care for patients with cancer at home. Are we meeting them? *J. Adv. Nurs.* **10**, 575–81.

Hinton, J. (1981). Sharing or withholding awareness of the dying between husband and wife. *J. Psychosom. Res.* **25**, 337–43.

Hinton, J. (1994). Can home maintain an acceptable quality of life for patients with terminal cancer and their relatives? *Pall. Med.* **8**, 183–96.

Hippocrates (1931). An English translation by W.H.S. Jones. William Heinemann, London.

Holder, G., Brand, S., Hatzinger, M., and Holsboer-Trachsler, E. (2002). Reduction of daytime sleepiness in a depressive patient during adjunct treatment with modafinil. *J. Psychiatry Res.* **36**, 49–52.

Honma, H., Kohsaka, M., Suzuki, I., Fukuda, N., Kobayashi, R., Sakakibara, S., Matubara, S., and Koyama, T. (1998). Motor activity rhythm in dementia with delirium. *Psychiatry Clin. Neurosci.* **52**, 196–8.

Hooten, W. and Pearlson, G. (1996). Delirium caused by tacrine and ibuprofen interaction [letter]. *Am. J. Psychiatry* **153**, 842.

Horowitz, M.J., Siegel, B., Holen, A., Bonanno, G.A., Milbrath, C., and Stinson, C. (1997). Diagnostic criteria for complicated grief disorder. *Am. J. Psychiatry* **154**, 904–10.

Houts, P.S., Rusenas, I., Simmonds, M.A., and Hufford, D.L. (1991). Information needs of families of cancer patients: a literature review and recommendations. *J. Cancer Educ.* **6**, 255–61.

Huang, S.C., Tsai, S.J., Chan, C.H., Hwang, J.P., and Sim, C.B. (1998). Characteristics and outcome of delirium in psychiatric inpatients, *Psychiatry Clin. Neurosci.* **52**, 47–50.

Hughes, R.J. (1980). Correlations between EEG and chemical changes in uremia. *Electroencephalogr. Clin. Neurophysiol.* **48**, 583–94.

Ildegarda di Bingen (1997). *Cause e cure delle infermità.* Sellerio, Palermo.

Inouye, S.K. (1998). Delirium in hospitalized older patients: recognition and risk factors. *J. Geriatr. Psychiatry Neurol.* **11**, 118–25.

Inouye, S.K. and Charpentier, P.A. (1996). Precipitating factors for delirium in hospitalized elderly persons. Predictive model and interrelationship with baseline vulnerability. *J. Am. Med. Assoc.* **275**, 852–7.

Inouye, S.K., van Dyck, C.H., Alessi, C.A., Balkin, S., Siegal, A.P., and Horwitz, R.I. (1990). Clarifying confusion: the confusion assessment method. A new method for detection of delirium. *Ann. Intern. Med.* **113**, 941–8.

Inouye, S.K., Viscoli, C.M., Horwitz, R.I., Hurst, L.D., and Tinetti, M.E. (1993). A predictive model for delirium in hospitalized elderly medical patients based on admission characteristics. *Ann. Intern. Med.* **119**, 474–81.

Inouye, S.K., Bogardus, S.T., Charpentier, P.A., Leo-Summers, L., Acampora, D., Holford, T.R., and Coeney, L.M. (1999*a*). A multicomponent intervention to prevent delirium in hospitalized older patients. *New Engl. J. Med.* **340**, 669–76.

Inouye, S.K., Schlesinger, M.J., and Lyndon, T.J. (1999*b*). Delirium: a symptom of how hospital care is failing older persons and a window to improve quality of hospital care. *Am. J. Med.* **106**, 565–73.

Inouye, S.K., Foreman, M.D., Mion, L.C., Katz, K.H., and Cooney, L.M.J. (2001). Nurses' recognition of delirium and its symptoms: comparison of nurse and researcher ratings. *Arch. Intern. Med.* **161**, 2467–73.

Itil, T. and Fink, M. (1968). EEG and behavioral aspects of the interaction of anticholinergic hallucinogens with centrally active compounds. *Prog. Brain Res.* **28**, 149–68.

Jackson, C.W., Markowitz, J.S., and Brewerton, T.D. (1995). Delirium associated with clozapine and benzodiazepine combination. *Ann. Clin. Psychiatry* **7**, 139–41.

Jackson, J.H. (1932). *Selected writings.* Hodder & Stoughton, London.

Jackson, T., Ditmanson, L., and Phibbs, B. (1997). Torsade de pointes and low-dose oral haloperidol. *Arch. Intern. Med.* **157**, 2013–15.

Jacobs, S. (1993). *Pathologic grief: maladaptation to loss.* American Psychiatric Press, Washington, DC.

Jacobs, S., Hansen, F., Kaasl, S., Ostfield, A., Berkman, L., and Kim, K. (1990). Anxiety disorders during acute bereavement: risk and risk factors. *J. Clin. Psychiatry* **51**, 269–74.

Jacobs, S., Mazure, C., and Prigerson, H. (2000). Diagnostic criteria for traumatic grief. *Death Stud.* **24**, 185–99.

Jacobson, S. and Jerrier, H. (2000). EEG in delirium. *Sem. Clin. Neuropsychiatry* **5**, 86–92.

Jacobson, S.A., Leuchter, A.F., and Walter, D.O. (1993*a*). Conventional and quantitative EEG in the diagnosis of delirium among the elderly. *J. Neurol. Neurosurg. Psychiatry* **56**, 153–8.

Jacobson, S.A., Leuchter, A.F., Walter, D.O., and Weiner, H. (1993*b*). Serial quantitative EEG among elderly subjects with delirium. *Biol. Psychiatry* **34**, 135–40.

Jacobson, S. and Schreibman, B. (1997). Behavioral and pharmacologic treatment of delirium. *Am. Fam. Physician* **56**, 2005–12.

Jellema, J.G. (1987). Hallucinations during sustained-release morphine and methadone administration. *Lancet* **i**, 392.

Jenkins, B.G. and Kraft, E. (1999). Magnetic resonance spectroscopy in toxic encephalopathy and neurodegeneration. *Curr. Opin. Neurol.* **12**, 753–60.

Jennings, M.T. (1995). Neurological complications of radiotherapy. In *Neurological complications of cancer* (ed. R.G. Wiley), pp. 219–40. Marcel Dekker Inc, New York.

Johns, M.W. (1993). Daytime sleepiness, snoring, and obstructive sleep apnea. The Epworth sleepiness scale. *Chest* **103**, 30–6.

Johnson, J.C., Kerse, N.M., Gottlieb, G., Wanich, C., Sullivan, E., and Chen, K. (1992). Prospective versus retrospective methods of identifying patients with delirium. *J. Am. Geriatr. Soc.* **40**, 316–19.

Johnson, L.C., Spinweber, C.L., Gomez, S.A., and Matteson, L.T. (1990). Daytime sleepiness, performance, mood, nocturnal sleep: the effect of benzodiazepine and caffeine and their relationship. *Sleep* **13**, 121–35.

Kagawa-Singer, M. and Blackhall, L.J. (2001). Negotiating cross-cultural issues at the end of life. *J. Am. Med. Assoc.* **286**, 2993–3001.

Karena, M., Meehan, K.M., Wang, H., David, S.R., Nisivoccia, J., Jones, B., Beasley, J., Feldman, P.D., Mintzer, J., Beckett, L., and Breier, A. (2002). Comparison of rapidly acting intramuscular olanzapine, lorazepam, and placebo: a double-blind, randomized study in acutely agitated patients with dementia. *Neuropsychopharmacology* **26**, 494–504.

Katirji, M.B. (1987). Visual hallucinations and cyclosporine. *Transplantation* **43**, 768–9.

Katz, L. and Chochinov, H.M. (1998). The spectrum of grief in palliative care. In *Topics in palliative care*, Vol 2 (ed. E. Bruera and R. Portenoy), pp. 295–310. Oxford University Press, New York.

Kaufer, D., Catt, K., Lopez, O., and De, K.S. (1998). Dementia with Lewy bodies: response of delirium-like features to donepezil. *Neurology* **51**, 1512.

Kawashima, T. and Yamada, S. (2002). Delirium caused by donepezil: a case study. *J. Clin. Psychiatry* **63**, 250–1.

Kay, D.C., Eisenstein, R.B., and Jasinski, D. (1969). Morphine effects on human REM state, waking state and NREM sleep. *Psychopharmacologia* **14**, 404–16.

Kesavan, S. and Sobala, G.M. (1999). Serotonin syndrome with fluoxetine plus tramadol. *J. R. Soc. Med.* **92**, 474–5.

Khawaja, I.S., Marotta, R.F., and Lippmann, S. (1999). Herbal medicine as a factor in delirium. *Psychiatr. Serv.* **50**, 969–70.

Khouzam, H.R., Donnelly, N.J., and Ibrahim, N.F. (1998). Psychiatric morbidity in HIV patients. *Can. J. Psychiatry* **43**, 51–6.

Kim, K.Y., McCartney, J.R., Kaye, W., Boland, R.J., and Niaura, R. (1996). The effect of cimetidine and ranitidine on cognitive function in postoperative cardiac surgery. *Int. J. Psychiatry Med.* **26**, 295–307.

Kinney, H.C., Korein, J., Panigrahy, A., Dikkes, P., and Goode, R. (1994). Neuropathological findings in the brain of Karen Ann Quinlan. *New Engl. J. Med.* **330**, 1469–75.

Kissane, D.W. and Bloch, S. (1994). Family grief. *Br. J. Psychiatry* **164**, 720–40.

Kissane, D.W., Bloch, S., Burns, W.I., McKenzie, D., and Posterino, M. (1994a). Psychological morbidity in the families of patients with cancer. *Psycho-Oncology* **3**, 47–56.

Kissane, D.W., Bloch, S., Burns, W.I., Patrick, J.D., Wallace, C.S., and McKenzie, D. (1994b). Perceptions of family functioning and cancer. *Psycho-Oncology* **3**, 259–69.

Kissane, D.W., Bloch, S., Onghena, P., McKenzie, D.P., Snyder, R.D., and Dowe, D.L. (1996). The Melbourne Family Grief Study, II: Psychosocial morbidity and grief in bereaved families. *Am. J. Psychiatry* **153**, 659–66.

Kissane, D.W., Bloch, S., McKenzie, D., McDowall, A., and Nitzan, R. (1998). Family grief therapy: a preliminary account of a new model to promote healthy family functioning during palliative care and bereavement. *Psycho-Oncology* **7**, 14–25.

Klagsbrun, S.C., Patient, family, amd staff suffering. *J. Pall. Care* **10**, 14–17.

Kloke, M., Bingel, U., and Seeber, S. (1994). Complications of spinal opioid therapy: myoclonus, spastic muscle tone and spinal jerking. *Support Care Cancer* **2**, 249–52.

Kobayashi, K., Takeuchi, O., Suzuki, M., and Yamaguchi, N. (1992). A retrospective study on delirium type. *Jpn J. Psychiatry Neurol.* **46**, 911–17.

Koponen, H., Partanen, J., Paakkonen, A., Mattila E., and Rikkinen, P.J. (1989). EEG spectral analysis in delirium. *J. Neurol. Neurosurg. Psychiatry* **52**, 980–5.

Koponen, H.J. and Riekkinen, P.J. (1993). A prospective study of delirium in elderly patients admitted to a psychiatric hospital. *Psychol. Med.* **23**, 103–9.

Kornblith, A.B. (2001). Does palliative care palliate? *J. Clin. Oncol.* **19**, 2111–13.

Kristjanson, L.J. (1997). The family as a unit of treatment. In *Topics in palliative care*, Vol. 1 (ed. R.K. Portenoy and E. Bruera), pp. 245–62. Oxford University Press, New York.

Kristjanson, L.J. and Ashercraft, T. (1994). The family's cancer journey: a literature review. *Cancer Nurs.* **17**, 1–17.

Kristjanson, L.J., Dudgeon, D., and Adaskin, E. (1996). Family members' perceptions of palliative cancer care: predictors of family functioning and family members' health. *J. Pall. Care* **12**, 10–20.

Kübler-Ross, E. (1969). *On death and dying.* Macmillan, New York.

Kupfer, A., Aeschlimann, C., and Cerny, T. (1996). Methylene blue and neurotoxic mechanism of ifosfamide encephalopathy. *Eur. J. Clin. Pharmacol.* **50**, 249–52.

Kurtz, M.E., Kurtz, J.C., Given, C.W., and Given, B. (1995). Relationship of caregiver reactions and depression to cancer patients' symptoms, functional states and depression. A longitudinal view. *Soc. Sci. Med.* **40**, 837–46.

Laccetti, M., Manes, G., Uomo, G., Lioniello, M., Rabitti, P.G., and Balzano, A. (2000). Flumazenil in the treatment of acute hepatic encephalopathy in cirrhotic patients: a double blind randomized placebo controlled study. *Dig. Liver Dis.* **32**, 335–8.

Lalonde, B., Uldall, K.K., and Berghuis, J.P. (1996). Delirium in AIDS patients: discrepancy between occurrence and health care provider identification. *AIDS Pat. Care STDS* **10**, 282–7.

Langenbucher, J., Martin, C.S., Labouvie, E., Sanjuan, P.M., Bavly, L., and Pollock, N.K. (2000). Toward the DSM-V: the Withdrawal-Gate Model versus the DSM-IV in the diagnosis of alcohol abuse and dependence. *J. Consult. Clin. Psychol.* **68**, 799–809.

Lapin, S.L., Auden, S.M., Goldsmith, L.J., and Reynolds, A.M. (1999). Effects of sevoflurane anaesthesia on recovery in children: a comparison with halothane. *Paediatr. Anaesth.* **9**, 283–6.

Lasagna, L. and DeKornfeld, T.J. (1961). Methotrimeprazine, a new phenothiazine derivative with analgesic properties. *J. Am. Med. Assoc.* **178**, 887–90.

Lawlor, P. (2002). The panorama of opioid-related cognitive dysfunction in patients with cancer: a critical literature appraisal. *Cancer* **94**, 1836–53.

Lawlor, P., Gagnon, B., Mancini, I., Pereira, J., and Bruera, E. (1998). Phenomenology of delirium and its subtypes in advanced cancer patients: a prospective study. *J. Pall. Care* **14**, 106.

Lawlor, P., Gagnon, B., Mancini, I.L., Pereira, J.L., Hanson, J., Suarez-Almazor, M.E., and Bruera, E. (2001). In reply to Davis *et al. Arch. Intern. Med.* **161**, 297–9.

Lawlor, P.G., Fainsinger, R.L. and Bruera, E.D. (2000*a*). Delirium at the end of life. Critical issues in clinical practice and research. *J. Am. Med. Assoc.* **284**, 2427–9.

Lawlor, P.G., Gagnon, B., Mancini, I.L., Pereira, J.L., Hanson, J., Suarez-Almazor, M.E., and Bruera, E.D. (2000*b*). Occurrence, causes and outcome of delirium in patients with advanced cancer. *Arch. Intern. Med.* **160**, 786–94.

Lawlor, P.G., Nekolaichuk, C., Gagnon, B., Mancini, I.L., Pereira, J.L., and Bruera, E.D. (2000*c*). Clinical utility, factor analysis and further validation of the Memorial Delirium Assessment Scale (MDAS) in advanced cancer patients. *Cancer* **88**, 2859–67.

Lederberg, M. (1998a). The family of the cancer patients. In *Psycho-Oncology* (ed. J. Holland), pp. 981–93. Oxford University Press, New York.

Lederberg, M. (1998b). Oncology staff stress and related interventions. In *Psycho-Oncology* (ed. J. Holland), pp. 1035–48. Oxford University Press, New York.

Lee, D.O. and Lee, C.D. (1999). Serotonin syndrome in a child associated with erythromycin and sertraline. *Pharmacotherapy* **19**, 894–6.

Leinonen, E., Koponen, H.J., and Lepola, U. (1993). Delirium during fluoxetine treatment. *Ann. Clin. Psychiatry* **5**, 255–7.

Leipzig, R.M., Goodman, H., Gray, G., Erle, H., and Reidenberg, M.M. (1987). Reversible, narcotic-associated mental status impairment in patients with metastatic cancer. *Pharmacology* **35**, 47–54.

Leis, A.M., Kristjanson, L., Koop, P., and Laizner, A. (1997). Family health and the palliative care trajectory: a cancer research agenda. *Cancer Prevent. Control* **1**, 352–60.

Lemkau, J.P., Mann, B., Little, D., Whitecar, P., Hershberger, P., and Schumm, J.A. (2000). A questionnaire survey of family practice physicians' perceptions of bereavement care. *Arch. Fam. Med.* **9**, 822–9.

Lemperiere, T. and Feline, A. (1977). *Psychiatrie de l'adulte.* Masson, Paris.

Leso, L. and Schwartz, T.L. (2002). Ziprasidone treatment of delirium. *Psychosomatics* **43**, 61–2.

Levenson, J.A. (1992). Should psychostimulants be used to treat delirious patients with depressed mood? *J. Clin. Psychiatry* **53**, 69.

Levenson, J.L. (1995). High-dose intravenous haloperidol for agitated delirium following lung transplantation. *Psychosomatics* **36**, 66–8.

Levin, T., Petrides, G., Weiner, J., Saravay, S., Multz, A.S., and Bailine, S. (2002). Intractable delirium associated with ziconotide successfully treated with electroconvulsive therapy. *Psychosomatics* **43**, 63–6.

Levine, P., Silberfarb, P., and Lipowski, Z. (1978). Mental disorders in cancer patients: a study of 100 psychiatric referrals. *Cancer* **42**, 1385–91.

Levkoff, S.E., Evans, D.A., Lipzin, B., Cleary, P.D., Lipsitz, L.A., Wetle, T.T., Reilly, C.H., Pilgrim, D.M., Schor, J., and Rowe, J. (1992). Delirium. The occurrence and persistence of symptoms among elderly hospitalized patients. *Arch. Intern. Med.* **152**, 334–40.

Levkoff, S.E., Lipzin, B., Cleary, P., Wetle, T., Evans, D., Rowe, J., and Lipsitz, L. (1996). Subsyndromal delirium. *Am. J. Geriatr. Psychiatry* **4**, 320–9.

Lewis, F.M. (1990). Strengthening family support: cancer and the family. *Cancer* **65**, 752–9.

Lindenbaum, J., Healton, E., Savage, D., Brust, J., Garrett, T., Podell, E., Marcell, P., Stabler, S., and Allen, R. (1988). Neuropsychiatric disorders caused by cobalamin deficiency in the absence of anemia or macrocytosis. *New Engl. J. Med.* **318**, 1720–8.

Lindesay, J. (1999). The concept of delirium. *Dement. Geriatr. Cogn. Disord.* **10**, 310–14.

Lipowski, Z.J. (1982). Differentiating delirium from dementa in the elderly. *Clin. Gerontol.* **1**: 3.

Lipowski, Z.J. (1980). Delirium: acute brain failure in man. Charles C. Thomas, Springfield Ill.

Lipowski, Z.J. (1990a). Etiology. In *Delirium: acute confusional states* (ed. Z.J. Lipowski), pp. 109–40. Oxford University Press, New York.

Lipowski, Z.J. (1990b). *Delirium: acute confusional states.* Oxford University Press, New York.

Lipowski, Z.J. (1992). Update on delirium. *Psychiatric Clin. N. Am.* **15**, 335–45.

Lipsitt, D.R. and Lipsitt, M.P. (1991). Guidelines for working with familes in consultation liaison psychiatry. In *Handbook of studies on general hospital psychiatry* (ed. F.K. Judd, G.D. Burrows, and D.R. Lipsitt), pp. 179–94. Elsevier, Amsterdam

Liptzin, B. (1999). What criteria should be used for the diagnosis of delirium? *Dement. Geriatr. Cogn. Dis.* **10**, 364–7.

Liptzin, B. and Levkoff, S.E. (1992). An empirical study of delirium subtypes. *Br. J. Psychiatry* **161**, 843–5.

Liptzin, B., Levkoff, S.E., Cleary, P.D., Pilgrim, D.M., Reilly, C.H., Albert, M., and Wetle, T.W. (1991). An empirical study of diagnostic criteria for delirium. *Am. J. Psychiatry* **148**, 454–7.

Liston, E. and Sones, D. (1990). Postictal hyperactive delirium in ECT: management with midazolam. *Convuls. Ther.* **6**, 19–25.

Litaker, D., Locala, J., Franco, K., Bronson, D.L., and Tannous, Z. (2001). Preoperative risk factors for postoperative delirium. *Gen. Hosp. Psychiatry* **23**, 84–9.

Lotsch, J., Kobal, G., Stockman, A., Brune, K., and Geisslinger, G. (1997). Lack of analgesic activity of morphine-6–glucuronide after short-term intravenous administration in healthy volunteers. *Anesthesiology* **87**, 1348–58.

Lynch, E.P., Lazor, M.A., Gellis, J.E., Orav, J., Goldman, L., and Marcantonio, E.R. (1998). The impact of postoperative pain on the development of postoperative delirium. *Anesth. Analgs.* **86**, 781–5.

MacDonald, A.J.D. (1999).Can delirium be separated from dementia? *Dement. Geriatr. Cogn. Disord.* **10**, 386–8.

Macdonald, G.A., Frey, K.A., Agranoff, B.W., Minoshima, S., Koeppe, R.A., Kuhl, D.E., Shulkin, B.L., and Lucey, M.R. (1997). Cerebral benzodiazepine receptor binding *in vivo* in patients with recurrent hepatic encephalopathy. *Hepatology* **26**, 277–82.

MacDonald, N., Der, L., Allan, S., and Champion, P. (1993). Opioid hyperexcitability: the application of alternate opioid therapy. *Pain* **53**, 353–5.

Mach, J.J., Kabat, V., Olson, D., and Kuskowski, M. (1996). Delirium and right-hemisphere dysfunction in cognitively impaired older persons. *Int. Psychogeriatr.* **8**, 373–82.

MacKenzie, T.B. and Popkin, M.K. (1980). Stress response syndrome occurring after delirium. *Am. J. Psychiatry* **137**, 1433–5.

Macleod, A.D. and Whitehead, L.E. (1997). Dysgraphia in terminal delirium. *Pall. Med.* **11**, 127–32.

Maddocks, I., Somogyi, A., Abbott, F., *et al.* (1996). Attenuation of morphine-induced delirium in palliative care by substitution with infusion of oxycodone. *J. Pain Symptom Manag.* **12**, 182–9.

Madi, S. and Langonnet, F. (1988). Postoperative agitation. A new cause [French]. *Cahiers d'Anesthesiologie* **36**, 509–12.

Maes, M., Vanoolaeghe, E., Degroote, J., Altamura, C., and Roels, C. (2000). Linear CT-scan measurement in alcohol-dependent patients without delirium tremens. *Alcohol* **20**, 117–23.

Magliano, L., Guarneri, M., Fiorillo, A., Marasco, C., Malangone, C., and Maj, M. (2001). A multicenter Italian study of patients' relatives' beliefs about schizophrenia. *Psychiatr. Serv.* **52**, 1528–30.

Magoun, H.W. (1952). An ascending reticular activating system in the brainstem. *Arch. Neurol. Psychiatry* **67**, 145–54.

Maguire, P. (2000). Communication with terminally ill patients and their families. In *Handbook of psychiatry in palliative medicine* (ed. H.M. Chochinov and W. Breitbart), pp. 291–301. Oxford University Press, New York.

Main, J. (2000). Improving management of bereavement in general practice based on a survey of recently bereaved subjects in a single general practice. *Br. J. Gen. Pract.* **50**, 863–6.

Makker, R. and Yanny, W. (2000). Postoperative delirium mimicking epilepsy. *Anaesthesia* **55**, 74–8.

Maltoni, M., Nanni, O., and Pirovano, M. (1999). Successful validation of the palliative prognostic score in terminally ill cancer patients. *J. Pain Symptom Manag.* **17**, 240–7.

Manepalli, J., Grossberg, G.T., and Mueller, C. (1990). Prevalence of delirium and urinary tract infections in a psychogeriatric unit. *J. Geriatr. Psychiatry Neurol.* **3**, 198–202.

Mann, T. (1994). *Buddenbrooks: the decline of a family* (transl. J.E. Woods). Everyman's Library, Alfred A. Knopf, New York.

Manos, P. and Wu, R. (1997). The duration of delirium in medical and postoperative patients referred for psychiatric consultation. *Ann. Clin. Psychiatry* **9**, 219–26.

Manzoni, A. (1972, English translation). *I promessi sposi [The betrothed]*. Penguin Books, London.

Marcantonio, E., Ta, T., Duthie, E., and Resnick, N. (2002). Delirium severity and psychomotor types: their relationship with outcomes after hip fracture repair. *J. Am. Geriatr. Soc.* **50**, 850–7.

Marcantonio, E.R., Goldman, L., Mangione, C.M., Ludwig, L.E., Muraca, B., Haslauer, C.M., Donaldson, M.C., Whittemore, A.D., Sugarbaker, D.J., Poss, R., Haas, S., Cook, E.F., Orav, E.J., and Lee, T.H. (1994*a*). A clinical prediction rule for delirium after elective noncardiac surgery. *J. Am. Med. Assoc.* **271**, 134–9.

Marcantonio, E.R., Juarez, G., Goldman, L., Mangione, C.M., Ludwig, L.E., Lind, L., Katz, N., Cook, E.F., Orav, J., and Lee, T.H. (1994*b*). The relationship of postoperative delirium with psychoactive medication. *J. Am. Med. Assoc.* **272**, 1518–22.

Marcantonio, E.R., Goldman, L., Orav, E.J., Cook, E.F., and Lee, T.H. (1998). The association of intraoperative factors with the development of postoperative delirium. *Am. J. Med.* **105**, 380–4.

Marcantonio, E.R., Flacker, J.M., Michaels, M., and Resnick, N.M. (2000). Delirium is independently associated with poor functional recovery after hip fracture. *J. Am. Geriatr. Soc.* **48**, 618–24.

Marcantonio, E.R., Flacker, J.M., Wright, R.J., and Resnick, N.M. (2001). Reducing delirium after hip fracture: a randomized trial. *J. Am. Geriatr. Soc.* **49**, 678–9.

Marder, S.R.A. (1998). Antipsychotic mediciations. In *Textbook of psychopharmacology* (ed. A.F. Schatzberg and C.B. Nemeroff), pp. 309–21. American Psychiatric Press, Washington, DC.

Margolese, H.C. and Chouinard, G. (2000). Serotonin syndrome from addition of low-dose trazodone to nefazodone. *Am. J. Psychiatry* **157**, 1022.

Mark, B.Z., Kunkel, E.J., Fabi, M.B., and Thompson, T.L.N. (1993). Pimozide is effective in delirium secondary to hypercalcemia when other neuroleptics fail. *Psychosomatics* **34**, 446–50.

Massie, M.J., Holland, J.C., and Glass, E. (1983). Delirium in terminally ill cancer patients. *Am. J. Psychiatry* **140**, 1048–50.

Matsuoka, Y., Miyake, Y., Arakaki, H., Tanaka, K., Saeki, T., and Yamawaki, S. (2001). Clinical utility and validation of the Japanese version of the Memorial Delirium Assessment Scale in a psychogeriatric inpatient setting. *Gen. Hosp. Psychiatry* **23**, 36–40.

Matsushima, E., Nakajima, K., Moriya, H., Matsuura, M., Motomiya, T., and Kojima, T. (1997). A psychophysiological study of the development of delirium in coronary care units. *Biol. Psychiatry* **41**, 1211–17.

Mayer, S.A., Chong, J.Y., Ridgway, E., Min, K.C., Commichau, C., and Bernardini, G.L. (2001). Delirium from nicotine withdrawal in neuro-ICU patients. *Neurology* **57**, 551–3.

Mayo-Smith, M.F. (1997). Pharmacological management of alcohol withdrawal. A meta-analysis and evidence-based practice guideline. American Society of Addiction Medicine Working Group on Pharmacological Management of Alcohol Withdrawal. *J. Am. Med. Assoc.* **278**, 144–51.

McAllister-Williams, R. and Ferrier, I. (2002). Rapid tranquillisation: time for a reappraisal of options for parenteral therapy, *Br. J. Psychiatry* **180**, 485–9.

McClement, S.E. and Woodgate, R.L. (1998). Research with families in palliative care: conceptual and methodological challenges. *Eur. J. Cancer Care* **7**, 247–54.

McCowan, C. and Marik, P. (2000). Refractory delirium tremens treated with propofol: a case, *Crit. Care Med.* **28**, 1781–4.

McCusker, J., Cole, M., Bellavance, F., and Primeau, F. (1998). Reliability and validity of a new measure of severity of delirium. *Int. Psychogeriatr.* **10**, 421–33.

McCusker, J., Cole, M., Abrahamowicz, M., Han, L., Podoba, J., and Ramman-Haddad, L. (2001*a*). Environmental risk factors for delirium in hospitalized older people. *J. Am. Geriatr. Soc.* **49**, 1327–34.

McCusker, J., Cole, M.G., Dendukuri, N., Belzile, E., and Primeau, F. (2001*b*). Delirium in older medical inpatients and subsequent cognitive and functional status: a prospective study. *Can. Med. Assoc. J.* **165**, 575–83.

McCusker, J., Cole, M., Abrahamowicz, M., Primeau, F., and Belzile, E. (2002). Delirium predicts 12–month mortality. *Arch. Intern. Med.* **162**, 457–63.

McDermott, J.L., Gideonse, N., and Campbell, J.W. (1991). Acute delirium associated with ciprofloxacin administration in a hospitalized elderly patient. *J. Am. Geriatr. Soc.* **39**, 909–10.

Meagher, D. and Trzepacz, P. (1998). Delirium phenomenology illuminates pathophysiology, management, and course. *J. Geriatr. Psychiatry Neurol.* **11**, 150–6; [discussion} 157–8.

Meagher, D., O'Hanlon, D., O'Mahony, E., and Casey, P. (1996). The use of environmental strategies and psychotropic medication in the management of delirium. *Br. J. Psychiatry* **168**, 512–15.

Meagher, D., O'Hanlon, D., O'Mahony, E., Casey, P., and Trzepacz, P. (1998). Relationship between etiology and phenomenologic profile in delirium. *J. Geriatr. Psychiatry Neurol.* **11**, 146–9; [discussion] 157–8.

Meagher, D., O'Hanlon, D., O'Mahony, E., Casey, P., and Trzepacz, P. (2000). Relationship between symptoms and motoric subtype of delirium. *J. Neuropsychiatry Clin. Neurosci.* **12**, 51–6.

Meagher, D.J. (2001). Delirium: optimizing management. *Br. Med. J.* **322**, 144–9.

Menza, M.A., Murray, G.B., Holmes, V.F., and Rafuls, W.A. (1987). Decreased extrapyramidal symptoms with intravenous haloperidol. *J. Clin. Psychiatry* **48**, 278–80.

Mercadante, S. (1995). Dantrolene treatment of opioid-induced myoclonus. *Anesth. Analges.* **81**, 1307–8.

Mercadante, S. (1997). Alkalinization is troublesome in advanced cancer patients with dyspnea [letter]. *J. Pain Symptom Manag.* **13**, 316–17.

Mercadante, S. (1998). Pilocarpine as an adjuvant to morphine therapy. *Lancet* **351**, 338–9.

Mercadante, S., De Conno, F., and Ripamonti, C. (1995). Propofol in terminal care. *J. Pain Symptom Manag.* **10**, 639–42.

Mermelstein, H. (1998). Clarithromycin-induced delirium in a general hospital. *Psychosomatics* **39**, 540–2.

Mesulam, M.-M. (1985). Attention, confusional states, and neglect. In *Principles of behavioral neurology*, Vol. 26 (ed. M.-M. Mesulam), pp. 125–68. F.A. Davis, Philadelphia.

Mesulam, M.-M., Waxman, S.G., Geschwind, N., and Sabin, T.D. (1976). Acute confusional state with right cerebral artery infarction. *J. Neurol. Neurosurg. Psychiatry* **39**, 84–9.

Metitieri, T., Bianchetti, A., and Trabucchi, M. (2000). Delirium as a predictor of survival in older patients with cancer. *Arch. Intern. Med.* **160**, 2866–8.

Meyer, H.P., Legemate, D.A., van den Brom, W., and Rothuizen, J. (1998). Improvement of chronic hepatic encephalopathy in dogs by the benzodiazepine receptor partial inverse agonist sarmazenil but not by the antagonist flumazenil. *Metab. Brain Dis.* **13**, 241–51.

Middleton, W., Burnett, P., Raphael, B. and Martinek, N. (1996). The bereavement response: a cluster analysis. *Br. J. Psychiatry* **169**, 167–71.

Miklowitz, D.J. and Hooley, J.M. (1998). Developing family psychoeducational treatments for patients with bipolar and other severe psychiatric disorders. A pathway from basic research to clinical trials. *J. Marital Fam. Ther.* **24**, 419–35.

Milisen, K., Foreman, M.D., Abraham, I.L., De Geest, S., Godderis, J., Vandermeulen, E., Fischler, B., Delooz, H.H., Spiessens, B., and Broos, P.L. (2001). A nurse-led interdisciplinary intervention program for delirium in elderly hip-fracture patients. *J. Am. Geriatr. Soc.* **49**, 523–32.

Minagawa, H., Yosuke, U., Yamawaki, S., and Ishitani, K. (1996). Psychiatric morbidity in terminally ill cancer patients. *Cancer* **78**, 1131–7.

Miotto, K., Darakjian, J., Basch, J., Murray, S., Zogg, J., and Rawson, R. (2001). Gamma-hydroxybutyric acid: patterns of use, effects and withdrawal. *Am. J. Addict* **10**, 232–41.

Monette, J., Galbaud du Fort, G., Fung, S.H., Massoud, F., Moride, Y., Arsenault, L., and Afilalo, M. (2001). Evaluation of the confusion assessment method (CAM) as a screening tool for delirium in the emergency room. *Gen. Hosp. Psychiatry* **23**, 20–5.

Montale, E. (1996). *Diario postumo: 66 poesie e altre.* Arnoldo Mondadori, Milano.

Morita, T., Otani, H., Tsunoda, J., Inoue, S., and Chihara, S. (2000). Successful palliation of hypoactive delirium due to multiorgan failure by oral methylphenidate. *Support Care Cancer* **8**, 134–7.

Morita, T., Tei, Y., Tsunoda, J., Inoue, S., and Chihara, S. (2002). Increased plasma morphine metabolites in terminally ill cancer patients with delirium: an intra-individual comparison. *J. Pain Symptom Manag.* **23**, 107–13.

Morita, T., Tsunoda, J., Inoue, S., and Chihara, S. (1999). The palliative prognostic index: a scoring system for survival prediction of terminally ill cancer patients. *Support Care Cancer* **7**, 128–33.

Morita, T., Tsunoda, J., Inoue, S., Chihara, S. and Oka, K. (2001). Communication Capacity Scale and Agitation Distress Scale to measure the severity of delirium in terminally ill cancer patients: a validation study. *Palliat. Med.*, **15**, 197–206.

Morita, T., Tsuneto, S., and Shima, Y. (2001a). Proposed definitions for terminal sedation. *Lancet* **358**, 335–6.

Morrison, R.S., Siu, A.L., Leipzig, R.M., Cassel, C.K., and Meier, D.E. (2000). The hard task of improving the quality of care at the end of life. *Arch. Intern. Med.* **160**, 743–7.

Moruzzi, G. and Magoun, H.W. (1949). Brain stem reticular formation and activation of the EEG. *Electroencephalogr. Clin. Neurophysiol.* **1**, 455–73.

Moss, J.H. (1995). Anileridine-induced delirium. *J. Pain Symptom Manag.* **10**, 318–20.

Muller, N., Klages, U., and Gunther, W. (1994). Hepatic encephalopathy presenting as delirium and mania. The possible role of bilirubin. *Gen. Hosp. Psychiatry* **16**, 138–40.

Mussi, C., Ferrari, R., Ascari, S., and Salvioli, G. (1999). Importance of serum anticholinerigic activity in the assessment of elderly patients with delirium. *J. Geriatr. Psychiatry Neurol.* **12**, 82–6.

Nakamura, J., Yoshimura, R., Okuno, T., Ueda, N., Yoshimura, R., Eto, S., Terao, T., Nakamura, J., Hachida, M., Yasumoto, K., Egami, H., Maeda, H., Nishi, M., and Aoyagi, S. (2001). Association of plasma free-3–methoxy-4–hydroxyphenyl (ethylene)glycol, natural killer cell activity and delirium in postoperative patients. *Int. Clin. Psychopharmacol.* **16**, 339–43.

Neumärker, K.J. (2001). Karl Bonhoeffer and the concept of symptomatic psychoses. *Hist. Psychiatry* **12**, 213–26.

Newman, J.P., Terris, D.J., and Moore, M. (1995). Trends in the management of alcohol withdrawal syndrome. *Laryngoscope* **105**, 1–7.

Nicholas, L.M. and Lindsey, B.A. (1995). Delirium presenting with symptoms of depression. *Psychosomatics* **36**, 471–9.

Nickell, P.V. (1991). Histamine-2 receptor blockers and delirium. *Ann. Intern. Med.* **115**, 658.

Nieves, A.V. and Lang, A.E. (2002). Treatment of excessive daytime sleepiness in patients with Parkinson's disease with modafinil. *Clin. Neuropharmacol.* **25**, 111–14.

Nijboer, C., Tempelaar, R., Sanderman, R., Triemstra, M., Spruijt, R.J., and Van den Bos, G. (1998). Cancer and caregiving: the impact on the caregiver's health. *Psycho-Oncology* **7**, 3–13.

Normann, C., Brandt, C., Berger, M., and Walden, J. (1998). Delirium and persistent dyskinesia induced by a lithium–neuroleptic interaction. *Pharmacopsychiatry* **31**, 201–4.

Northouse, L.L. (1988). Family issues in cancer care. In *Psychiatric aspects of cancer* (ed. R.J. Goldberg), pp. 82–101. Karger, Basel.

Norton, J.W. (2001). Gabapentin withdrawal syndrome. *Clin. Neuropharmacol.* **24**, 245–6.

O'Dowd, M.A. and McKegney, F.P. (1990). AIDS patients compared with others seen in psychiatric consultation. *Gen. Hosp. Psychiatry* **12**, 50–5.

O'Keeffe, S.T. (1994). Rating the severity of delirium: the delirium assessment scale. *Int. J. Geriatr. Psychiatry* **9**, 551–6.

O'Keeffe, S.T. (1999). Clinical subtypes of delirium in the elderly. *Dement. Geriatr. Cogn. Disord.* **10**, 380–5.

O'Keeffe, S.T. and Chonchubhair, A. (1995). Postoperative delirium in the elderly. *Br. J. Anaesth.* **73**, 673–87.

O'Keeffe, S.T. and Devlin, J.G. (1994). Delirium and dexamethasone suppression test in the elderly. *Neuropsychobiology* **30**, 153–6.

O'Keeffe, S.T., Tormey, W.P., Glasgow, R., and Lavan, J.N. (1994). Thiamine deficiency in hospitalized elderly patients. *Gerontology* **40**, 18–24.

Olofson, S.M., Weitzener, M.A., Valentine, A.D., Baile, W.F., and Meyers, C.A. (1996). A retrospective study of the psychiatric management and outcome of delirium in the cancer patient. *Support Care Cancer* **4**, 351–7.

Osmon, D.C. (1984). Luria–Nebraska neuropsychological battery case study: a mild drug related confusional state. *Int. J. Clin. Neuropsychol.* **6**, .

Osse, B.H., Vernooij-Dassen, M.J., de Vree, B.P., Schade, E., and Grol, R.P. (2000). Assessment of the need for palliative care as perceived by individual cancer patients and their families: a review of instruments for improving patient participation in palliative care. *Cancer* **88**, 900–11.

Owens, M.J. and Riscj, S.C. (1998). Atypical antipsychotics. In *Textbook of psychopharmacology* (ed. A.F. Schatzberg and C.B. Nemeroff), pp. 323–48. American Psychiatric Press, Washington, DC.

Palmstierna, T. (2001). A model for predicting alcohol withdrawal delirium. *Psychiatr. Serv.* **52**, 820–3.

Papersack, T., Garbusinski, J., Robberecht, J., Beyer, I., Willems, D., and Fuss, M. (1999). Clinical relevance of thiamine status amongst hospitalized elderly patients. *Gerontology* **45**, 96–101.

Parkes, C.M. (1998*a*). Bereavement. In *Oxford textbook of palliative medicine*, 2nd edn (ed. D. Doyle, G.W.C. Hanks, and N. MacDonald), pp. 995–1010. Oxford University Press, New York.

Parkes, C.M. (1998*b*). *Bereavement: studies of grief in adult life*, 3rd edn. Pelican, Harmondsworth,.

Parkes, C.M. (1998*c*). Coping with loss—bereavement in adult life. *Br. Med. J.* **316**, 856–9.

Parkh, S.S. and Chung, F. (1995). Postoperative delirium in the elderly. *Anesth. Analges.* **80**, 1223–32.

Passik, S.D. and Cooper, M. (1999). Complicated delirium in a cancer patient successfully treated with olanzapine. *J. Pain Symptom Manag.* **17**, 219–23.

Patten, S.B., Williams, J.V., Haynes, L., Mc Cruden, J., and Arboleda-Flórez, J. (1997). The incidence of delirium in psychiatric inpatient units. *Can. J. Psychiatry* **42**, 858–63.

Payne, S. and Relf, M. (1990). The assessment of need for bereavement follow-up in palliative and hospice care. *Pall. Med.* **8**, 291.

Perry, E., Walker, M., Grace, J., and Perry, R. (1999). Acetylcholine in mind: a neurotransmitter correlate of consciousness. *Trends Neurosci.* **22**, 273–80.

Perry, N.K. (2000). Venlafaxine-induced serotonin syndrome with relapse following amytriptiline. *Postgrad. Med. J.* **76**, 254–6.

Peruselli, C., Paci, E., Franceschi, P., *et al.* (1997). Outcome evaluation in a home palliative care service. *J. Pain Symptom Manag.* **13**, 158–67.

Petterson, K. and Rottemberg, D.A. (1997). Radiation damage to the brain. In *Handbook of clinical neurology*, Vol. 23 (ed. C.J. Vecht), pp. 325–51. Elsevier, Amsterdam.

Pirovano, M., Maltoni, M., Nanni, O., Marinari, M., Indelli, M., Zaninetta, G., Petrella, V., Barni, S., Zecca, E., Scarpi, E., Labianca, R., Amadori, D., and Luporini, G. (1999). A new palliative prognostic score: a first step for the staging of terminally ill cancer patients. *J. Pain Symptom Manag.* **17**, 231–9.

Platt, M.M., Breitbart, W., Smith, M., Marotta, R., Weisman, H., and Jacobsen, P.B. (1994). Efficacy of neuroleptics in hypoactive delirium. *J. Neuropsychiatry Clin. Neurosci.* **6**, 66–7.

Plum, F. and Posner, J. (1980*a*). Psychogenic unresponsiveness. In *The diagnosis of stupor and coma*, pp. 305–12. F.A. Davis, Philadelphia.

Plum, F. and Posner, J.B. (1980*b*). *The diagnosis of stupor and coma*, Vol. 19. F.A. Davis, Philadelphia.

Pollio, D.E., North, C.S., Osborne, V., Kap, N., and Foster, D.A. (2001). The impact of psychiatric diagnosis and family system relationship on problems identified by families coping with a mentally ill member. *Fam. Process* **40**, 199–209.

Pompei, P., Foreman, M., Rudberg, M.A., Inouye, S.K., Braund, V., and Cassel, C.K. (1994). Delirium in hospitalized older persons: outcomes and predictors. *J. Am. Geriatr. Soc.* **42**, 809–15.

Pompei, P., Foreman, M., Cassel, C., Alessi, C., and Cox, D. (1995). Detecting delirium among hospitalized older patients. *Arch. Intern. Med.* **155**, 301–7.

Portenoy, R.K. (2000). Physical symptom management in the terminally ill. In *Handbook of psychiatry in palliative medicine* (ed. H.M. Chochinov and W. Breitbart), pp. 99–129. Oxford University Press, New York.

Posner, J.B. (1995). *Neurologic complications of cancer*, Vol. 45. F.A. Davis, Philadelphia.

Posner, J. and Plum, F. (1967). Spinal-fluid pH and neurologic symptoms in systemic acidosis. *New Engl. J. Med.* **277**, 605–15.

Posner, J., Swanson, A.G.. and Plum, F. (1965). Acid–base balance in cerebrospinal fluid. *Arch. Neurol.* **12**, 479–96.

Potter, J.M., Reid, D.B., Shaw, R.P., Hackett, P., and Hickman, P.E. (1989). Myoclonus associated with treatment with high doses of morphine: the role of supplemental drugs. *Br. Med. J.* **299**, 150–3.

Pourcher, E., Filteau, M., Bouchard, R.H., and Baruch, P. (1994). Efficacy of the combination of buspirone and carbamazepine in early post-traumatic delirium. *Am. J. Psychiatry* **151**, 150–1.

Prigerson, H., Frank, E., Kasl, S., Reynolds, C.r., Anderson, B., Zubenko, G., Houck, P., George, C., and Kupfer, D. (1995). Complicated grief and bereavement-related depression as distinct disorders: preliminary empirical validation in elderly bereaved spouses. *Am. J. Psychiatry* **152**, 22–30.

Prigerson, H.G., Bierhals, A.J., Kasl, S.V., Reynolds, C.F.r., Shear, M.K., Newsom, J.T., and Jacobs, S. (1996). Complicated grief as a disorder distinct from bereavement-related depression and anxiety: a replication study. *Am. J. Psychiatry* **153**, 1484–6.

Prigerson, H.G., Bierhals, A.J., Kasl, S.V., Reynolds, C.F.R., Shear, M.K., Day, N., Beery, L.C., Newsom, J.T., and Jacobs, S. (1997). Traumatic grief as a risk factor for mental and physical morbidity. *Am. J. Psychiatry* **154**, 616–23.

Prigerson, H.G., Shear, M.K., Jacobs, S.C., Reynolds, C.F.R., Maciejewski, P.K., Davidson, J.R., Rosenheck, R., Pilkonis, P.A., Wortman, C.B., Williams, J.B., Widiger, T.A., Frank, E., Kupfer, D.J., and Zisook, S. (1999). Consensus criteria for traumatic grief. A preliminary empirical test. *Br. J. Psychiatry* **174**, 67–73.

Quill, T.E., Byock, I.R., and for the ACP–ASIM end of life consensus panel (2000). Responding to intractable terminal suffering. the role of terminal sedation and voluntary refusal of food and fluids. *Ann. Intern. Med.* **132**, 408–14.

Rabins, P.V. (1991). Psychosocial and management aspects of delirium. *Int. Psychogeriatr.* **3**, 319–24.

Rabow, M.W., Hardie, G., Fair, J.M., and McPhee, S.J. (2000). End of life care content in 50 textbooks from multiple specialties. *J. Am. Med. Assoc.* **283**, 771–8.

Rahakonen, T., Luukkainen-Markkulla, R., Paanila, S., Sivenius, S., and Sulkava, R. (2000). Delirium episode as a sign of undetected dementia among community dwelling elderly subjects: a 2 year follow-up study. *J. Neurol. Neurosurg. Psychiatry* **69**, 519–21.

Ramirez, A., Addington-Hall, J., and Richards, M. (1998). ABC of palliative care: the carers. *Br. Med. J.* **316**, 208–11.

Rammonah, K.W., Rosenberg, J., Lynn, D.J., Blumenfeld, A.M., and Pollak Nagaraja, H.N. (2002). Efficacy and safety of modafinil (Provigil) for the treatment of fatigue in multple sclerosis: a two centre phase 2 study. *J. Neurol. Neurosurg. Psychiatry* **72**, 179–83.

Rando, T.A. (1988). Anticipatory grief: the term is a misnomer but the phenomenon exists. *J. Pall. Care* **4**, 70–3.

Rao, V. and Lyketsos, C. (2000). The benefits and risks of ECT for patients with primary dementia who also suffer from depression. *Int. J. Geriatr. Psychiatry* **15**, 729–35.

Ravona-Springer, R., Dolberg, O.T., Hirschmann, S., and Grunhaus, L. (1998). Delirium in elderly patients treated with risperidone: a report of three cases. *J. Clin. Psycopharmacol.* **18**, 171–2.

Resnick, M. and Burton, B.T. (1984). Droperidol vs haloperidol in the initial management of acutely agitated patients. *J. Clin. Psychiatry* **45**, 298–9.

Richtie, J., Steiner, W., and Abramowicz, M. (1996). Incidence and risk factors for delirium among psychiatric inpatients. *Psychiatr. Serv.* **47**, 727–30.

Riker, R.R., Fraser, G.L., and Cox, P.M. (1994). Continuous infusion of haloperidol controls agitation in critically ill patients, *Crit. Care Med.* **22**, 433–40.

Rinck, G.C., van den Bos, A.M., Kleijnen, J., de Haes, H.J.C.J.M., Schade, E., and Veenhof, C.H.N. (1997). Methodologic issues in effectiveness research on palliative cancer care: a systematic review. *J. Clin. Oncol.* **15**, 1697–707.

Ripamonti, C. and Bruera, E. (1997). CNS adverse effects of opioids in cancer patients. Guidelines for treatment. *CNS Drugs* **8**, 21–37.

Ripamonti, C., Filiberti, A., Totis, A., De Conno, F., and Tamburini, M. (1999). Suicide among patients with cancer cared for at home by palliative-care teams. *Lancet* **354**, 1877–8.

Robbins, T.W. and Everitt, B.J. (1995). Arousal systems and attention. In *The cognitive neuroscience* (ed. M. Gazzaniga), pp. 703–20. MIT Press, Cambridge, Massachusetts.

Robertsson, B. (1999). Assessment scales in delirium. *Dement. Geriatr. Cogn. Dis.* **10**, 368–79.

Robertsson, B., Karlsson, I., Styrud, E., and Gottfries, C. (1997). Confusional State Evaluation (CSE): an instrument for measuring severity of delirium in the elderly. *Br. J. Psychiatry* **170**, 565–70.

Robertsson, B., Blennow, K., Gottfries, C., and Wallin, A. (1998). Delirium in dementia. *Int. J. Geriatr. Psychiatry* **13**, 49–56.

Robertsson, B., Olsson, L., and Wallin, A. (1999). Occurrence of delirium in different regional brain syndromes. *Dement. Geriatr. Cogn. Disord.* **10**, 278–83.

Robertsson, B., Blennow, K., Brane, G., Edman, A., Karlsson, I., Wallin, A., and Gottfries, C. (2001). Hyperactivity of the hypothalamic-pituitary-adrenal axis in demented patients with delirium. *Int. J. Clin. Psychopharmacol.* **16**, 39–47.

Robinson, L. and Stacy, R. (1994). Palliative care in the community: setting practice guidelines for primary care teams. *Br. J. Gen. Pract.* **44**, 461–4.

Robinson, L.A., Nuamh, I.F., Lev, E., and McCorkle, R. (1995). A prospective longitudinal investigation of spousal bereavement examining Parkes and Weiss' Bereavement Risk Index. *J. Pall. Care* **11**, 5–13.

Rockwood, K. (1999). Educational interventions in delirium. *Dement. Geriatr. Cogn. Dis.* **10**, 426–9.

Rockwood, K., Cosway, S., Stolee, P., Kydd, D., Carver, D., Jarret, P., and O'Brien, B. (1994). Increasing recognition of delirium in elderly patients. *J. Am. Geriatr. Soc.* **42**, 252–6.

Rockwood, K., Goodman, J., Flynn, M., and Stolee, P. (1996). Cross-validation of the delirium rating scale in older patients. *J. Am. Geriatr. Soc.* **44**, 839–42.

Rolfson, D.B., McElhaney, J.E., Rockwood, K., Finnegan, B.A., Entwistle, L.M., Wong, J.F., and Suarez-Almazor, M.E. (1999). Incidence and risk factors for delirium and other adverse outcomes in older adults after coronary artery bypass graft surgery. *Can. J. Cardiol.* **15**, 771–6.

Rolland, J.S. (1994). *Families, illness, and disability. An integrative model.* Basic Books, New York.

Rosebush, P.I., Margetts, P., and Mazurek, M.F. (1999). Serotonin syndrome as a result of clomipramine monotherapy, *J. Clin. Pharmacol.* **19**, 285–7.

Rosen, J., Sweet, R., Mulsant, B., Rifai, A.H., Pasternak, R., and Zubenko, G. (1994). The delirium rating scale in psychogeriatric inpatient setting. *J. Neuropsychiatry Clin. Neurosci.* **6**, 30–5.

Rosenbraugh, C.J., Flockart, D.A., Yasuda, S.U., and Woosley, R.L. (2001). Visual hallucination and tremor induced by sertraline and oxycodone in a bone marrow transplant recipient. *J. Clin. Pharmacol.* **41**, 224–7.

Rosenfeld, M. and Dalmau, J. (2001). The clinical spectrum and pathogenesis of paraneoplastic disorders of the central nervous system. *Hematol. Oncol. Clin. N. Am.* **15**, 1109–28.

Ross, C.A. (1991). Etiological models and their phenomenological variants. CNS arousal systems: possible role in delirium. *Int. Psychogeriatr.* **3**, 353–71.

Ross, C.A., Peyser, C.E., Shapiro, I., and Folstein, M.F. (1991). Delirium: phenomenologic and etiologic subtypes. *Int. Psychogeriatr.* **3**, 135–47.

Roth-Romer, S., Fann, J., and Syrjala, K. (1997). The importance of recognizing and measuring delirium. *J. Pain Symptom Manag.* **13**, 125–7.

Rothschild, A.J. (1995). Delirium: an SSRI–benztropine adverse effect? *J. Clin. Psychiatry* **56**, 492–5.

Sales, E., Shulz, R. and Biegel, D. (1992). Predictors of strain in families of cancer patients: a review of the literature. *J. Psychosoc. Oncol.* **10**, 1–26.

Salkind, A.R. (2000). Acute delirium induced by intravenous trimethoprim–sulfamethoxazole therapy in a patient with acquired immunodeficiency syndrome. *Hum. Exp. Tox.* **19**, 149–51.

Sandberg, O., Gustafson, Y., Brännström, B., and Bucht, G. (1999). Clinical profile of delirium in older patients. *J. Am. Geriatr. Soc.* **47**, 315–18.

Sandberg, O., Franklin, K., Bucht, G., and Gustafson, Y. (2001). Sleep apnea, delirium, depressed mood, cognition, and ADL ability after stroke. *J. Am. Geriatr. Soc.* **49**, 391–7.

Sasajima, Y., Sasajima, T., Uchida, H., Kawai, S., Haga, M., Akasaka, N., Kusakabe, M., Inaba, M., Goh, K., and Yamamoto, H. (2000). Postoperative delirium in patients with lower limb ischemia: what are the specific markers? *Eur. J. Vasc. Endovasc. Surg.* **20**, 132–7.

Saunderson, E.M. and Ridsdale, L. (1999). General practitioners' beliefs and attitudes about how to respond to death and bereavement: a qualitative study. *Br. Med. J.* **319**, 293–6.

Scammell, T.E., Estabrooke, I.V., McCarthy, M.T., Chemelli, R.M., Yanagishawa, M., Miller, M.S., and Saper, C.B. (2000). Hypothalamic arousal regions are activated during modafinil induced wakefulness. *J. Neurosci.* **20**, 8620–8.

Schachter, S. (1992). Quality of life for families in the management of home care patients with advanced cancer. *J. Pall. Care* **8**, 61–6.

Schachter, S.R. and Coyle, N. (1998). Palliative home care. Impact on families. In *Psycho-Oncology* (ed. J. Holland), pp. 1004–15. Oxford University Press, New York.

Schaefer, C., Queensbury, C.P., and Wi, S. (1995). Mortality following conjugal bereavement and the effects of shared environment. *Am. J. Epidemiol.* **141**, 1142–51.

Schor, J.D., Levkoff, S.E., Lipsitz, L.A., Reilly, C.H., Cleary, P.D., Rowe, J.W., and Evans, D.A. (1992). Risk factors for delirium in hospitalized elderly. *J. Am. Med. Assoc.* **267**, 827–31.

Schumacher, L., Pruitt, J.N., and Phillips, M. (2000). Identifying patients 'at risk' for alcohol withdrawal syndrome: a treatment protocol. *J. Neurosci. Nurs.* **32**, 158–63.

Schwab, R.A. and Bachhuber, B.H. (1991). Delirium and lactic acidosis caused by ethanol and niacin coingestion. *Am. J. Emerg. Med.* **9**, 363–5.

Schwartz, T.L. and Masand, P. (2000). Treatment of delirium with quetiapine. *J. Clin. Psychiatry Prim. Care Companion* **2**, 10–12.

Scott, J.C. and Stanski, D.R. (1987). Decreased fentanyl and alfentanil dose requirements with age. A simultaneous pharmacokinetic and pharmacodynamic evaluation. *J. Pharmacol. Clin. Ther.* **240**, 159–66.

Scott, J.C., Cooke, J.E., and Stanski, D.R. (1991). Electroencephalographic quantitation of opioid effect: comparative pharmacodynamics of fentanyl and sufentanil. *Anesthesiology* **74**, 34–42.

Sellal, F. and Collard, M. (2001). Sindrome confusionale. In *Encyclopédie médico-chirugicale*, Vol. 17–044–C-30, Editions Scientifiques et Médicales. Elsevier SAS, Paris.

Seltzer, B. and Mesulam, M. (1990). Confusional states and delirium as a disorder of attention. In *Handbook of neuropsychology*, Vol. 1 (ed. F. Boller and J. Grafman), pp. 165–74. Elsevier, Amsterdam.

Serdaru, M., Hausser-Hauw, C., Laplane, D., Buge, A., Castaigne, P., Goulon, M., Lhermitte, F., and Hauw, J. (1988). The clinical spectrum of alcoholic pellagra encephalopathy: a retrospective analysis of 22 cases studied pathologically. *Brain* **111**, 829–42.

Settle, E.C. and Ayd, F.J. (1983). Haloperidol: a quarter century of experience. *J. Clin. Psychiatry* **44**, 440–8.

Shapiro, B.A., Warren, J., Egol, A.B., Greenbaum, D.M., Jacobi, J., Nasraway, S.A., Schein, R.M., Spevetz, A., and Stone, J.R. (1995). Practice parameters for intravenous analgesia and sedation for adult patients in the intensive care unit: an executive summary. Society of Critical Care Medicine [see comments]. *Crit. Care Med.* **23**, 1596–600.

Sharma, N.D., Rosman, H.S., Padhi, I.D., and Tisdale, J.E. (1998). Torsades de pointes associated with intravenous haloperidol in critically ill patients. *Am. J. Cardiol.* **81**, 238–40.

Sheldon, F. (1998). ABC of palliative care: bereavement. *Br. Med. J.* **316**, 456–8.

Shelly, M.P., Sultan, M.A., Bodenham, A., and Park, G.R. (1991). Midazolam infusions in critically ill patients. *Eur. J. Anaesthesiol.* **8**, 21–7.

Siegel, K., Ravis, V.H., Houts, P., and Mor, V. (1991). Caregiver burden and unmet patient needs. *Cancer* **68**, 1131–40.

Silber, M.H. and Rye, D.B. (2001). Solving the mystery of narcolepsy. The hypocretin story. *Neurology* **56**, 1616–18.

Silverman, G.K., Jacobs, S.C., Kasl, S.V., Shear, M.K., Maciejewski, P.K., Noaghiul, F.S., and Prigerson, H.G. (2000). Quality of life impairments associated with diagnostic criteria for traumatic grief. *Psychol. Med.* **30**, 857–62.

Simon, L., Jewell, N. and Brokel, J. (1997). Management of acute delirium in hospitalised elderly: a process of improvement project. *J. Geriatr. Nurs.* **18**, 150–4.

Sipahimalani, A. and Masand, P. (1997). Use of risperidone in delirium: case reports. *Ann. Clin. Psychiatry* **9**, 105–7.

Sipahimalani, A. and Masand, P. (1998). Olanzapine in the treatment of delirium. *Psychosomatics* **39**, 422–30.

Sivilotti, M.L., Burns, M.J., Aaron, C.K., and Greenberg, M.J. (2001). Pentobarbital for severe gamma-butyrolactone withdrawal. *Ann. Emerg. Med.* **38**, 660–5.

Sjogren, P. and Banning, A. (1989). Pain sedation and reaction time during long-term treatment of cancer patients with oral and epidural opioids. *Pain* **39**, 5–11.

Sjogren, P., Dragsted, L., and Christensen, C.B. (1993a). Myoclonic spasms during treatment with high doses of intravenous morphine in renal failure. *Acta Anaesthesiol. Scand.* **37**, 780–2.

Sjogren, P., Jonsson, T., Jensen, N.H., Drenck, N.E., and Jensen, T.S. (1993b). Hyperalgesia and myoclonus in terminal cancer patients treated with continuous intravenous morphine. *Pain* **55**, 93–7.

Sjogren, P., Jensen, N.-H., and Jensen, T.S. (1994). Disappearance of morphine induced hyperalgesia after discontinuing or substituting morphine with other opioid agonists. *Pain* **59**, 313–16.

Sjogren, P., Thunedborg, L.P., Christrup, L., Hansen, S.H., and Franks, J. (1998). Is development of hyperalgesia, allodynia and myoclonus related to morphine metabolism during long-term administration? *Acta Anaesthesiol. Scand.* **42**, 1070–5.

Sjogren, P., Olsen, A.K., Thomsen, A.B., and Dalberg, J. (2000). Neuropsychological performance in cancer patients: the role of oral opioids, pain and performance status. *Pain* **86**, 237–45.

Skinner Cook, A. and Dworkin, D.S. (1992). *Helping the bereaved. Therapeutic interventions for children, adolescents, and adults.* Basic Books, New York.

Slatkin, N.E., Rhiner, M. and Bolton, T.M. (2001). Donezepil in the treatment of opiate induced sedation. *J. Pain Symptom Manag.* **21**, 425–38.

Smith, D.L. and Wenegrat, B.G. (2000). A case report of serotonin syndrome associated with combined nefazodone and fluoxetine. *J. Clin. Psychiatry* **61**, 146.

Smith, M.J., Breitbart, W.S., and Platt, M.M. (1994). A critique of instruments and methods to detect, diagnose, and rate delirium. *J. Pain Symptom Manag.* **10**, 35–77.

Snyder, S., Reyner, A., Schmeidler, J., Bogursky, E., Gomez, H., and Strain, J.J. (1992). Prevalence of mental disorders in newly admitted medical inpatients with AIDS. *Psychosomatics* **33**, 166–70.

Spinetta, J.J. (1984). Measurement of family function, communication and cultural effect. *Cancer* **53**, 2330–7.

Spunberg, J.J., Chang, C.H., Goldman, M., Auricchio, E., and Bell, J.J. (1981). Quality of long-term survival following irradiation for intracranial tumors in children under the age of two. *Int. J. Rad. Oncol. Biol. Phys.* **7**, 727–36.

Stahl, S.M. (2000). *Essentials of psychopharmacology.* Cambridge University Press, Cambridge.

Stanford, B.J. and Stanford, S.C. (1999). Postoperative delirium indicating an adverse drug interaction involving the selective serotonin reuptake inhibitor, paroxetine? *J. Psychopharmacol.* **13**, 313–(1999)17.

Stanilla, J.K., de Leon, J., and Simpson, G.M. (1997). Clozapine withdrawal resulting in delirium with psychosis: a report of three cases. *J. Clin. Psychiatry* **58**, 252–5.

Stefano, G.B., Bilfinger, T.V., and Fricchione, G.L. (1994). The immune neuro-link and the macrophage: postcardiotomy delirium, HIV associated dementia and psychiatry. *Prog. Neurobiol.* **42**, 475–88.

Steg, R.E. and Garcia, E.G. (1991). Complex visual hallucinations and cyclosporine neurotoxicity. *Neurology* **41**, 1156.

Steinberg, R.B., Gilman, D.E., and Johnson, F.I. (1992). Acute toxic delirium in a patient using transdermal fentanyl. *Anesth. Analges.* **75**, 1014–16.

Steinmetz, D., Walsh, M., Gabel, L.L., and Williams, P.T. (1993). Family physicians' involvement with dying patients and thier families. Attitudes, difficulties and strategies. *Arch. Fam. Med.* **2**, 753–61.

Sternbach, H. (1991). The serotonin syndrome. *Am. J. Psychiatry* **148**, 705–13.

Stiefel, F. and Bruera, E. (1991). Psychostimulants for hypoactive–hypoalert delirium? *J. Pall. Care* **7**, 25–6.

Stiefel, F. and Morant, R. (1991). Morphine intoxication during acute reversible renal insufficiency. *J. Pall. Care* **7**, 45–7.

Stiefel, F., Fainsinger, R., and Bruera, E. (1992). Acute confusional states in patients with advanced cancer. *J. Pain Symptom Manag.* **7**, 94–8.

Stiefel, F.C., Breitbart, W.S., and Holland, J.C. (1989). Corticosteroids in cancer: neuropsychiatric complications. *Cancer Invest.* **7**, 479–91.

Stoudemire, A., Anfinson, T. and Edwards, J. (1996). Corticosteroid-induced delirium and dependency. *Gen. Hosp. Psychiatry* **18**, 196–202.

Stroebe, M.S. and Stroebe, W. (1993). The mortality of bereavement. In *Handbook of bereavement: theory, research, and intervention* (ed. M.S. Stroebe, W. Stroebe, and R.O. Hansson), pp. 175–95. Cambridge University Press, New York.

Stroebe, M.S., van Son, M., Stroebe, W., Kleber, R., Schut, H., and van den Bout, J. (2000). On the classification and diagnosis of pathological grief. *Clin. Psychol. Rev.* **20**, 57–75.

Strouse, T.B., El-Saden, S., Bonds, C., Ayars, N., and Busuttil, W. (1998). Immunosuppressant neurotoxicity in liver transplant recipients. *Psychosomatics* **39**, 124–33.

Suc, E., Kalifa, C., Brauner, R., Hambrand, J.L., Terrier-Lacombe, M.J., Vassal, G., and Lemerle, J. (1990). Brain tumors under the age of three: the price of survival. A retrospective study of 20 long-term survivors. *Acta Neurochir.* **106**, 93–8.

Sweeting, H.N. and Gilhooly, M.L. (1990). Anticipatory grief: a review. *Soc. Sci. Med.* **30**, 1073–80.

Szeto, H.H., Inturrisi, C.E., Houde, R., Saal, R., Cheigh, J., and Reidengerg, M.M. (1977). Accumulation of normeperidine, an active metabolite of meperidine, in patients with renal failure or cancer. *Ann. Intern. Med.* **86**, 738–4l.

Szymanski, S., Jody, D., Leipzig, R., Masiar, S., and Lieberman, J. (1991). Anticholinergic delirium caused by retreatment with clozapine. *Am. J. Psychiatry* **148**, 1752.

Tavcar, R. and Dernovsek, M.Z. (1998). Risperidone-induced delirium. *Can. J. Psychiatry* **43**, 194.

Tejera, C.A., Saravay, S.M., Goldman, E., and Gluck, L. (1994). Diphenhydramine-induced delirium on elderly hospitalized patients with mild dementia. *Psychosomatics* **35**, 399–402.

Teseo, P.J., Thaler, H.T., Lapin, J., Inturrisi, C.E., Portenoy, R.K., and Foley, K.M. (1995). Morphine-6–glucuronide concentrations and opioid-related side effects: a survey in cancer patients. *Pain* **61**, 46–54.

Thomas, H., Schwartz, E., and Petrilli, R. (1992). Droperidol versus haloperidol for chemical restraint of agitated and combative patients. *Ann. Emerg. Med.* **21**, 407–13.

Tombaugh, T.N. and McIntyre, N.J. (1992). The mini-mental state examination: a comprehensive review. *J. Am. Ger. Soc.* **40**, 922–35.

Torres, R., Mittal, D. and Kennedy, R. (2001). Use of quetiapine in delirium. Case reports. *Psychosomatics* **42**, 347–9.

Towne, A.R., Waterhouse, E.J., Boggs, J.G., Garnett, L.K., Brown, A.J., Smith, J.R.J., and De Lorenzo, R.J. (2000). Prevalence of non-convulsive status epilepticus in comatose patients. *Neurology* **54**, 340–5.

Trachman, S.B., Begun, D.L., and Kirch, D.G. (1991). Delirium in a patient with meningeal carcinomatosis. *Psychosomatics* **32**, 455–7.

Treloar, A. and Macdonald, A. (1997*a*). Outcome of delirium: part 1. Outcome of delirium diagnosed by DSM-III-R, ICD-10 and CAMDEX and derivation of the Reversible Cognitive Dysfunction Scale among acute geriatric inpatients. *Int. J. Geriatr. Psychiatry* **12**, 609–13.

Treloar, A. and Macdonald, A. (1997*b*). Outcome of delirium: part 2. Clinical features of reversible cognitive dysfunction—are they the same as accepted definitions of delirium?. *Int. J. Geriatr. Psychiatry* **12**, 614–18.

Trill, M.D. and Holland, J. (1993). Cross-cultural differences in the care of patients with cancer. A review. *Gen. Hosp. Psychiatry* **15**, 21–30.

Trzepacz, P.T., Teague, G.B., Lipowski, Z.J. (1985). Delirium and other organic mental disorders in a general hospital. *Gen. Hosp. Psychiatry* **7**, 101.

Trzepacz, P. and Dew, M.A. (1995). Further analysis of the delirium rating scale. *Gen. Hosp. Psychiatry* **17**, 75–9.

Trzepacz, P., Ho, V., and Mallavarapu, H. (1996). Cholinergic delirium and neurotoxicity associated with tacrine for Alzheimer's dementia. *Psychosomatics* **37**, 299–301.

Trzepacz, P., Mulsant, B., Amanda, D.M., Pasternak, R., Sweet, R., and Zubenko, G. (1998). Is delirium different when it occurs in dementia? A study using the delirium rating scale. *J. Neuropsychiatry Clin. Neurosci.* **10**, 199–204.

Trzepacz, P.T. (1994a). The neuropathogenesis of delirium. A need to focus our research. *Psychosomatics* **35**, 374–91.

Trzepacz, P.T. (1994b). A review of delirium assessment instruments. *Gen. Hosp. Psychiatry* **16**, 397–495.

Trzepacz, P.T. (1999). Update on the neuropathogenesis of delirium. *Dement. Geriatr. Cogn. Disord.* **10**, 330–4.

Trzepacz, P.T. and DiMartini, A. (1992). Survival of 247 liver transplant candidates. Relationship to pretransplant psychiatric variables and presence of delirium. *Gen. Hosp. Psychiatry* **14**, 380–6.

Trzepacz, P.T., Baker, R.W., and Greenhouse, J. (1988a). A symptom rating scale for delirium. *Psychiatry Res.* **23**, 89–97.

Trzepacz, P.T., Brenner, R.P., Coffman, G.C., and van Thiel, D.H. (1988b). Delirium in liver transplantation candidates: discriminant analysis of multiple test variables. *Biol. Psychiatry* **24**, 3–15.

Trzepacz, P.T., Brenner, R., and Van Thiel, D.H. (1989a). A psychiatric study of 247 liver transplantation candidates. *Psychosomatics* **30**, 147–53.

Trzepacz, P.T., Sclabassi, R.J., and Van Thiel, D.H. (1989b). Delirium a subcortical phenomenon? *J. Neuropsychiatry* **1**, 283–90.

Trzepacz, P.T., DiMartini, A., and Tringall, R.D. (1993). Psychopharmacologic issues in organ transplantation. *Psychosomatics* **34**, 290–8.

Trzepacz, P.T., Tarter, R., Shah, A., *et al.* (1994). SPECT scan and cognitive findings in subclinical hepatic encephalopathy. *J. Neuropsychiatry Clin. Neurosci.* **6**, 170–5.

Trzepacz, P.T., Mittal, D., Torres, R., Kanary, K., Norton, J., and Jimerson, N. (2001). Validation of the delirium rating scale-revised-98: comparison with the delirium rating scale and the cognitive test for delirium. *J. Neuropsychiatry Clin. Neurosci.* **13**, 229–42.

Tucker, G.J. (1999). The diagnosis of delirium and DSM-IV. *Dement. Geriatr. Cogn. Disord.* **10**, 359–63.

Tuma, R. and DeAngelis, L.M. (2000). Altered mental status in patients with cancer. *Arch. Neurol.* **57**, 1727–31.

Tune, L., Carr, S., Hoag, E., and Cooper, T. (1992). Anticholinergic effects of drugs commonly prescribed for the elderly: potential means for assessing risk of delirium. *Am. J. Psychiatry* **149**, 1393–4.

Tune, L., Carr, S., Cooper, T., Klug, B., and Golinger, R.C. (1993). Association of anticholinergic activity of prescribed medications with postoperative delirium. *J. Neuropsychiatry Clin. Neurosci.* **5**, 208–10.

Twycross, R. (1992). Corticosteroids in advanced cancer [editorial; comment]. *Br. Med. J.* **305**, 969–70.

Twycross, R. and Lichter, I. (1998). The terminal phase. In *Oxford textbook of palliative medicine*, 2nd edn (ed. D. Doyle, G.W.C. Hanks, and N. MacDonald), pp. 977–92. Oxford University Press, New York.

Tyler, H.R. (1968). Neurologic disorders in renal failure. *Am. J. Med.* **44**, 734–48.

Uchiyama, M., Tanaka, K.K.I., and Toru, M. (1996). Efficacy of mianserin for symptoms of delirium in the aged: an open trial study. *Prog. Neuropsychopharmacol. Biol. Psychiatry* **20**, 651–6.

Uldall, K.K. and Berghuis, J.P. (1997). Delirium in AIDS patients: recognition and medication factors. *AIDS Pat. Care STDS* **11**, 435–41.

Uldall, K.K., Harris, V.L., and Lalonde, B. (2000*a*). Outcomes associated with delirium in acutely hospitalized acquired immune deficiency syndrome patients. *Comprehens. Psychiatry* **41**, 88–91.

Uldall, K.K., Ryan, R., Berghuis, J.P., and Harris, V.L. (2000*b*). Association between delirium and death in AIDS patients. *AIDS Pat. Care STDS* **14**, 95–100.

Unseld, E., Ziegle, G., Gemeinhardt, A., Janssen, V., and Klotz, U. (1990). Possible interaction of fluoquinolones with the benzodiazepine–GABA-receptor complex. *Br. J. Clin. Pharmacol.* **30**, 63–70.

Vachon, M.L.S. (1998). The emotional problems of the patient. In *Oxford textbook of palliative medicine*, 2nd edn (ed. D. Doyle, G.W.C. Hanks, and N. MacDonald), pp. 883–907. Oxford University Press, New York.

van der Mast, R.C. (1999). Postoperative delirium. *Dement. Geriatr. Cogn. Dis.* **10**, 401–5.

van der Mast, R.C. and Fekkes, D. (2000). Serotonin and aminoacids: partners in delirium. *Sem. Clin. Neuropsychiatry* **5**, 125–31.

van der Mast, R.C. and Roest, F.H.J. (1996). Delirium after cardiac surgery: a review of the literature. *J. Psychosom. Res.* **41**, 109–13.

van der Mast, R.C., Fekkes, D., Moleman, P., and Pepplinkhizen, L. (1991). Is postoperative delirium related to reduced plasma tryptophan? *Lancet* **338**, 851–2.

van der Mast, R.C., van den Broek, W.W., Fekkes, D., Pepplinkhuizen, L., and Habbema, J.D.F. (1999). Incidence of and preoperative predictors for delirium after cardiac surgery. *J. Psychosom. Res.* **46**, 479–83.

van der Mast, R.C., van den Broek, W.W., Fekkes, D., Pepplinkhuizen, L., and Habbema, J.D. (2000). Is delirium after cardiac surgery related to plasma amino-acids and physical conditions? *J. Neuropsychiatry Clin. Neurosci.* **12**, 57–63.

van der Molen-Eijgenraam, M., Blanken-Meijs, J.T., Heeringa, M., and van Grootheest, A.C. (2001). Delirium due to increase in clozapine level during an inflammatory reaction [in Dutch]. *Ned. Tijdschr. Geneesk.* **145**, 427–30.

Van Deurzen-Smith, E. (1997). *Everyday mysteries.* Routledge, London.

van Hemert, A.M., van der Mast, R.C., Hengeveld, M.W., and Vorstenbosch, M. (1994). Excess mortality in general hospital patients with delirium: a 5–year follow-up of 519 patients seen in psychiatric consultation. *J. Psychosom. Res.* **38**, 339–46.

van Leeuwen, A., Molders, J., Sterkmans, P., Mielants, P., Martens, C., Toussaint, C., Hovent, A., Desseilles, M., Koch, H., Devroye, A., and Parent, M. (1977). Droperidol in acutely agitated patients. A double-blind placebo-controlled study. *J. Nerv. Ment. Dis.* **164**, 280–3.

Van Praag, H., Falcon, M., Guendelman, D., and Frenk, H. (1993). The development of analgesic, pro- and anticonvulsant opiate effect in the rat. *Ann. Istituto Sup. Sanita* **29**, 419–29.

van Steijn, J., Nieboer, P., Hospers, G., de Vries, E., and Mulder, N. (2001). Delirium after interleukin-2 and alpha-interferon therapy for renal cell carcinoma. *Anticancer Res.* **21**, 3699–700.

Vasconcelos, M., Silva, K., Vidal, G., Silva, A., Domingues, R., and Berditchevsky, C. (1999). Early diagnosis of pediatric Wernicke's encephalopathy. *Ped. Neurol.* **20**, 289–94.

Ventafridda, V., Ripamonti, C., De Conno, F., Tamburini, M., and Cassileth, B.R. (1990*a*). Symptom prevalence and control during cancer patients' last days of life. *J. Pall. Care* **6**, 7–11.

Ventafridda, V., Spoldi, E., and De Conno, F. (1990*b*). Control of dyspnea in advanced cancer patients [letter]. *Chest* **98**, 1544–5.

Venturini, I., Corsi, L., Avallone, R., Farina, F., Bedogni, G., Baraldi, C., Baraldi, M., and Zeneroli, M.L. (2001). Ammonia and endogenous benzodiazepine-like compounds in the pathogenesis of hepatic encephalopathy. *Scand. J. Gastroenterol.* **36**, 423–35.

Vidal, S., Andrianjatovo, J.J., Dubau, B., Winnok, S., and Maurette, P. (2001). Encephalopathies postoperatoires: la carence en thiamine, une étiologie a ne pas meconnaitre. *Ann. Fr. Anesth. Reanim.* **20**, 40–3.

Viganò, A., Dorgan, M., Buckingham, J., Bruera, E., and Suarez-Almazor, M.E. (2001). Survival prediction in terminal cancer patients: a systematic review of the literature. *Pall. Med.* **14**, 363–74.

Vitiello, M.V., Bliwise, D.L., and Prinz, P.N. (1992). Sleep in Alzheimer's disease and the sundown syndrome. *Neurology* **46**, 83–93.

Voltz, R. (2002). Paraneoplastic neurological syndromes: an update on diagnosis, pathogenesis and therapy. *Lancet Neurology* **1**, 294–305.

Voltz, R., Gultekin, H., Rosenfeld, M.R., Gerstner, E., Eichen, J., Posner, J., and Dalmau, J. (1999). A serologic marker of paraneoplastic limbic and brain-stem encephalitis in patients with testicular cancer. *New Engl. J. Med.* **340**, 1788–95.

Wada, Y. and Yamaguchi, N. (1993). Delirium in the elderly: relationship of clinical symptoms to outcome. *Dementia* **4**, 113–16.

Wallesch, C.W. and Hundsaltz, A. (1994). Language function in delirium: a comparison of single word processing in acute confusional state and probable Alzheimer's disease. *Brain Lang.* **46**, 592–606.

Wasserstrom, W.R., Glass, J.P., and Posner, J.B. (1982). Diagnosis and treatment of leptomeningeal metastasis from solid tumors: experience with 90 patients. *Cancer* **49**, 759–72.

Webster, R. and Holroyd, S. (2000). Prevalence of psychotic symptoms in delirium. *Psychosomatics* **41**, 519–22.

Weed, H.G., Lutman, C.V., Young, D.C., and Schuller, D.E. (1995). Preoperative identification of patients at risk for delirium after major head and neck cancer surgery. *Laryngoscope* **105**, 1066–8.

Weiner, A.L. (1999). Meperidine as a potential cause of serotonin syndrome in the emergency department. *Acad. Emerg. Med.* **6**, 156–8.

Weitzener, M.A., Olofson, S.M., and Forman, A.D. (1995). Patients with malignant meningitis presenting with neuropsychiatric manifestations. *Cancer* **76**, 1804–8.

Welborn, L.G., Hannallah, R.S., Norden, J.M., Ruttimann, U.E., and Callan, C.M. (1996). Comparison of emergence and recovery characteristics of sevoflurane, desflurane, and halothane in pediatric ambulatory patients. *Anesth. Analges.* **83**, 917–20.

Welch-McCaffery, D. (1988). Family issues in cancer care: current dilemmas and future directions. *J. Psychosoc. Oncol.* **6**, 199–211.

Wellisch, D.K. (2000). Family issues in palliative care. In *Handbook of psychiatry in palliative medicine* (ed. H.M. Chochinov and W. Breitbart), pp. 275–89. Oxford University Press, New York.

Wellisch, D.K., Wolcott, D.L., Pasnau, R.O., Fawzy, F.I., and Landsverk, J. (1989). An evaluation of the psychosocial problems of the homebound cancer patient: relationship of patient adjustment to family problems. *J. Psychosoc. Oncol.* **7**, 55–76.

Wengel, S., Roccaforte, W., and Burke, W. (1998). Donepezil improves symptoms of delirium in dementia: implications for future research., *J. Geriatr. Psychiatry Neurol.* **11**, 159–61.

Wengs, W.J., Talwar, D., and Bernard, J. (1993). Ifosfamide-induced nonconvulsive status epilepticus. *Arch. Neurol.* **50**, 1104–5.

Werz, M.A. and MacDonald, R.L. (1982). Opiate alkaloids antagonize postsynaptic glycine and GABA responses: correlation with convulsant action. *Brain Res.* **236**, 107–19.

Whyte, J. (1992). Neurologic disorder of attention and arousal: assessment and treatment. *Arch. Phys. Med. Rehabil.* 1094–103.

Wilkins-Ho, M. and Hollander, Y. (1997). Toxic delirium with low-dose clozapine. *Can. J. Psychiatry* **42**, 429–30.

Williams, J.B.W. (1999). Psychiatric classification. In *Textbook of psychiatry* (ed. R.E. Hales, S.C. Yudofsky, and J.A. Talbott), pp. 227–52. American Psychiatric Press, Washington, DC.

Williams-Russo, P., Urquhart, B.L., Sharrock, N.E., and Charlson, M.E. (1992). Postoperative delirium: predictors and prognosis in elderly orthopedics patients. *J. Am. Geriatr. Soc.* **40**, 759–67.

Wilt, J.L., Minnema, A.M., Johnson, R.F., and Rosenblum, A.M. (1993). Torsade de pointes associated with the use of intravenous haloperidol. *Ann. Intern. Med.* **119**, 391–4.

Winawer, N. (2001). Postoperative delirium. *Med. Clin. N. Am.* **85**, 1229–39.

Wise, M.G. and Trzepacz, P.T. (1996). Delirium (confusional states). In *Textbook of consultation–liaison psychiatry* (ed. J.R. Rundell and M.G. Wise), pp. 259–74. American Psychiatric Press, Washington, DC.

Wise, M.G., Gray, K.F., and Seltzer, B. (1999). Delirium, dementia and amnestic disorders. In *Textbook of psychiatry* (ed. R.E. Hales, S.C. Yudofsky, and J.A. Talbott), pp. 317–62. American Psychiatric Press, Washington, DC.

Wojnar, M., Bizon, Z., and Wasilewski, D. (1999). The role of somatic disorders and physical injury in the development and course of alcohol withdrawal delirium. *Alcohol Clin. Exp. Res.* **23**, 209–13.

Wolf, H.G. and Curran, D. (1935). Nature of delirium and allied states. The dysergastic reaction. *Arch. Neurol. Psychiatry* **33**, 1175–215.

Woof, W.R. and Carter, Y.H. (1997*a*). The grieving adult and the general practitioner: a literature review in two parts (part 1). *Br. J. Gen. Pract.* **47**, 443–8.

Woof, W.R. and Carter, Y.H. (1997*b*). The grieving adult and the general practitioner: a literature review in two parts (part 2). *Br. J. Gen. Pract.* **47**, 509–14.

Worden, J.W. (1991). *Grief counseling and grief therapy.* A handbook for the mental health practitioner. Springer, New York.

World Health Organization (1992). *The ICD-10 classification of mental and behavioral disorders: clinical descriptions and diagnostic guidelines.* WHO Publications, Geneva.

World Health Organization (1993). *The ICD-10 classification of mental and behavioral disorders: diagnostic criteria for research.* World Health Organization, Geneva,.

World Health Organization (1996). *Diagnostic and management guidelines for mental disorders in primary care. ICD-10.* Chapter V, Primary Care Version. Hogrefe and Huber, Gottingen.

World Health Organization (2001). *International classification of functioning and disability* (ICDH-2), full draft version, World Health Organization, Geneva.

Yaksh, T.L., Harty, G.J., and Onofrio, B.M. (1986). High doses of spinal morphine produce a nonopiate receptor mediated hyperesthesia: clinical and theoretic implications. *Anesthesiology* **64**, 590–7.

Yancik, R. (1984*a*). Coping with hospice work stress. *J. Psychosoc. Oncol.* **2**, 19–35.

Yancik, R. (1984*b*). Source of work stress for hospice staff. *J. Psychosoc. Oncol.* **2**, 21–31.

Young, G.B. (1998). Major syndromes of impaired consciousness. In *Coma and impaired consciousness. A clinical perspective* (ed. G.B. Young, A.H. Ropper, and C.F. Bolton), pp. 39–78. McGraw-Hill, New York.

Young, G.B., Leung, L.S., Campbell, V., DeMelo, J., Schieven, J., and Tilsworth, R. (1992). The electroencephalogram in metabolic/toxic coma. *Am. J. Electroencephalogr. Technol.* **32**, 243–59.

Young, G.B., McLachlan, R.S., Kreeft, J.H., and DeMelo, J. (1997). An electroencephalographic classification system for coma. *Can. J. Neurol. Sci.* **24**, 320–5.

Yue, M., Faisinger, R.L., and Bruera, E. (1994). Cognitive impairment in a patient with a normal mini-mental state examination (MMSE). *J. Pain Symptom Manag.* **9**, 51–3.

Zacny, J.P. (1995). A review of the effects of opioids on psychomotor and cognitive functioning in humans. *Exp. Clin. Psychopharmacol.* **3**, 432–66.

Zalsman, G., Hermesh, H., and Munitz, H. (1998). Alprazolam withdrawal delirium: a case report. *Clin. Neuropharmacol.* **21**, 201–2.

Zarate, C.A., Baldessarini, R.J., Siegel, A.J., Nakamura, A., McDonald, J., Muir-Hutchinson, L.A., Cherkerzian, T., and Tohen, M. (1997). Risperidone in the elderly: a pharmacoepidemiologic study. *J. Clin. Psychiatry* **58**, 311–17.

Zeimer, H. (2000). Paraneoplastic limbic encephalitis should not be overlooked as a possible cause of delirium in cancer patients. *Arch. Intern. Med.* **160**, 2866.

Zeitlin, S.V. (2001). Grief and bereavement. *J. Pall. Care* **28**, 415–25.

Zeman, A. (2001). Consciousness. *Brain* **124**, 1263–89.

Ziske, C.G., Schottker, B., Gorschuler, M., Mey, U., Kleinschmidt, R., Schlegel, U., Sauerbruck, T., and Schmidt-Wolf, G.H. (2002). Acute transient encephalopathy after paclitaxel infusion. Report of three cases. *Ann. Oncol.* **13**, 629–31.

Zisook, S. (2000). Understanding and managing bereavement in palliative care. In *Handbook of psychiatry in palliative medicine* (ed. H.M. Chochinov and W. Breitbart), pp. 321–4. Oxford University Press, New York.

Zou, Y., Cole, M., Primeau, F., McCusker, J., Bellavance, F., and Laplante, J. (1998). Detection and diagnosis of delirium in the elderly: psychiatrist diagnosis, confusion assessment method, or consensus diagnosis? *Int. Psychogeriatr.* **10**, 303–8.

Appendix 1

Mini-Mental State Examination (MMSE) (Folstein *et al.* 1975)

	Score	Maximum score
What is the year, season, date, day, month?	( )	5
Where are we: state (region), country, town, hospital, floor?	( )	5
Name three objects; then ask the patient all 3 after you have said them.	( )	3
Give one point for each correct answer.		
Serial 7s subtracting from 100 for 5 consecutive times	( )	5
(93, 86, 79, 72, 65). One point for each correct answer.		
Ask patient to repeat the three objects named before.	( )	3
Ask patient to name a pencil and a watch.	( )	2
Ask patient to repeat the following: 'No ifs, ands, or buts.'	( )	1
Ask patient to follow a three-stage command: 'Take a paper in your right hand. Fold it and put it on the floor.'	( )	3
Ask patient to read and obey the following command: 'Close your eyes.'	( )	1
Ask patient to write a sentence.	( )	1
Ask patient to copy designs (two pentagons overlapping over two sides).	( )	1
Total	( )	30
Assess consciousness level along a visual analogue:		

Hypervigilant	Alert	Drowsy	Stupor	Coma

Appendix 2

The Confusion Assessment Method (CAM)

This CAM instrument is reprinted with permission from Inouye *et al.* (1990, table 1), Copyright 1990, American Medical Association.

The CAM instrument

Acute onset

1.   Is there evidence of an acute change in mental status from the patient's baseline?

Inattention

The questions listed under this topic were repeated for each topic where applicable.

2 (a).   Did the patient have difficulty focusing attention, for example, being easily distractable, or having difficulty keeping track of what was being said?

Not present any time during interview.

Present at some time during interview, but in mild form.

Present at some time during interview, in marked form.

Uncertain.

2 (b).   (If present or abnormal) Did this behaviour fluctuate during the interview, that is, tend to come and go or increase and decrease in severity?

Yes.

No.

Uncertain.

Not applicable.

2 (c).   (If present or abnormal) Please describe this behaviour.

Disorganized thinking

3.   Was the patient's thinking disorganized or incoherent, such as rambling or irrelevant conversation, unclear or illogical flow of ideas, or unpredictable switching from subject to subject?

Altered level of consciousness

4.   Overall, how would you rate this patient's level of consciousness?

Alert (normal).

Vigilant (hyperalert, overly sensitive to environmental stimuli, startled very easily).

Lethargic (drowsy, easily aroused).

Stupor (difficult to arouse).

Coma (unarousable).

Uncertain.

Disorientation

5.   Was the patient disoriented at any time during the interview, such as thinking that he or she was somewhere other than the hospital, using the wrong bed, or misjudging the time of day?

Memory impairment

6.   Did the patient demonstrate any memory problems during the interview, such as inability to remember events in the hospital or difficulty remembering instructions?

Perceptual disturbances

7.   Did the patient have any evidence of perceptual disturbances, for example, hallucinations, illusions, or misinterpretations (such as thinking something was moving when it was not)?

Psychomotor agitation

8.   (Part 1) At any time during the interview, did the patient have an unusually increased level of motor activity, such as restlessness, picking at bedclothes, tapping finger, or making frequent sudden changes of position?

Psychomotor retardation

8.   (Part 2) At any time during the interview, did the patient have an unusually decreased level of motor activity, such as sluggishness, staring into space, staying in one position for a long time, or moving very slowly?

Altered sleep–wake cycle

9.   Did the patient have evidence of disturbance of the sleep–wake cycle, such as excessive daytime sleepiness with insomnia at night?

The Confusion Assessment Method (CAM) diagnostic algorithm

The diagnosis of delirium by CAM requires the presence of features 1 and 2 and either of features 3 or 4.

Feature 1   Acute onset and fluctuating course

This feature is usually obtained from a family member or nurse and is shown by positive responses to the following questions. Is there evidence of an acute change in mental status from the patient's baseline? Did the (abnormal) behaviour fluctuate during the day, that is, tend to come and go or increase and decrease in severity?

Feature 2   Inattention

This feature is shown by a positive response to the following question. Did the patient have difficulty focusing attention, for example, being easily distractable or having difficulty keeping track of what was being said?

Feature 3   Disorganized thinking

This feature is shown by a positive response to the following question. Was the patient's thinking disorganized or incoherent, such as rambling or irrelevant conversation, unclear or illogical flow of ideas, or unpredictable switching from subject to subject?

Feature 4   Altered level of consciousness

This feature is shown by any answer other than 'alert' to the following question. Overall, how would you rate this patient's level of consciousness? Possible answers are: alert (normal); vigilant (hyperalert); lethargic (drowsy, easily aroused); stupor (difficult to arouse); or coma (unarousable).

Appendix 3

The Confusion Assessment Method for the intensive care unit (CAM–ICU)

The following is reprinted with permission from Ely *et al.* (2001a); copyrighted 2001, American Medical Association. Features are scored as absent or present on the basis of the following assessment. See also Ely *et al.* (2001b) for more details.

Features and descriptions

I   Acute onset or fluctuating course

    A   Is there evidence of an acute change in mental status from baseline?

    B   Or, did the (abnormal) behaviour fluctuate during the past 24 hours, that is, tend to come and go or increase and decrease in severity as evidenced by fluctuations on the Richmond Agitation Sedation Scale (RASS)* or the Glasgow Coma Scale?

II   Inattention[†]

Did the patient have difficulty focusing attention as evidenced by a score of fewer than 8 correct answers on either the visual or auditory components of the Attention Screening Examination (ASE)?

III   Disorganized thinking

Is there evidence of disorganized or incoherent thinking as evidenced by incorrect answers to 3 or more of the 4 questions and inability to follow the commands?

Questions

    1   Will a stone float on water?

    2   Are there fish in the sea?

    3   Does 1 pound weigh more than 2 pounds?

    4   Can you use a hammer to pound a nail?

Commands

    1   Are you having unclear thinking?

    2   Hold up this many fingers. (Examiner holds 2 fingers in front of the patient.)

    3   Now do the same thing with the other hand (without holding the 2 fingers in front of the patient).

(If the patient is already extubated from the ventilator, determine whether the patient's thinking is disorganized or incoherent, such as rambling or irrelevant conversation, unclear or illogical flow of ideas, or unpredictable switching from subject to subject.)

IV Altered level of consciousness

Is the patient's level of consciousness anything other than alert, such as being vigilant or lethargic or in a stupor, or coma?

Alert   *Spontaneously fully aware of environment and interacts appropriately.*

Vigilant   Hyperalert.

Lethargic   Drowsy but easily aroused; unaware of some elements in the environment or not spontaneously interacting with the interviewer; becomes fully aware and appropriately interactive when prodded minimally.

Stupor   Difficult to arouse; unaware of some all elements in the environment or not spontaneously interacting with the interviewer; becomes incompletely aware when prodded strongly; can be aroused only by vigorous and repeated stimuli and, as soon as the stimulus ceases, stuporous subject lapses back into unresponsive state.

Coma   Unarousable; unaware of all elements in the environment with no spontaneous interaction or awareness of the interviewer so that the interview is impossible even with maximal prodding.

Overall CAM-ICU assessment (features 1 and 2 and either feature 3 or 4)   Yes __   No __

---

* The score included 10–point RASS range from a high of 4 (combative) to a low of –5 (comatose and unresponsive). Under the RASS system, patients who were spontaneously alert, calm, and not agitated were scored at 0 (neutral zone). Anxious or agitated patients received a range of scores depending on their level of anxiety: 1, anxious; 2, agitated (fighting ventilator); 3, very agitated (pulling on or removing catheters); 4, combative (violent and dangerous to staff). The scores –1 to –5 were assigned to patients with varying degrees of sedation based on their ability to maintain eye contact for: –1, more than 10 seconds; –2, less than 10 seconds; –3, eye opening but no eye contact. If physical stimulation was required, the patient were scored as either –4 for eye opening or movements with physical or painful stimulation or –5 for no response to physical or painful stimulation,. The RASS has excellent interrater reaibility and intraclass correlation coefficients of 0.95 and 0.97, respectively, and has been validated against a visual analogue scale and geropsychiatric diagnoses in 2 intensive care unit studies.

† In completing the visual ASE, the patients were shown 5 simple pictures (previously published) (Ely *et al.* 2001b) at 3 second intervals and asked to remember them. They were then immediately shown 10 subsequent pictures and asked to nod 'yes' or 'no' to indicate whether they had just seen each of the pictures. Since 5 pictures had been shown to them already, for which the correct response was to nod 'yes' and 5 others were new, for which the correct response was to shake their heads 'no', patients scored perfectly if they achieved 10 correct responses. Scoring accounted for either errors of omission (indicating 'no' for a previously shown picture) or for errors of commission (indicating 'yes' for a picture not previously shown). In completing the auditory ASE, patients were asked to squeeze the rater's hand whenever they heard the letter A during the recitation of a series of 10 letters. The rater then read 10 letters from the following list in a normal tone at a rate of 1 letter per second: S, A, H, E, V, A, A, R, A, T. A scoring method similar to that of the visual ASE was used for the auditory ASE testing.

Appendix 4

The Delirium Rating Scale (DRS)

The following is reprinted from Trzepacz *et al.* (1988*a*), copyright 1988, with permission from Elsevier Science.

Item 1   Temporal onset of symptoms

This item addresses the time course over which symptoms appear. The maximum rating is for the most abrupt onset of symptoms—a common pattern of delirium. Dementia is usually more gradual in onset (Lipowski 1982). Other psychiatric disorders, such as affective disorders, might be scored with 1 or 2 points on this item. Sometimes delirium can be chronic (e.g. in geriatric nursing home patients), and, unfortunately, only 1 or 2 points would be assessed in that situation.

0   Gradual-onset change from longstanding behaviour, essentially a chronic or chronic–recurrent disorder

1   Gradual onset of symptoms, occurring within a 6-month period

2   Acute change in behaviour or personality occurring over a month

3   Abrupt change in behaviour, usually occurring over a 1- to 3-day period

Item 2   Perceptual disturbances

This item rates most highly the extreme inability to perceive differences between internal and external reality, while intermittent misperceptions such as illusions are given 2 points. Depersonalization and derealization can be seen in other organic mental disorders and thus are given only 1 point.

0   None evident by history or observation

1   Feelings of depersonalization or derealization

2   Visual illusions or misperceptions including macropsia, micropsia, e.g. may urinate in wastebasket or mistake bedclothes for something else

3   Evidence that the patient is markedly confused about external reality, e.g. not discriminating between dreams and reality

Item 3   Hallucination type

The presence of any type of hallucination is rated. Auditory hallucinations alone are rated with less weight because of their common occurrence in primary psychiatric disorders. Visual hallucinations are generally associated with organic mental syndromes, although not exclusively, and are given 2 points. Tactile hallucinations are classically described in delirium, particularly due to anticholinergic toxicity, and are given the most points.

0   Hallucinations not present

1   Auditory hallucinations only

2   Visual hallucinations present by patient's history or inferred by observation, with or without auditory hallucinations

3   Tactile, olfactory, or gustatory hallucinations present with or without auditory hallucinations

Item 4   Delusions

Delusions can be present in many different psychiatric disorders, but tend to be better organized and more fixed in non-delirious disorders and thus are given less weight. Chronic fixed delusions are probably most prevalent in schizophrenic disorders. New delusions may indicate affective and schizophrenic disorders, dementia, or substance intoxication but should also alert the clinician to possible delirium and are given 2 points. Poorly formed delusions, often of a paranoid nature, are typical of delirium. (Lipowski 1980).

0   Not present

1   Delusions are systematized, i.e. well-organized and persistent

2   Delusions are new and not part of a pre-existing primary psychiatric disorder

3   Delusions are not well circumscribed; are transient, poorly organized, and mostly in response to misperceived environmental cues, e.g. are paranoid and involve persons who are in reality care-givers, loved ones, hospital staff, etc.

Item 5   Psychomotor behaviour

This item describes degrees of severity of altered psychomotor behaviour. Maximum points can be given for severe agitation or severe withdrawal to reflect either the hyperactive or hypoactive variant of delirium (Lipowski 1980).

0   Not present

1   Mild restlessness, tremulousness, or anxiety evident by observation and a change from patient's usual behaviour

2   Moderate agitation with pacing, removing intravenous tubes, etc.

3   Severe agitation, needs to be restrained, may be combative; or has significant withdrawal from the environment, but not due to major depression or schizophrenic catatonia

Item 6   Cognitive status during formal testing

Information from the cognitive portion of a routine mental status examination is needed to rate this item. The maximum rating of 4 points is given for severe cognitive deficits while only 1 point is given for mild inattention which could be attributed to pain and fatigue seen in medically ill persons. Two points are given for a relatively isolated cognitive deficit, such as memory impairment, which could be due to dementia or organic amnestic syndrome as well as to early delirium.

0 No cognitive deficits, or deficits that can be alternatively explained by lack of education or mental retardation

1 Very mild cognitive deficits that might be attributed to inattention due to acute pain, fatigue, depression, or anxiety associated with having a medical illness

2 Cognitive deficit largely in one major area tested, e.g. memory, but otherwise intact

3 Significant cognitive deficits that are diffuse, i.e. affecting many different areas tested. They must include periods of disorientation to time or place at least once in each 24-h period. Registration and/or recall are abnormal; concentration is reduced

4 Severe cognitive deficits, including motor or verbal perseverations, confabulations, disorientation to person, remote and recent memory deficits, and inability to cooperate with formal mental tests

Item 7   Physical disorder

Maximum points are given when a specific lesion or physiological disturbance can be temporally associated with the altered behaviour. Dementias are often not found to have a specific underlying medical cause, while delirium usually has at least one identifiable physical cause (Trzepacz et al. 1985).

1 None present or active

2 Presence of any physical disorder that might affect mental state

3 Specific drug, infection, metabolic, central nervous system lesion, or other medical problem that can be temporally implicated in causing the altered behaviour or mental status

Item 8   Sleep–wake cycle disturbance

Disruption of the sleep–wake cycle is typical in delirium, with the demented person generally having significant sleep disturbance much later in their course (Lipowski 1982). Severe delirium is on a continuum with stupor and coma, and persons with a resolving coma are likely to be delirious temporarily.

0 Not present; awake and alert during the day, and sleep without significant disruption at night

1 Occasional drowsiness during the day and mild sleep continuity disturbance at night; may have nightmares but can readily distinguish them from reality

2 Frequent napping and unable to sleep at night, constituting a significant disruption of or a reversal of the usual sleep–wake cycle

3 Drowsiness prominent, difficulty staying alert during the interview, loss of self-control over alertness and somnolence

4 Drifts into stuporous or comatose periods

Item 9   Lability of mood

Rapid shifts in mood can occur in various organic mental syndromes, perhaps due to a disinhibition of one's normal control. The patient may be aware of this lack of emotional control and may behave inappropriately relative to the situation or to his/her thinking state, e. g. crying for no apparent reason. A delirious patient may score points on any of these items depending upon the severity of the delirium and upon how their underlying psychological state 'colours' their delirious presentation. Patients with borderline personality disorder might score 1 or 2 points on this item.

0   Not present; mood stable

1   Affect/mood somewhat altered and changes over the course of hours; patient states that mood changes are not under self-control

2   Significant mood changes that are inappropriate to situation, including fear, anger, or tearfulness; rapid shifts of emotion, even over several minutes

3   Severe disihibition of emotions, including temper outbursts, uncontrolled inappropriate laughter, or crying

Item 10   Variability of symptoms

The hallmark of delirium is waxing and waning of symptoms, which is given 4 points on this item. Demented as well as delirious patients, who become more confused at night when environmental cues are decreased, could score 2 points.

0   Symptoms stable and mostly present during daytime

1   Symptoms worsen at night

2   Fluctuating intensity of symptoms, such that they wax and wane during 24-hr period

Total score _____

Appendix 5

Delirium Rating Scale, revised 1998 (DRS-R-98)

This is a revision of the Delirium Rating Scale (Trzepacz *et al.* 1998*a*; see Appendix 4). It is used for initial assessment and repeated measurements of delirium symptom severity. The sum of the scores of the 13 items provides a severity score. In all available ratings of delirium severity, reasonable time frames should be chosen between ratings to document meaningful changes because delirium symptom severity can fluctuate without interventions.

The DRS-R-98 severity scale

1 Sleep–wake cycle disturbance

Rate the sleep–wake pattern using all sources of information, including family, care-givers, nurses' reports, and patient. Try to distinguish sleep from resting with eyes closed.

0 Not present

1 Mild sleep continuity disturbance at night or occasional drowsiness during the day

2 Moderate disorganization of sleep–wake cycle (e.g. falling asleep during conversations, napping during the day, or several brief awakenings during the night with confusion/behavioural changes, or very little night-time sleep)

3 Severe disruption of sleep–wake cycle (e.g. day–night reversal of sleep–wake cycle or severe circadian fragmentations with multiple periods of sleep and wakefulness or severe sleeplessness)

2 Perceptual disturbances and hallucinations

Illusions and hallucinations can be of any sensory modality. Misperceptions are 'simple' if they are uncomplicated, such as a sound, noise, colour, spot, or flash and 'complex' if they are multidimensional, such as voices, music, people, animals, or scenes. Rate if reported by patient or care-giver, or inferred by observation.

0   Not present

1   Mild perceptual disturbances (e.g. feelings of derealization or depersonalization; or patient may not be able to discriminate dreams from reality)

2   Illusions present

3   Hallucinations present

3   Delusions

Delusions can be of any type, but are most often persecutory. Rate if reported by patient, family, or care-givers. Rate as delusional if ideas are unlikely to be true yet are believed by the patient who cannot be dissuaded by logic. Delusional ideas cannot be explained by the patient's cultural or religious background.

0   Not present

1   Mildly suspicious, hypervigilant, or preoccupied

2   Unusual or overvalued ideation that does not reach delusional proportions or could be plausible

3   Delusional

4   Lability of affect

Rate the patient's affect as the outward presentation of emotion and not as a description of what the patient feels.

0   Not present

1   Affect somewhat altered or incongruent to situation; changes over the course of hours; emotions are mostly under self-control

2   Affect is often inappropriate or incongruent to situation; changes over the course of minutes; emotions are not consistently under self-control, though they respond to redirection by others

3   Severe and consistent disinhibition of emotions; affect changes rapidly, is inappropriate to context, and does not respond to redirection by others

5   Language

Rate abnormalities of spoken, written, or sign language that cannot be otherwise attributed to dialect or stuttering. Assess fluency, grammar, comprehension, semantic content, and naming. Test comprehension and naming non-verbally, if necessary, by having patient follow commands or point.

0   Normal language

1   Mild impairment including word-finding or problems with naming or fluency

2   Moderate impairment including comprehension difficulties or deficit in meaningful communication (semantic content)

3   Severe impairment including nonsensical semantic content, word salad, muteness, or severely reduced comprehension

6 Thought process abnormalities

Rate abnormalities of thinking processes based on verbal or written output. If a patient does not speak or write, do not rate this item.

0 Normal thought process

1 Tangential or circumstantial

2 Associations loosely connected occasionally, but largely comprehensible

3 Associations loosely connected most of the time

7 Motor agitation

Rate by observation, including observation by others such as visitors, family, and clinical staff. Do not include dyskinesia, tics, or chorea.

0 No restlessness or agitation

1 Mild restlessness of gross motor movements or mild fidgeting

2 Moderate motor agitation including dramatic movements of the extremities, pacing, fidgeting, removing intravenous lines, etc.

3 Severe motor agitation, such as combativeness or a need for restraint or seclusion

8 Motor retardation

Rate movements by direct observation or using other sources such as family, visitors, and clinical staff. Do not rate components of retardation that are caused by parkinsonian symptoms. Do not rate drowsiness or sleep.

0 No slowness of voluntary movements

1 Mildly reduced frequency, spontaneity, or speed of motor movements, to a degree that may interfere somewhat with the assessment

2 Moderately reduced frequency, spontaneity, or speed of motor movements, to the extent that it interferes with participation in activities of self-care

3 Severe motor retardation with few spontaneous movements

9 Orientation

For patients who cannot speak there can be a visual or auditory presentation of multiple-choice answers. Allow patient to be wrong by up to 7 days instead of 2 days for patients hospitalized more than 3 weeks. Disorientation to person means not recognizing familiar persons and may be intact even if the person has naming difficulty but recognizes the person. Disorientation to person is most severe when one doesn't know one's own identity and is rare. Disorientation to person usually occurs after disorientation to time and/or place.

0 Oriented to person, place, and time

1 Disoriented to time (e.g. by more 2 days or wrong month or wrong year) or to place (e.g. name of building, city, state), but not both

2 Disoriented to time and place

3 Disoriented to person

10   Attention

Patients with sensory deficits or who are intubated or whose hand movements are constrained should be tested using an alternative modality to writing. Attention can be assessed during the interview (e.g. verbal perseverations, distractability, and difficulty with set shifting) and/or through use of specific tests, e.g. digit span.

0   Alert and attentive

1   Mildly distractable or mild difficulty sustaining attention, but able to refocus with cueing. On formal testing makes only minor errors and is not significantly slow in responses

2   Moderate inattention with difficulty focusing and sustaining attention. On formal testing, makes numerous errors and requires prodding to focus or finish the task

3   Severe difficulty focusing and/or sustaining attention with many incorrect or incomplete responses or inability to follow instructions. Distractable by other noises or events in the environment

11   Short-term memory

Defined as recall of information (e.g. 3 items presented either verbally or visually) after a delay of about 2 to 3 minutes. When formally tested, information must be registered adequately before recall is tested. The number of trials to register as well as the effect of cueing can be noted on scoresheet. Patient should not be allowed to rehearse during the delay period and should be distracted during this time. Patient may speak or nonverbally communicate to the examiner the identity of the correct items. Short-term deficits noticed during the course of the interview can be used also.

0   Short-term memory intact

1   Recalls 2/3 items; may be able to recall third item after category cueing

2   Recalls 1/3 items; may be able to recall other item after category cueing

3   Recalls 0/3 items

12   Long-term memory

Can be assessed formally through interviewing for recall of past personal (e.g. past medical history or experiences that can be corroborated from another source) or general information that is culturally relevant. When formally tested, use a verbal and/or visual modality for 3 items that are adequately registered and recalled after at least 5 minutes. The patient should be not allowed to rehearse during the delay period during formal testing. Make allowances for patients with less than 8 years of education or who are mentally retarded regarding general information question. Rating of the severity of deficits may involve a judgement about all the ways in which long-term memory is assessed, including recent and/or remote long-term memory ability informally tested during the interview as well as any formal testing of recent long-term memory using 3 items.

0   No significant long-term memory deficits

1 Recalls 2/3 items and/or has minor difficulty recalling details of other long-term information

2 Recalls 1/3 items and/or has moderate difficulty recalling other long-term information

3 Recalls 0/3 items and/or has severe difficulty recalling other long-term information

13 Visuospatial ability

Assess informally and formally. Consider patient's difficulty navigating one's way around living areas or environment (e. g. getting lost). Test formally by drawing or copying a design, by arranging puzzle pieces, or by drawing a map and identifying major cities, etc. Take into account any visual impairments that may affect performance.

0 No impairment

1 Mild impairment such that overall design and most details or pieces are correct; and/or little difficulty navigating in his/her surroundings

2 Moderate impairment with distorted appreciation of overall design and/or several errors of details or pieces, and/or needing repeated redirection to keep from getting lost in a newer environment; trouble locating familiar object in immediate environment

3 Severe impairment on formal testing; and/or repeated wandering or getting lost in environment

DRS-R-98 optional diagnostic items

These three items can be used to assist in the differentiation of delirium from other disorders for diagnostic and research purposes. They are added to the severity score for the total scale score, but are *not* included in the severity score.

14 Temporal onset of symptoms

Rate the acuteness of onset of the initial symptoms of the disorder or episode being currently assessed, not their duration. Distinguish the onset of symptoms attributable to delirium when it occurs concurrently with a different pre-existing psychiatric disorder. For example, if a patient with major depression is rated during a delirium episode due to an overdose, then rate the 'Onset of the delirium symptoms'.

0 No significant change from usual or longstanding baseline behaviour

1 Gradual onset of symptoms, occurring over a period of several week to a month

2 Acute change in behaviour or personality occurring over days to a week

3 Abrupt change in behaviour occurring over a period of several hours to a day

15 Fluctuation of severity of symptoms

Rate the waxing and waning of an individual symptom or cluster of symptoms over the time frame being rated. Usually applies to cognition, affect, intensity of hallucinations, thought disorder, language disturbance. Take into consideration that perceptual disturbances usually occur intermittently, but might cluster in periods of greater intensity when other symptoms fluctuate in severity.

0   No symptom fluctuation

1   Symptom intensity fluctuates in severity over hours

2   Symptom intensity fluctuates in severity over minutes

16   Physical disorders

Rate the degree to which a psychological, medical, or pharmacological problem can be specifically attributed as the cause of the symptom being assessed. Patients may have such a problem but the problem may or may not have a causal relationship to the symptoms being rated.

0   None present or active

1   Presence of any physical disorder that might affect mental state

2   Drug, infection, metabolic disorder, CNS lesion, or other medical problem that can be specifically implicated in causing the altered behaviour or mental state

The DRS-R-98 scoresheet

The DRS-R-98 scoresheet is shown in Fig. A5.1.

DRS-R-98 SCORESHEET

Name of patient: _____ Date: ___/___/___ Time: _____

Name of Rater: _____

SEVERITY SCORE: [   ]   TOTAL SCORE: [   ]

Severity Item	Item Score				Optional Information
Sleep-wake cycle	0	1	2	3	Naps Nocturnal disturbance only Day-night reversal
Perceptual disturbances	0	1	2	3	Sensory type of illusion or hallucination: Auditory visual olfactory tactile Format of illusion or hallucination: simple complex
Delusions	0	1	2	3	Type of delusion: persecutory Nature: poorly formed systematized
Lability of affect	0	1	2	3	Type: angry anxious dysphoric Elated irritable
Language	0	1	2	3	Check here intubated, mute, etc.
Thought process	0	1	2	3	Check here intubated, mute, etc.
Motor agitation	0	1	2	3	Check here if restrained *Type of restraints:*
Motor retardation	0	1	2	3	Check here if restrained *Type of restraints:*
Orientation	0	1	2	3	Date: Place: Person:
Attention	0	1	2	3	
Shot-term memory	0	1	2	3	Record # of trials for registration of items: Check here if category cueing helped
Long-term memory	0	1	2	3	Check here if category cueing helped
Visuospatial ability	0	1	2	3	Check here if unable to use hands
Diagnostic Item	**Item Score**				
Temporal onset of symptom	0	1	2	3	Check here if symptoms appeared on a background of other psychopathology
Fluctuation of symptom severity	0	1	2		Check here if symptoms only appeared during the night

Fig. A5.1 The Delirium Rating Scale, revised, 1998 (DRS-R-98) scoresheet. (Reprinted with permission from Trzepacz et al. (2001). Copyright 2001 American Psychiatric Association)

Appendix 6

Memorial Delirium Assessment Scale (MDAS)

The following is reprinted by permission of Elsevier Science from Breitbart *et al.* (1997), copyright 1997 by the US Cancer Pain Relief Committee.

Instructions: Rate the severity of the following symptoms of delirium based on current interaction with subject or assessment of his/her behaviour or experience over past several hours (as indicated in each time).

Item 1   Reduced level of consciousness (awareness)

Rate the patient's current awareness of and interaction with the environment (interviewer, other people/object in the room; for example, ask patients to describe their surroundings).

☐   0: none   (Patient spontaneously fully aware of environment and interacts appropriately)

☐   1: mild   (Patient is unaware of some elements in the environment, or not spontaneously interacting appropriately with the interviewer; becomes fully aware and appropriately interactive when prodded strongly; interview is prolonged but not seriously disrupted)

☐   2: moderate   (Patient is unaware of some or all elements in the environment, or not spontaneously interacting appropriately with the interviewer; becomes incompletely aware and appropriately interactive when prodded strongly; interview is prolonged but not seriously disrupted)

☐   3: severe   (Patient is unaware of all elements in the environment with no spontaneous interaction or awareness of the interviewer; so that the interview is difficult-to-impossible, even with maximal prodding)

Item 2   Disorientation

Rate current state by asking the following 10 orientation items: date; month; day; year; season; floor; name of hospital; city; state; and country.

☐   0: none   (Patient knows 9–10 items)

☐   1: mild   (Patient knows 7–8 items)

☐   2: moderate   (Patient knows 5–6 items)

☐   3: severe   (Patient knows no more than 4 items)

Item 3   Short-term memory impairment

Rate current state by using repetition and delayed recall of 3 words [patient must immediately repeat and recall words 5 min later after an intervening task. Use alternate sets of 3 words for successive evaluations (for example, apple, table, tomorrow; sky, cigar, justice)].

☐ 0: none   (All 3 words repeated and recalled)

☐ 1: mild   (All 3 words repeated; patient fails to recall 1)

☐ 2: moderate   (All 3 words repeated; patient fails to recall 2–3)

☐ 3: severe   (Patient fails to repeat 1 or more words)

Item 4   Impaired digit span

Rate current performance by asking subjects to repeat first 3, then 4, and then 5 digits forward and then 3, then 4 backwards; continue to the next step only if patient succeeds at the previous one.

☐ 0: none   (Patient can do at least 5 numbers forward and 4 backward)

☐ 1: mild   (Patient can do at least 5 numbers forward and 3 backward)

☐ 2: moderate   (Patient can do 4–5 numbers forward; cannot do 3 backward)

☐ 3: severe   (Patient can do no more than 3 numbers forward)

Item 5   Reduced ability to maintain and shift attention

As indicated during the interview by questions needing to be rephrased and/or repeated because patient's attention wanders, patient loses track, patient is distracted by outside stimuli or over-absorbed in a task.

☐ 0: none   (None of the above; patient maintains and shifts attention normally)

☐ 1: mild   (Above attentional problems occur once or twice without prolonging the interview)

☐ 2: moderate   (Above attentional problems occur often, prolonging the interview without seriously disrupting it)

☐ 3: severe   (Above attentional problems occur constantly, disrupting and making the interview difficult-to-impossible)

Item 6   Disorganized thingking

As indicated during the interview by rambling, irrelevant, or incoherent speech, or by tangential, circumstantial, or faulty reasoning. Ask patient a somewhat complex question (for example, 'Describe your current medical condition.').

☐ 0: none   (Patient's speech is coherent and goal-directed)

☐(1: mild   (Patient's speech is slightly difficult to follow; responses to questions are slightly off target but not so much as to prolong the interview)

☐ 2: moderate   (Disorganized thought or speech are clearly present, such that interview is prolonged but not disrupted)

☐ 3: severe   (Examination is very difficult or impossible due to disorganized thinking or speech)

Item 7   Perceptual disturbance

Misperceptions, illusions, hallucinations inferred from inappropriate behaviour during the interview or admitted by subject, as well as those elicited from nurse/family/chart accounts of the past several hours or of the time since last examination:

☐ 0: none   (No misperceptions, illusions, hallucinations)

☐ 1: mild   (Misperceptions, or illusions related to sleep; fleeting hallucinations on

                       1–2 occasions without inappropriate behaviour)

☐   2: moderate   (Hallucinations or frequent illusions on several occasions with minimal inappropriate behaviour that does not disrupt the interview)

☐   3: severe   (Frequent or intense illusions or hallucinations with persistent inappropriate behaviour that disrupts the interview or seriously interferes with medical care)

Item 8   Delusions

Rate delusions inferred from inappropriate behaviour during the interview or admitted by patient, as well as delusions elicited from nurse/family/chart accounts of the past several hours or of the time since the previous examination.

☐   0: none   (No evidence of misinterpretations or delusion)

☐   1: mild   (Misperceptions, or suspiciousness without clear delusional ideas or inappropriate behaviour)

☐   2: moderate   (Delusions admitted by the patient or evidenced by his/her behaviour that do not or only marginally disrupt the interview or interfere with medical care)

☐   3: severe   (Persistent and/or intense delusions resulting in inappropriate behaviour, disrupting the interview or seriously interfering with medical care)

Item 9   Decreased or increased psychomotor activity

Rate activity over past several hours, as well as activity during the interview, by cycling (a) hypoactive, (b) hyperactive, or (c) elements of both present:

☐   0: none   (Normal psychomotor activity)

☐   1: mild   (Hypoactivity is barely noticeable, expressed as slightly slowing of movement. Hyperactivity is barely noticeable or appears as simple restlessness)
      a b c

☐   2: moderate   (Hypoactivity is undeniable, with marked reduction in the number of movements or marked slowness of movement; subject rarely spontaneously moves or speaks. Hyperactivity is undeniable: subject moves almost constantly. In both cases, exam is prolonged as a consequence)
      a b c

☐   3: severe   (Hypoactivity is severe: patient does not move or speak without prodding; is catatonic. Hyperactivity is severe: patient is constantly moving, overreacts to stimuli, requires surveillance and or restraint; getting through the exam is difficult or impossible)
      a b c

Item 10   Sleep–wake cycle disturbance (disorder of arousal)

Rate patient's ability to either sleep or stay awake at the appropriate times. Utilize direct observation during the interview, as well as reports from nurses, family, patient, or charts describing sleep–wake cycle disturbance over the past several hours or since last examination. Use observations of the previous night for morning evaluations only.

☐   0: none   (At night sleeps well; during the day, has no trouble staying awake)

☐   1: mild   (Mild deviation from appropriate sleep and wakefulness states: at night, difficulty falling asleep or transient night awakening, needs medication to sleep well; during the day, reports periods of drowsiness or, during the interview, is drowsy but can easily awaken him/herself)

☐   2: moderate   (Moderate deviations from appropriate sleep and wakefulness states: at night, sleeplessness; during the day, patient spends most of the time sleeping or, during the interview, can only be roused to complete wakefulness by strong stimuli)

☐   3: severe   (Severe deviations from appropriate sleep and wakefulness states: at night, repeated and prolonged night awakening; during the day, reports of frequent and prolonged napping or, during the interview, cannot be roused to full wakefulness by any stimuli)

Appendix 7

Confusion State Evaluation Rating scale for assessment of delirium

Instructions

The main purpose of this rating scale is to assess degree of delirium. The scale may also, to a certain extent, to be useful in diagnostic contexts, as it covers the symptoms that, in the literature, are judged to be central to or generally associated with delirium.

The assessment is mainly based on the patient's condition during the interview. This means that the judgements rely on the rater's own observations. For some items, however, information is also required from a key person or staff members who know the patient well. For these items, the length of observation period is stated in the text. As the degree of delirium fluctuates, the observation period should not be too long.

Assessment of the degree of delirium may be difficult or even impracticable if the patient is also suffering from advanced dementia, severe personality disorder, hearing or visual handicaps, or aphasia. If a patient has one or more of these complications, it is important to try to judge to what extent they would hamper the rating and to consider whether the scale can be confidently used for that patient.

The scale consists of three parts, in all including twenty-two items. One part of the scale covers symptoms that have been judged to be key symptoms both in the diagnosis of delirium and in the assessment of the degree of delirium. This part of the scale includes the following symptoms: disorientation to person, time, space, and situation, thought and memory disturbances, disturbance of the sleep–wake pattern, and perceptual disturbances. Another part of the scale includes symptoms that occur frequently with delirium: irritability, emotional lability, mental uneasiness, and increased and reduced psychomotor activity. The third part includes items relating to duration and intensity of the delirium. There is no clear division between the three parts, as the items have been arranged to allow a natural flow of the interview.

Most items have a short introductory note, stating what is intended to be assessed. Each item has five well-defined scale points. The rater ticks off the point that best corresponds to the patient's state. If the state of the patient is not in accordance with any of the definitions of the scale points but seems to fall in between it is possible to score half points. Scores on the symptoms that make up the delirium syndrome—the key symptoms—are added together. This sum represents the patient's degree of delirium, the delirium score. For symptoms associated with delirium but not included in the syndrome, that scores are not added together; they are evaluated individually.

(Barbro Robertsson, AnnaLena Nyth, and CG Gottfries, Göteborg University, Dept. of Clinical Neurosciences, Section of Psychiatry and Neurochemistry, Mölndal Hospital, S-431, Mölndal, Sweden)

1   Disorientation to person

Refers to deficits in the awareness of one's own identity and circumstances.

Is fully orientated to person.	Is a little uncertain about own exact age: may misjudge it by a few years.	Is occasionally mistaken when describing current personal circumstances: whether married, has any children, is young or old.	Is usually mistaken when describing current personal circumstances: whether married, has any children, is young or old.	Is completely disorientated to person.

0	0.5	1	1.5	2	2.5	3	3.5	4

2   Disorientation to time

Refers **primarily** to deficits in the awareness of the time of day.

Is fully orientated to time.	Knows approximately what *time of day* it is: may misjudge it by a couple of hours.	Is occasionally uncertain about what *time of day* it is: may misjudge it by several hours, but can tell whether it is day or night.	Is usually uncertain about what *time of day* it is: may misjudge it by several hours, but can tell whether it is day or night.	Cannot tell whether it is day or night.

0	0.5	1	1.5	2	2.5	3	3.5	4

3   Disorientation to space

Refers to deficits both in the ability to describe a familiar environment, for instance, how the dining/bedroom and the toilet are located in relation to each other, and in the ability to find one's way in a familiar environment. This can be tested by asking the patient to sketch part of the place where he/she lives and/or show the way.

Is fully orientated to space.	Finds the way around the nearest environment, but cannot explain the relation between the rooms in own environment.	For short spells has obvious difficulty in finding the way in nearest environment.	Most often has obvious difficulty in finding the way in the nearest environment.	Is completely disorientated to space. Needs help to find the way.
0 0.5	1 1.5	2 2.5	3	3.5 4

4   Disorientation to situation

Refers to deficits in the awareness of one's own context and situation and of the roles that other individuals have in this context. Such deficits become apparent from the patient's answers to direct questions, and also from his *behaviour* on the ward and during the interview. For instance, he/she may pack up his things, want to leave, believe he/she is somewhere else, mix up people and the past and the present, take pictures for real, or urinate in the waste-paper basket.

Is fully orientated to situation.	Is a little uncertain and lost in the current situation.	For short spells is somewhat disorientated to situation, and then has difficulty in understanding own situation. Mixes up roles or the past and present. Can be given insight.	Is usually disorientated to situation. Has difficulty in understanding own situation. For instance, mixes up roles. May be given some insight, but this is short-lived.	Is completely disorientated to situation. Efforts to explain the situation are unsuccessful.
0 0.5	1 1.5	2 2.5	3	3.5 4

5 Thought disturbance

Thought disturbance can manifest itself as muddled/incoherent speech with breaks of association or excessive associations. The assessment may be difficult or impracticable if severe aphasia/dysphasia is present.

Has no thought disturbance.	May occasionally lose the thread or reveal irrelevant thought during conversation.	Sometimes reveals illogical, irrelevant thought which are manifest as muddled/ incoherent speech.	Speech is usually incoherent, with unpredictable shifts from one subject to another because of an irrelevant, unclear flow of thoughts.	Speech is completely incoherent— words muddled/ nonsensical— because of thought disturbance.

0	0.5	1	1.5	2	2.5	3	3.5	4

6 Memory disturbance

Refers to deficits in the ability to give an account of the last few hours'events and their relationship. The patient should first be encouraged to give his own account of what occurred earlier in the day (or the previous day). Next, the rater may help by asking questions and, lastly, by reminding the patient of the events. The assessment may be difficult or impracticable if severe aphasia/dysphasia is present.

Has no memory disturbance.	May have forgotten a single event from the last few hours, but remembers when reminded.	For short spells has unclear recollections about what has happened in the last few hours/days. May remember single events. Remembers better when reminded.	Usually has unclear recollections of what has happened in the last few hours. May remember single events. Reminders are of no great value.	Remembers nothing of what has happened during the last few hours.

0	0.5	1	1.5	2	2.5	3	3.5	4

7   Disturbance of the ability to concentrate

Normal ability to concentrate means ability to adjust the degree of attention to the requirements of a given task or situation. It *may* be of help for the rater to observe how the patient performs a task, such as describing his home, drawing a figure, spelling word, or reciting the days of the week forwards and backwards. To be rated here, the behavioural disturbance has to be due to difficulty in concentrating, not to lack of interest or deficient intellectual capacity, for instance because of memory disturbance.

Has normal ability to concentrate.	Has some difficulty in collecting thoughts and/or describes difficulty in concentrating.	Questions/ instructions must sometimes be repeated. Has difficulty in collecting thoughts and reduced staying power.	Only very simple conversation is possible— questions often have to be repeated. Tries unsuccessfully to collect thoughts and perform given tasks.	Conversation is practically impossible. Is completely unable to collect thoughts and perform tasks for short spells.
0 0.5	1 1.5	2 2.5	3	3.5 4

8   Increased distractibility

Refers to deficits in the ability to adequately shift one's attention from one stimulus to another. This disturbance manifests itself as a tendency to respond to new stimuli and to shift form one stimulus to another far too readily, i.e. to be easily distracted.

Is not easily distracted.	Is occasionally distracted by irrelevant things or events.	Somewhat poor in attention and then distracted by irrelevant stimuli which makes it difficult to conduct the interview.	Is easily distracted. Often shifts the attention and is distracted by irrelevant stimuli. The interview can hardly be conducted.	Constantly wanders from one subject to another. Is very easily disturbed. Even the tiniest irrelevant stimulus causes interruption.
0 0.5	1 1.5	2 2.5	3	3.5 4

9   Perseveration, prolonged latency

Refers to deficits in the ability to notice changes in the environment. In a conversation, the disturbance is often evident from the patient's absent-mindedness, his not noticing all stimuli, his repeating of phrases or clinging to a favourite subject or a previous train of thought, or from a prolonged latency when answering questions. The patient is difficult to divert and distract.

Has no increased tendency to perseveration.	Occasionally perseveres or returns to the 'favourite subject', or in unreasonably slow in answering questions.	Perseveres repeatedly or clings to own trains of thought, which disturbs the conversation, or is absent-minded; the latency before answers is markedly prolonged.	Makes perseveration the rule rather then the exception or is constantly markedly absent-minded. Can hardly be influenced or distracted.	Cannot be diverted.

0	0.5	1	1.5	2	2.5	3	3.5	4

10   Irritability

Refers to one's possible negative attitude towards the environment or oneself, as reflected in the choice of words an expressions, intonation, gestures, or postures.

Shows no signs of irritability.	Shows signs of irritability.	Answers somewhat peevishly occasionally falls silent, or talks spontaneously in an exasperated tone about episodes that have caused irritation.	Often answers peevishly, remains silent, or takes up an unresponsive posture, but can be diverted. It is difficult to conduct the interview.	Is very irritated during the whole interview Cannot be diverted.

0	0.5	1	1.5	2	2.5	3	3.5	4

11 Emotional lability

Refers to sudden changes related to mood, for instance, between laughter and crying, anger, and fit of rage.

Shows no sudden uncalled-for mood swings.	Occasionally shows sudden mood swings, for instance from fits of laughter to seriousness.	Repeatedly shows sudden mood swings.	Sometimes shows unrestrained and uncalled-for swings from one outburst of feeling to another.	Shows unrestrained and uncalled-for swings from one outburst of feeling to another during the entire interview.

0	0.5	1	1.5	2	2.5	3	3.5	4

12 Wakefulness disturbance

Shows no signs of tiredness during the entire interview.	Shows slight signs of tiredness during the entire interview, such as occasional sighs or yawns.	It is markedly tired. Yawns and sighs repeatedly, or complains about tiredness.	Sometimes falls asleep, but wakes up easily when spoken to and then continues the conversation.	Falls asleep. Is roused with great difficulty, but very soon falls asleep again.

0	0.5	1	1.5	2	2.5	3	3.5	4

13 Increased psychomotor activity

Refers to presence of restlessness, fidgetiness, and stereotyped movements. In rating this item, allowance should be made for physical handicaps, if any.

Shows no increase in psychomotor activity.	Displays slight restlessness. Occasionally fiddles at various objects, changes position, or scratches head.	Displays slight restlessness during the entire interview: wrings hands, changes position, scratches head.	Sometimes also shows signs of more severe restlessness or uneasiness. Makes effort to rise, and, occasionally actually rises.	Displays severe restlessness during the whole interview. Is unable to keep still.

0	0.5	1	1.5	2	2.5	3	3.5	4

14   Reduced psychomotor activity

In ratings this item, allowance should be made for physical handicaps, if any. Note that the lack of facial expressions may coexist with *increased* psychomotor activity.

Displays no reduction in psychomotor activity.	Displays lack of facial expressions, gestures and reduced co-movements during the interview.	Displays moderately reduced psychomotor activity.	Displays markedly reduced psychomotor activity. Moves only when absolutely necessary.	Is totally inhibited: neither eats nor goes to the toilet without assistance.

0	0.5	1	1.5	2	2.5	3	3.5	4

15   Mental uneasiness

Mental uneasiness occurs with anxiety, apprehension, helplessness and despair, but also with over-excitement, tension, and mania like-states.

Shows no signs of mental uneasiness.	Shows diffuse signs of mental uneasiness or helplessness, but does not actively seek help.	Shows clear signs of mental uneasiness. May seek help, or be tense, but can be diverted or reassured.	Displays severe mental uneasiness. Seeks staff members or relatives. Is difficult to divert, must often be reassured.	Displays extremely severe mental uneasiness. Desperately seeks help, or is over-excited, but cannot accept help and cannot be diverted. Cannot stay alone.

0	0.5	1	1.5	2	2.5	3	3.5	4

16   Impaired contact

Refers to degree of contact than can be established with the patient, *irrespective* of his intellectual capacity. The degree of contact is reflected in the concord that can be achieved and in the patient's response in the form of eye contact, smiles or effort to keep up the conversation, as well as his ability to cooperate and follow instructions. Contact may *also* be impaired if the patient misinterprets the interviewer's intention and emotional expression, or if he/she continuous talking without caring whether the interviewer understand or not. Before rating this item, it is important to try to compensate for obstacles to contact by disturbances of sense organs, language and other external conditions.

Rapport can be established.		Contact wavers for occasional short spells when the patient lapses into reveries.		Contact sometimes wavers while the patient shuts himself off. The concord is disturbed and there is a tendency to emotional mis-interpretations.		Contact can be established only for occasional short spells. Concord is lacking: emotional mis-interpretations occur.		No contact can be established. The patient is totally shut off.
0	0.5	1	1.5	2	2.5	3	3.5	4

17   Paranoid delusion

Refers to unfounded experiences of being observed or alluded to, or the patient believes without cause that other people have evil designs on him or that hostile acts are aimed at him, for instance unfaithfulness, and theft of his money or possessions.

Has no delusions.		Slow slight signs of casual suspiciousness.		Sometimes has clear experience of other people's wishing him/her harm, going behind his/her back and so on.		Has more obtrusive paranoid delusions that tend to recur rapidly. Can be given insight, but this is short of duration.		Has continuous and disabling paranoid delusions.
0	0.5	1	1.5	2	2.5	3	3.5	4

18   Hallucinations

Refers to perceptions in the absence of external stimuli, i.e. the patient sees, hears, or feels pictures, sounds or object that do not actually exist.

Has no hallucinations.		Shows slight signs of casual hallucinations.		Has occasional distinct hallucinations.		Has recurrent distinct hallucinations.		Has constantly recurrent or lasting distinct hallucinations.	
0	0.5	1	1.5	2	2.5	3	3.5	4	

19   Disturbance of the sleep–wake pattern

Refers to disturbance at night or drowsiness in the daytime. The observation period should cover **the last 24 hours**. Rating on this item should be done together with staff members or a key person.

Has no disturbance of the sleep–wake pattern.		Has mild sleep disturbance. Has difficulty in falling asleep or occasionally wakes up in the night.		Has had sleep disturbance during the last 24 hours. Sometimes wakes up in the night.		Has severe sleep disturbance with long periods of wakefulness in the night.		Severe disturbance of the sleep–wake pattern. Only sleeps for short spells both day and night. Normal diurnal rhythm is absent.	
0	0.5	1	1.5	2	2.5	3	3.5	4	

20   Sudden impairment and/or fluctuations

Are there signs (reported by relatives or staff) that the patient's mental status has sudden impairment from the normal condition and/or that the abnormal behaviour fluctuates (varies) during a 24-hour period, comes and goes, or increase or decreases in severity?

No sudden impairment or fluctuations.				It is doubtful whether impairment or fluctuations have occurred.				Yes, impairment and/or fluctuations have occurred or are currently present.	
0	0.5	1	1.5	2	2.5	3	3.5	4	

21 Intensity of the current episode

This should be a global assessment of the patient's delirium; the scale steps are not defined in detail. Only the severity of the delirium should be assessed; the duration of the episode should be disregarded.

Is not delirious.	Has a tendency towards delirium.	Is mildly delirious.	Is markedly delirious.	Is completely delirious.

0	0.5	1	1.5	2	2.5	3	3.5	4

22 Frequency and intensity of the episodes

For each of the categories A–C, mark on the scale for how long the condition in question has been present. The observation period should cover a predefined period of time. The assessment should be made together with staff members or a key person.

The assessment applies to .... number of days.

	Never occurs	Occasionally for short spells: <2 hours and <2 times in 24 hours	Several times and longer: >2 hours and/or >3 times in 24 hours	More or less the whole time except: <2 hours and <2 times in 24 hours	All day and all night
	0	1	2	3	4
A. Lucid or almost lucid*	☐	☐	☐	☐	☐
B. Mild delirium	☐	☐	☐	☐	☐
C. Severe delirium	☐	☐	☐	☐	☐

* does not meet the DSM-III-R criteria for delirium.

Delirium scale summary sheet

Central disturbances in the delirium syndrome

1.	Disorientation to person	0	0.5	1	1.5	2	2.5	3	3.5	4
2.	Disorientation to time	0	0.5	1	1.5	2	2.5	3	3.5	4
3.	Disorientation to space	0	0.5	1	1.5	2	2.5	3	3.5	4
4.	Disorientation to situation	0	0.5	1	1.5	2	2.5	3	3.5	4
5.	Thought disturbance	0	0.5	1	1.5	2	2.5	3	3.5	4
6.	Memory disturbance	0	0.5	1	1.5	2	2.5	3	3.5	4
7.	Disturbance of the ability to concentrate	0	0.5	1	1.5	2	2.5	3	3.5	4
8.	Distractibility	0	0.5	1	1.5	2	2.5	3	3.5	4
9.	Perseveration	0	0.5	1	1.5	2	2.5	3	3.5	4
16.	Impaired contact	0	0.5	1	1.5	2	2.5	3	3.5	4
17.	Paranoid delusions	0	0.5	1	1.5	2	2.5	3	3.5	4
18.	Hallucinations	0	0.5	1	1.5	2	2.5	3	3.5	4

Total score for the delirium syndrome _____

Symptoms often occurring with delirium

10.	Irritability	0	0.5	1	1.5	2	2.5	3	3.5	4
11.	Emotional lability	0	0.5	1	1.5	2	2.5	3	3.5	4
12.	Wakefulness disturbance	0	0.5	1	1.5	2	2.5	3	3.5	4
13.	Increased psychomotor activity	0	0.5	1	1.5	2	2.5	3	3.5	4
14.	Reduced psychomotor activity	0	0.5	1	1.5	2	2.5	3	3.5	4
15.	Mental uneasiness	0	0.5	1	1.5	2	2.5	3	3.5	4
19.	Disturbance of the sleep–wake pattern	0	0.5	1	1.5	2	2.5	3	3.5	4

Extent and course of the delirium

20.	Sudden impairment and/or fluctuations	0				2				4
21.	Intensity of the current episode	0	0.5	1	1.5	2	2.5	3	3.5	4
22.	Frequency and intensity of the episode									
	A	0		1		2		3		4
	B	0		1		2		3		4
	C	0		1		2		3		4

Index

Note: References to figures are indicated by 'f' and references to tables are indicated by 't' when they fall on a page not covered by the text reference.